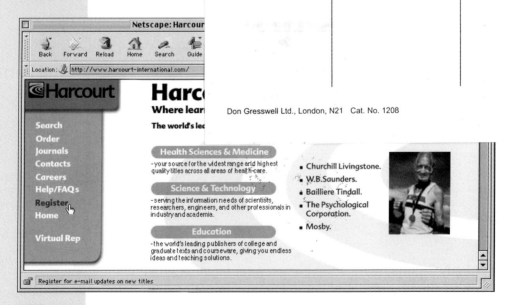

The use of
COMPUTERS
in general practice

To Margot

Commissioning Editor: Ellen Green
Project Manager: Fiona Conn
Design direction: Judith Wright

The use of COMPUTERS in general practice

John Preece

Consultant Editor, *Health Service Computing* magazine
Formerly Editor, *Practice Computing Magazine*
GP Principal
Honorary Research Fellow, Exeter University

Fourth edition

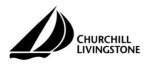
CHURCHILL
LIVINGSTONE

EDINBURGH LONDON NEW YORK PHILADELPHIA ST LOUIS SYDNEY TORONTO 2000

CHURCHILL LIVINGSTONE
An imprint of Harcourt Publishers Limited

© Harcourt Publishers Limited 2000

⬚ is a registered trademark of Harcourt Publishers Limited

The right of John Preece to be identified as author of this work has been asserted by him in accordance with the Copyright, Designs and Patents Act 1988

First edition 1983
Second edition 1990
Third edition 1994
Fourth edition 2000

ISBN 044306394X

British Library Cataloguing in Publication Data
A catalogue record for this book is available from the British Library

Library of Congress Cataloging in Publication Data
A catalog record for this book is available from the Library of Congress

NOTE
Medical knowledge is constantly changing. As new information becomes available, changes in treatment, procedures, equipment and the use of drugs become necessary. The authors and the publishers have taken care to ensure that the information given in this text is accurate and up-to-date. However, readers are strongly advised to confirm that the information, especially with regard to drug usage, complies with the latest legislation and standards of practice.

The
publisher's
policy is to use
**paper manufactured
from sustainable forests**

Typeset by IMH(Cartrif), Loanhead, Scotland
Printed in China

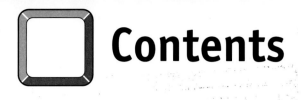

Contents

Preface and Acknowledgements

This book originated from a series of 14 research studies which I undertook over a period of as many years, the purpose of which was to enquire into the underlying principles of computer design in general practice. Early design work had to be tested on prototype systems at a time when prototypes were expensive luxuries, and I am particularly grateful to IBM, whose investigations showed that the 1970 experimental system which they supported was in fact the first use of real-time computing in general practice. Through Ed Lippmann's accomplished software we were able to experience and describe the benefits of the new electronic record.

I would also like to thank Philips of Holland, Update Software, Plessey, the ABPI Exeter University Joint Drug Intelligence Project, Syntex, Boehringer Ingelheim and the many other individual members of the pharmaceutical industry who have fostered this research. Their good faith and generous help is acknowledged with warm gratitude.

The book also takes account of other people's published experience in the field of general practice computing and areas related to it – a debt reflected in the Further Reading lists at the end of many of the chapters. Although these lists are not comprehensive, they endeavour to represent those contributions in each field which might be considered significant and interesting to general practitioners. The design of currently marketed systems has stemmed from this earlier corporate research, but is now refined in the light of field experience through user groups. This process of refinement has also been noted in the book's content.

Of the many friends I have made along the way, the following have influenced my views. Ed Lippmann, John Ashford, Ceese Klap, Abraham Marcus, David Holmes, Ian Herbert, Keith Watson, Bill Gerard, Eric Snell, Alan Pitchford, Carol Beaumont, Emily Donnelly, John Hearson, Lesley Shirt, and Chris Whitt. To these and to all others who put their shoulder to the wheel in the common cause of general practice computer development, I am duly grateful. Finally my thanks are due to John Fry, Anthony Gresford, Ellen Green and Fiona Conn for their help and encouragement in compiling the book, and to my wife for preparing the typescript with unfailing patience.

John Preece 1999

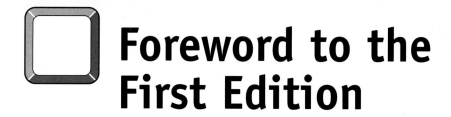

Foreword to the First Edition

In the past few years general practice records have advanced from the dark ages to the jet age. The speed of change has been breathtaking and frightening.

From antiquated small medical record envelopes with unattractive continuation cards, general practice records passed through a tentative stage of A4 records, with only a few practices taking them up, to the computer.

Many practitioners, especially those over 50, are uncertain and afraid of computers as applied to practice records and analyses. They tend to adopt King-Canute-type attitudes and seek to hold back the tide of progress. They will find it impossible to prevent advances of technology being applied to general practice. Younger practitioners and particularly the coming generations will take the application of computers to everyday practice in their stride.

The microchip evolution has been breathtakingly rapid with better and cheaper equipment. Soon many ordinary households will have their own personal computers. Can general practice be left behind?

The computer is for the future. General practice needs to be taken firmly by the hand, led and guided through the microchip jungle to a realistic and practical use of computers.

There can be no better guide than John Preece. A pioneer in this field, he has been using and researching with computers in his Exeter practice for almost 20 years. His many papers and demonstrations have charted one passage from then to now.

It is fortunate for us that he has brought together his experience in this book. It is written clearly and concisely with a minimum of technological jargon. It is intended to reassure and encourage those moving into the computer age in general practice. Undoubtedly this book will be essential reading for all practitioners seeking to learn and understand about computers for their practices.

January 1983
John Fry

1 A general introduction to computers

1.1 A DEVELOPMENTAL INTERACTION BETWEEN MAN AND MACHINE

The computer is harbinger to a new epoch in the conduct of human affairs. Its impact is similar in magnitude to that produced by the change from Stone Age to Bronze Age, to the introduction of the wheel, the adoption of writing, the discovery of electricity – all changes that have altered the direction and increased the speed of the development of civilization.

The heralds of change have commonly had a hostile reception. Galileo was forced to recant in prison when he suggested that the earth travelled around the sun, Darwin was accused of blasphemy and the Tolpuddle martyrs were deported. Socrates and Rousseau were both persecuted for their innovations.

For a long time after their invention computers were viewed with general distrust. They had a mistaken public image, which smacked of political police or visitors from outer space. Their true role is that of servants, punctilious in their obedience. Basically, the computer is a capsule of electronic reflexes comparable with the nervous system of some primitive animals. In its more advanced forms it possesses virtually limitless, unfailing memory, and may be conditioned with reflexes of lightning speed and considerable complexity. Like primitive animals it fails to innovate, to use artistic expression, to produce analogy or humour. It is an automaton.

The critical phase in human evolution at which the human prototype diverged from the African ape was marked by a threefold increase in brain size, with corresponding enhancement of organizational ability and the acquisition of speech. Humans as the planet's supreme toolmakers have now created the computer, a device that extends their own organizational and communicative skills far beyond that achieved by natural selection.

1.2 DEVELOPMENTAL PATHWAYS THAT LED TO THE COMPUTER

The immediate precursor of the computer is the calculating machine, which in turn derives from simpler calculating devices such as the abacus, introduced to take man past the finger count of 10 for which he was anatomically equipped.

However, the developmental pathway has not been quite straight. Counting with tens, hundreds and thousands as a milometer does is electronically difficult. The smallest unit of electronic storage, called a 'bit' (as a contraction of 'binary digit') is capable of either positive or negative polarity but no third state. The need to record a number as a succession of positively or negatively polarized bits involves binary numbering. When the two states of polarization in a bit have been used to represent 0 and 1, any further increase must be shown as a change of polarity in the next adjacent bit; the two bits are then read together as an entity. Successive increases invoke further bits in sequence, in a chain reaction (Fig. 1.1). Special arithmetical rules, and special algebraic rules (*Boolean algebra*) apply to binary operations.

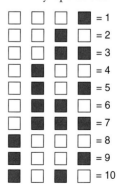

Fig. 1.1 The representation of the numbers 1–10 by binary code

The need to manipulate and store text and, therefore, letters called for the formation of an internal storage alphabet of characters. Here a group of 8 bits in fixed relationship to each other is read as a single entity or *byte* (probably a contraction of 'by eight'; Fig. 1.2).

Assemblies of 8 bits to a byte allow 128 individual characters to be represented by different combinations in the commonly used ASCII code (American Standard Code for Information Interchange). All letters of the conventional alphabet in both upper and lower case may thus be accommodated, along with numerals and a limited selection of special characters (this form of coding is sometimes referred to as *alphanumeric*). If numerals are stored in ASCII, they must be translated into binary for the purposes of arithmetical computation, and retranslated afterwards.

Greater versatility is, of course, obtainable by increasing the number of bits in the byte capsule, and '16-bit' (Fig. 1.3), '32-bit' and '64-bit' operations are now commonplace.

Storage capacity is measured by the number of 8-bit bytes that can be accommodated. A *kilobyte* is the term for 2^{10} bytes, a *megabyte* represents 2^{20} bytes and a *gigabyte* is 2^{30} bytes. A kilobyte of text typed with double spacing would cover an A4 page.

1.3   AN OVERVIEW OF COMPUTER FUNCTIONALITY

Very simply, the computer accepts one sort of data (input), causes it to react with pre-stored processive data (a program) and produces resultant data (output). This is a close parallel to the way we put numbers into a calculator, process them by addition, subtraction, multiplication or division and produce a result. Just as calculators have function keys to invoke the four arithmetical rules, so the computer has command keys to invoke one or other programmed function. The computer also possesses straightforward number and letter keys, in common with the typewriter, for text input.

The term *computer system* is applied to the fully functioning unit incorporating *hardware* (the equipment), *software* (the programs), electricity supply, communication provision and consumables (such as printer ink and paper). The basic hardware components are:

- A *central processing unit* (*CPU*) with provision for the electronic interaction of input data and program data in an area called *memory*.

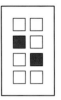

Fig. 1.2   A 'byte' composed of 8 bits

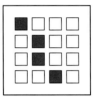

Fig. 1.3   A 'byte' composed of 16 bits, sometimes referred to as a double byte electronic word

- *Disk storage* – rotating circular plates whose surfaces are coated with magnetic material read by pickup heads. *Hard disks* are integral sealed units housed in a hard disk drive. *Floppy disks* are interchangeable lightweight flexible magnetic plates (*diskettes*) that are fed into the port of a floppy disk drive by the user. Some processors have two floppy disk ports. *CD-ROM* disks and drives provide high-volume unalterable storage for access to data sources such as encyclopaedic reference or elaborate programmes. All drives, the CPU and relevant circuitry are housed in a casing (*the base unit*) placed on the desk or on the floor (*tower unit*). The base unit is usually cooled by an air fan.
- The means to communicate with peripheral equipment and other computers in the immediate vicinity – a *serial port* and communication '*card*' circuitry housed in the base unit. Messages are conveyed through suitable interconnecting wiring.
- The means to communicate with remote computers through telephone channels – a *modem* (or a *terminal adapter* for ISDN), which may or may not be housed in the base unit.
- A typewriter-like *keyboard*, with added command keys, and a *mouse* or *tracker ball*.
- A *visual display unit* (*VDU*) – a television-type screen to show text, charts, images, animation and video – usually in colour.
- An *electricity supply* with provision for protection of the computer against harmful variations in voltage.

- A *printer* – in a PC usually connected to the *parallel port* in the base unit (parallel ports transmit multiple flows of data simultaneously; serial ports transmit a single flow).
- A *'backup' unit*, which accepts reduplicated electronic copies of the contents of disk storage as a provision against possible corruption or loss of the primary copy.
- Optional extra components may include *speakers* to provide for *multimedia*, or a *microphone* to allow voice input.

Figure 1.4 represents the assembled components of a basic computer system.

1.4 INTERACTION OF DATA

When the computer is switched on, programs are read from disk storage into processor memory (a procedure known as *booting up* derived from 'pulling oneself up by one's own boot straps'). 'New' data entered through the keyboard appear on the screen and, when a command key is depressed, interact with the programs in the processor. Resultant data now appear on the screen in place of the 'new' data and, if the user approves them, s/he presses a further command key, whereupon the resultant data are removed from the screen and will now be added to any data previously held in disk storage. The contents of the screen may also be printed out as *hard copy* (i.e. on paper) if the appropriate command key is activated, or alternatively transmitted as a communication. Data previously stored may be recalled, and viewed and amended on the screen.

Dictionaries

A further source of interactive data in modern computer systems is the dictionary or directory to which both the programs and the new data can be referred

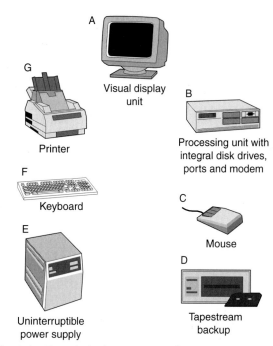

Fig. 1.4 The principal components of a computer system (a) Visual display unit (b) Processing unit with integral hard disk, modem and serial port (c) Mouse (d) Tapestream backup (e) Uninterruptible power supply (f) Keyboard (g) Printer

during data processing. These are also stored on the hard disk. Familiar examples in general practice are the Read codes, drug dictionaries and protocol libraries. A schematic representation of data relationships is shown in Figure 1.5.

1.5 SYSTEM CONFIGURATIONS

The overall plan of arrangement of a computer system is referred to as its configuration. Broadly speaking,

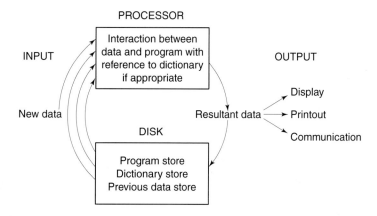

Fig. 1.5 Data relationships in a computer

computers are either used as single units in small offices or at home, or in multiples connected by a network in which one computer (the *server*) dominates (Box 1.1).

While large corporate tasks may call for more powerful *mini* or larger *mainframe* computers, and highly sophisticated mathematical research may require *supercomputers*, most routine work is now carried out on *microcomputers*, of which there are two main varieties. Although Apple Macintosh ('Mac') microcomputers are often used for high-quality graphics and publishing applications, the lion's share of the rest of the market belongs to IBM-compatible machines (the so called personal computer or 'PC'). In either case the equipment (the *hardware*) used has required its own brand-specific programs (*software*) to provide motivation. After years of fierce market competition, kits are now available that will operate both Mac and PC software – the *power PC*.

Networks may be set up using cables if the links are within the same building (a *local area network* or *LAN*). For intercommunication at a distance, linkage through modems or terminal adapters and telecommunications will be needed, and networks so arranged are referred to as *wide area networks* (*WANs*). Examples of WANs are the Racal HealthLink and NHSnet, which link NHS users.

Strictly speaking, the term 'local area network' is reserved for a configuration in which individual terminals have their own processing power (and are known as *intelligent workstations*), although usually dominated by a master processor (the *fileserver*). The term *multiuser* is reserved for a configuration in which individual terminals have no processing power (*dumb terminals*) and are motivated solely by the fileserver to which they are wired.

Intelligent workstations are PCs in their own right, but a more recent development, the *network station*, has been introduced in which processing power, though integral, has been stripped to the bone for purposes of economy.

In addition to the basic housekeeping software that drives an individual computer (the *operating system*) and the programs that perform tasks for specific types of use (*application software*), networks have to use network software (*netware*) to coordinate their activities.

Electronic mail (*e-mail*) usually employs *nodes* or *depots* where mail is stored while awaiting onward transmission to the recipient – *store and forward* operations. Where direct e-mail access between sender and recipient can be achieved without an intermediary, data intended for transmission are stored, until called for, in an area of the sender's computer. In

---

Box 1.1 Common uses of computers

Common uses of standalone computers
Word processing, spreadsheets, database management, personal organizer, games, desktop publishing, digital photography, CD-ROM reference, computer-aided design, accounts (cash flow, payroll, VAT, tax)

And with added telecommunications
e-mail, e-banking, e-shopping, Internet access

Common uses of networked computers
Manufacturing, commerce, stock market, banking, education, publishing, insurance, defence, control of air, sea and road traffic, public services, central and local government, law, architecture, engineering, advertising

---

either case the place where data are stored for transmission is known as the intended recipient's *mailbox*.

1.6 THE COMPUTER'S COMPONENTS IN GREATER DETAIL

Processors

Processors are rated according to their principal chip technology, their speed and their memory capacity. A *chip* is a miniaturized circuit board implanted on a sliver of silicon. The development of progressively more powerful principal chips ('286', '386', '486', Pentium I, II or III, with suffixes such as NMX or SX denoting further enhancement) has allowed GP computing to keep pace with rapidly increasing data processing demands.

Processors have speed ratings, quoted in megahertz (MHz): 1 MHz equals 1 000 000 cycles (basic electronic operations) per second. Pentiums started at 75 MHz, and now exceed 600 MHz. Xeon, Merced and McKinley processors are under development and offer even more power.

A computer's price tag is related to its speed. Processor chips manufactured by Intel predominated in IBM-compatible PCs during the 1990s, but are now facing stiff competition.

Memory capacity is described in megabytes and has two components, ROM and RAM. ROM (*read-only memory*) is the area of processor memory that, like the brain stem, houses basic housekeeping instructions, which cannot be overwritten nor erased and are not deleted when the computer is switched off. RAM (*random access* or *read-and-write memory*) is the amount of processor memory available to process user data and programs, which data will be lost when the computer is switched off unless they are first stored on disk or printed out. The *motherboard* is the scaffolding circuitry of the base unit on which are lodged the processor chip, ROM and RAM, and the *BIOS* (the basic input–output system that regulates data flow to and from the processor). A motherboard provides additional connectivity with external equipment through *expansion slots*. Users wishing to upgrade their processor chips are best advised to upgrade their motherboard at the same time, whereas RAM can often be upgraded independently (check with your GP system supplier).

Visual display units (VDUs, monitors)

VDUs are monochrome or colour cathode ray display screens upon which the text, and still or moving images, that are the subject of the computer's processing are presented to the user.

VDUs vary in quality according to their size, dot pitch, resolution and scan rate, factors that are reflected in their cost. Standard monitor sizes are 14, 15 or 17 inches measured diagonally, and these are suitable for GP work; reception appointment applications may benefit from the use of larger screens. 14-inch screens characteristically accommodate 80 characters in each of 20–24 horizontal lines.

VDUs display their data by the use of closely packed light-emitting dots, which are activated by regular and rapid refreshment. *Dot pitch* is the size of each dot, which should be no greater than 0.26 mm if fuzziness is to be avoided. Resolution is measured as the number of dots across and down the screen, with a greater density of dots providing finer details. A good minimum standard is SVGA, which equates with 640 horizontal dots and 480 vertical dots.

The *scan rate* refreshes the image at frequent, regular intervals, and not only helps to determine picture quality but, if insufficiently rapid, will cause eye strain. In order to avoid undue technicality it will suffice to recommend that *interlaced* monitors should be avoided, and that a vertical scan rate of not less than 72 Hz is required.

Power saving features are worth having, and will be noted in the sales literature. Certification standards for minimal stray radiation are TCO-92, TCO-95 and MPRIL.

VDUs must be adjustable for brightness and contrast, and must be capable of tilt or swivel positioning. Liquid crystal display (LCD) is used in portable computers (see Chapter 24).

Keyboards

Keyboards accommodate two types of key – data entry and command keys. *Data entry keys* are alpha-betic, with a typewriter layout (with shift keys for upper or lower case), and numeric, which may or may not be arranged as an additional, separate numeric cluster or *numeric key pad*. The most important command keys in general use are: those controlling cursor movements; the *enter/return* key, which signifies the acceptance of data that have just been entered and motivates the next step in processing; the *escape* key (which conventionally allowed return to the main menu screen from any point in the system); the *help* key, which summons textual advice for the user on how to proceed in a given situation; the *insert* and *delete* keys; and special numbered *function keys* (which are allocated special tasks when user software is written). *Control* and *Alt* keys are also accorded special tasks.

Keyboards should display characters of sufficient size and contrast to be easily legible, the surface of the keys should be matt to avoid glare, and the board must be adjustable for tilt from front to back. A pad to support the wrists may be incorporated, or purchased as an optional extra.

Disk drives

Hard disk units are usually housed within the body of the base unit, although earlier models were freestanding. The platters are enclosed in a sealed, dust-free capsule (*hard disk drive*), which also contains the motor and reading head. The reading head of a hard disk drive, in contrast to diskette drives, is not in physical contact with the platter surface, so that wear does not occur. Hard disk drives are easily damaged if dropped, and some computers provide safe locking mechanisms that can be invoked while the base unit is being relocated.

Hard disk capacity is measured in megabytes or gigabytes, and its size is always critical to the accommodation of an application, which nowadays must often allow for the use of large databases, dictionaries and software modules. Interchangeable hard disks are available, as are hard disk expansion cards – self-contained miniaturized drives on circuit cards that can be inserted into existing circuitry.

Floppy disk (diskette) drives allow the diskette to be loaded through a port in the processor, and there may be two such drives. Industry-standard diskettes are 3½ inches in diameter, accommodating 1.44 Mb of data, and this is the only size now encountered in GP systems.

New blank diskettes must be formatted before use – the provision for this comes with all generic and GP software. Formatting structures the surface of the diskette electronically into the radial and circumferential subdivisions used to address data. Diskettes can be purchased preformatted for use in DOS and Windows applications.

As the reading head of the diskette drive makes contact with the surface of the diskette (in contrast to hard disks), degradation takes place with constant use. It is therefore essential to make working copies of all diskettes that contain key programs, and to keep the original diskettes in safe custody. Diskettes may also be corrupted if their surface is damaged by touch or abrasion via the aperture in the protective sleeve that exists to allow reading head access. Degradation may occur as the result of other types of physical abuse, such as overheating or exposure to the magnetic field of much electrical equipment, (though, fortunately, not as a rule to that of the computer terminal itself). Working programs on diskette should be protected by occlusion of the 'overwrite slot' situated on the edge of the diskette casing; a small sliding panel exists to allow this. It is important to use only diskettes of reputable make and source and to institute a strict discipline to prevent the use of any unauthorized diskette on the practice system, in order to minimize the threat of computer virus infection.

Optical disk drives (laser, CD-ROM, WORM) are provided for computers, and their massive 640 Mb storage capacity makes them suitable for applications involving large amounts of reference material such as is required in providing access to voluminous electronic text books, encyclopaedias, directories or computer programs. A reflected laser beam allows minute indentations to be detected on the surface of the platter. Because there is no physical contact, degradation does not occur.

Normally, optical disks allow reading only, because recording etches the surface of the disk and cannot be overwritten. However, as the disk capacity often far exceeds the reading requirements of some applications, a head that writes as well as reads allows empty tracks on the disk to be used while outdated ones are ignored. Optical disks that allow a generous but finite number of recordings (rewritable CD) are also available and, though a more expensive option, constitute a suitable medium for regular security backup.

When listing the computer's components, it is conventional to arrange the order of drives so that the hard disk is preceded by the floppy and followed by the CD-ROM. If there is only one of each, then these would be shown as A drive (floppy), C drive (hard), and D drive (CD-ROM). If two floppy drives and two hard disk drives are present, then the CD-ROM drive becomes drive E.

Printers

There are three main categories of printer.

- *Dot matrix* printers employ print heads that house fine metal rods in a cluster of slots. Characters are formed by the protrusion of selected rods to form a pattern, and the protruding rods press the printer ribbon against the paper. Dot matrix printers are cheap, noisy and comparatively slow (80–300 characters per second), and the print quality depends upon the number of rods in the print head. 9-pin and 24-pin machines are commonly available but the former do not achieve 'near-letter quality' (NLQ). Fonts are easily varied, and graphs and charts can be produced, but a change of colour requires a change of ribbon. The print head tends to get hot with prolonged use.
- *Inkjet* (including *bubble jet*) printers can now be obtained inexpensively, although some of the cheapest models have proved unreliable. Inkjet printers are quiet, fast, have good print quality and font variety, and can produce graphs and charts. Colour printing is possible, although there are sometimes problems with ink smudging. The printer uses a jet of ink to form the characters on the paper, and the cartridge employed to do this must be replaced regularly, adding to running costs.
- *Laser printers.* Top-quality printing is the prerogative of the laser printer, which, like a photocopier, uses a light-sensitive drum to record the pattern of the image to be transferred. The drum's light sensitivity is translated into an electrostatic charge, which attracts toner, and the toner is transferred to the copy paper. Unlike a photocopier, the laser printer uses its programmed laser beam to write the image to the drum. Laser printers are fast, quiet, relatively expensive, and versatile as regards font variety, graphics and colour. They also use cartridges.

Combination machines are now available that can alternatively provide laser printing, copying, faxing and scanning, with input–output to a workstation.

Table 1.1 compares the principal features of the three types of printer.

It is essential to ensure that the following factors are taken into account when selecting a printer.

- The system software must be compatible and also possess the appropriate printer control program.
- The system hardware must be compatible.
- The stationery accepted by the printer must allow for the practice's requirements – continuous stationery ('tractor-feed'), individual sheets of

Table 1.1   Printers compared

	Cost	Noise	Speed	Print quality	Graphs and statistical charts	Colour capability	Font variety
Dot matrix 9-pin	L	H	–	–	+	–	+
Dot matrix 24-pin or 48-pin	L	H	–	+	+	–	+
Inkjet	H	L	+	+	+	(+)	+
Laser	H	L	+	++	+	+	+

L = Low; H = High; + = Good feature; - = Poor feature
Inkjet colour printing tends to smudge

paper ('friction feed'), labels, envelopes and paper of varying sizes. Printer feeds that 'push' rather than 'pull' the paper tend to waste less. Practices frequently site a continuous stationery printer in the reception area for batch work, such as repeat medication and mailmerge, and a single sheet printer in the consulting room for single prescriptions and patient advice leaflets.

- The printer must have an adequate *print buffer* – an electronic reservoir for data waiting to be printed, which can receive the practice system's printer message very rapidly and free the computer for other tasks.
- Noisy printers will need a sound-insulating *acoustic hood* if they are to be placed in a working area. Some high-quality printers now emit hardly any noise.
- Printouts of illustrations that are more complex than graphs and charts will require a high-quality laser printer or a special printer called a *digital plotter*, and special software. Printouts of spreadsheets larger than A4 will require wide-bodied printers.

Communication requirements

Computers can communicate with other remote computers through telecommunication, but in order to do so must be provided with special communications software, a circuit-board called a *communications controller*, a serial port in the processor casing into which cables can be plugged, a modem or terminal adapter, and special cabling. The need for compatibility between all the foregoing items is absolute.

The term *modem* is an abbreviation for 'modulator–demodulator'. Because older telephone lines are specifically designed to carry sound signals, the electronic binary signals used in computers must be translated into suitable wave-form (analogue) frequencies for transmission and reconverted to binary on reception. Modems carry out signal conversion, carry out integrity checks on received data to ensure accuracy of transmission, and compact data so that these may be transmitted more rapidly, with potential economy in line charges (a potential unrealized if the carrier charges by volume instead of time). Some modems can send and receive simultaneously. A modem's speed is measured by the number of kilobytes that it can transmit per second (kb/s). Earlier ratings for modems used a scale prefixed by the letter V in which V34+, for instance, referred to a modem that could transmit 32 600 bytes per second. The highest-speed transmissions require the use of special data communications service agencies, as will increasingly be the case within the NHS. Many computers now have modem facilities built in as circuit boards within the processor.

As with digital television, newer telephone systems transmit digital signals that accommodate the requirements of both voice and data. Digital telephony needs a *codec* (coder-decoder), also known as a *terminal adapter*, in place of a modem.

Clean electricity

The demands of other local electrical equipment, and sometimes the vagaries of the central source, may subject computer equipment to voltage variation that is beyond its tolerance. The result may be corruption of data or equipment failure. It is vital therefore that safeguards should be built in to the computer's electricity supply at installation, and the following options are available.

- The provision of a separate ring main in the premises in which the computer is housed (this leaves the system vulnerable to central supply faults).
- A *surge buffer* (constant voltage transformer) that filters out harmful 'spikes' and 'surges' in voltage. The surge buffer is both cheap and effective, but cannot protect against power cuts.

- An *uninterruptible power supply* (UPS), an independent electricity supply using a system of batteries continuously charged from the mains. This is a more expensive option, but one that can bridge a gap in mains supply at least long enough to allow orderly shut down of the system. It is therefore a standard component of all GP systems.

Backup

Security copies of the data recorded on the hard disk should be taken and stored in a fireproof safe, so that in the event of system failure involving loss of data, reconstruction can take place. Data may be copied to magnetic tape (a *tape streamer*), to a second and independent hard disk or to a rewritable compact disk. Miniaturized tapes (digital audio tapes) are often employed. Compact CDs (*minidisks*) may be used for this purpose in future.

So vital is backup that it is now common practice to carry out the procedure daily as an automated routine, retaining the security copies for as many as five successive working days in safe custody, and overwriting the oldest in each day's backup. The member of staff appointed as computer manager should be held responsible by contract for all his/her duties, and this must include backup. A backup security copy must always be taken as a precaution when software enhancements are introduced, when the system engineer is due to make a visit on site, or when software maintenance repairs ('patching') are carried out through modems.

Suppliers' maintenance contracts specifically exclude responsibility for data loss in the event of system failure.

Software architecture

Software that manipulates data at the finest level of bits and bytes is called *machine* (or *object*) *code*. To write each new piece of software starting afresh at this elementary level would be needlessly repetitive – for example coordinating instructions required for system 'housekeeping' will always be required, regardless of the overall application. These coordinating instructions, which contain a myriad of hierarchical commands and subroutines, are packaged as an *operating system*. Examples of operating systems are MS-DOS (Microsoft Disk Operating System), Windows 95, 98 and 2000 (a higher-level operating system that works over MS-DOS), UNIX (a Bell Laboratory design) and MUMPS (Massachusetts General Hospital Utility Multiprogramming System).

Programmers also employ smaller preconstructed subunits of software (*macros*) that they have built or borrowed for repetitive situations in their work.

Using the operating system that the programmers judge best suited to the application they plan, they now construct the suite of *application programs* that will allow the user to perform specified tasks. Some application programs are devoted to tasks commonly undertaken, such as book-keeping or payroll, for which generic commercial software (called *off-the-shelf* or *shrink-wrapped*) is available. In other cases the task will be highly specialized, as it is in general medical practice, and *bespoke* (tailor-made) software will have to be written. The finished application software package is known as *source code*, and reputable software companies are increasingly placing a copy of their source code in *ESCROW* with an independent legally appointed referee, whose function would be to release the code to users in the event of company bankruptcy.

Until the advent of the IBM Personal Computer, most software was hardware-specific, forcing users to purchase both software and hardware as a package. Now, much hardware is interchangeable – the IBM PC has had many imitators, known as *clones*. Application programs cannot as a rule be moved to another operating system, nor are networking and 'multiuser' operating systems usually compatible with each other. The number of 'off-the-shelf' application programs for MS-DOS and Windows is very extensive, but care should be taken not to purchase one written for a later version than that held on the system.

Licence fees included in the purchase price are payable for the use of both the operating system and 'off-the-shelf' application programs. Sometimes the application program and operating system will be included on the same diskette or CD-ROM, but at other times the two must be loaded separately. *Shareware* is a form of marketing whereby users can try out software in a limited form for a small, or no, fee, and pay the residue if they wish to obtain the full package and updates.

Although the user is permitted to make his/her own working copy of a program diskette, the copyright law forbids the taking of copies for third parties – a law not always respected.

The term *fourth-generation software* (4GL) is usually applied to very powerful software packages such as: *structured query languages* (SQL) for interrogating complex databases; application software generators, which take over much of the programmer's work; and decision-support software. A *toolkit* is an assembly of various software packages that the programmer uses when constructing software. *Fifth-generation software* is already being developed, especially in Japan, and is likely to be able to make value judgements and highly complex decisions.

Apart from application programs, specialist software for general practice includes morbidity dictionaries (in particular the Read codes), drug dictionaries (such as the Multilex group) and protocols for data entry and decision support such as PRODIGY, MENTOR, SOPHIE and ISIS. Historically, licence fees have been payable for the use of these packages but in future PRODIGY will be freely available to NHS users.

Interfaces

The following interfaces between the computer and user are available.

Typewriter-configuration keyboard, VDU with cursor, cursor vector keys or joystick

This has a maximum speed of input of 60 words per minute – about half the speed of speech.

Stenographic keyboard

This has keys representing phonetic syllables supported by automatic spelling checks and is used in law courts – it runs at the speed of speech.

Graphical user interface (GUI)

This employs displayed symbols and option lists (*menus*) that can be selected by moving cursor to target and pressing a command key.

WIMPS stands for:

- *Windows* – subsections of the screen highlighted to attract attention
- *Icons* – symbols
- *Mouse* – a hand-held box made to move across a flat surface: a ball housed on the undersurface of the box rotates as the user slides the mouse, and two-dimensional vectors are translated into cursor movement on the screen
- *Pull-down menus* – cursor activation on a trigger point at the top of the screen causes a list of options to unravel; trigger points for alternative menus are usually arranged in series along a horizontal line at the top of the screen – the *menu bar*. The menu bar is sometimes displayed across the bottom of the screen, in which case menus unravel upwards (*pop-up menus*).

A *dialogue box* is a window that appears on the screen while a dialogue is taking place between the user and the system, and which contains questions and answers appropriate to the current transaction. The screen may be subdivided into a number of such boxes concurrently open for access (*tiling*). Alternatively, a series of subdecisions may invoke a succession of 'chained' boxes partially superimposed on each other on the screen (*cascade display*). The mouse has one or more command keys built into its upper surface, the use of which activates selection. Single depression of these keys, double successive depressions and sustained depression with or without accompanying mouse movement all convey unique signals to the system. *Tracker balls* are also vector-sensing devices, but in these the rotating ball faces upwards in its socket for activation by the user's palm.

Sensitive screens

Selection of options displayed on the screen may also be made in other ways. *Touch screens* sense the presence and coordinates of the selecting finger. Hand-held pens, which may be connected by cable to the processor, are also used as pointers to items displayed on a sensitive screen, and here the process that logs the screen coordinates is usually initiated by depression of a small command key in the nose, or on the back, of the pen. Pen technology is under vigorous development and the pen's movements across the screen can now be memorized. As a result of this, signatures, handwritten block capitals and basic handwritten command signals (such as X or O) can all be recognized by the system. The parallel development of pen technology and a sensitive flat screen have been combined to produce an integral *process and display* unit the size of a telephone directory for which no keyboard is needed (NCR 3125 and equivalent models). The machine has an A4-sized screen and allows facsimile forms to be completed.

Optical recognition

This may involve:

- *mark sense readers* (used for single pencil stroke answers to multiple choice questionnaires on paper)
- *optical character recognition* (OCR), which can turn printed text into binary code
- *scanners*, which translate both text (with the help of OCR) and images into binary code (scanners may also be used to transmit or file X-rays)
- *magnetic ink character recognition* (used on cheques)
- *bar codes* (as used in supermarkets and dispensing stock control).

Handwriting recognition

Handwriting recognition using a small graphics pad has been used in pilot schemes to submit claims to the health authority.

Voice recognition

By far the easiest form of input, this is currently undergoing intensive development.

A system may employ two types of interface in combination. It is common for a conventional keyboard to augment mouse or touch screen input.

2 'Off-the-shelf' software packages

2.1 INTRODUCTION

In 1981 IBM's launch of the concept of the personal computer, and its collaboration with the software house Microsoft who designed the MS-DOS operating system for use with that computer, had far-reaching results for the computer industry. Because standards for performance and compatibility had at last been established, software could be moved around between many different makes of hardware, and competitive price reduction in both hardware and software rapidly followed. An extensive range of 'off-the-shelf' commercial packages based on DOS became available during the 1980s, with businesses as the principal customer. Word processing started to replace the typewriter, spreadsheets took over from ledgers and calculators, and database management software replaced filing cabinets. 'Off-the-shelf' software is now most plentiful and cheapest for DOS and Windows use, less varied for Mac OS (the Apple Macintosh operating system) and UNIX, and very limited for less widely used operating systems.

'Off-the-shelf' software cannot be used as a substitute for bespoke software. Although commercial database management packages have often been the starting point for the development of a GP system, several years of customization are needed to produce the finished product – a task well beyond most enthusiastic amateurs. 'Off-the-shelf' packages may be used as adjuncts to the practice system for the purpose for which they were designed, although written approval from the GP system supplier must then be obtained, and must specify whether the third party software is to be included in the maintenance agreement. Word processing will already be offered as an option by the GP supplier, and it is an important advantage for a GP system to possess word processing facilities at all levels of textual data input (full integration). 'Off-the-shelf' software is most competitively priced in mail order catalogues.

Principal 'off-the-shelf' packages that may be of use in general practice are as follows.

2.2 ENHANCED WORD PROCESSING

Word processing began as an aid to typists – an advance on the facilities provided by the typewriter and the electric typewriter. Basically it assists in the assembly and refinement of text before the finished product is committed to paper or electronic mail. Because of its widespread application and importance, word processing has become one of the main foci of system development, and its extensions and ramifications influence, and in some cases dominate, computer use in many areas other than the typist's desk.

It is convenient to consider the wide range of functions provided by word processing by subdividing the more important ones into the areas of work in which they provide assistance.

Typing aids

- Automatic paper feed and alignment in printer
- Automatic carriage return, line spacing; print of uniform density
- Automatic scroll up when display is filled with text, with subsequent new data being entered in lowest lines
- Controlled left-hand margin with indentation at start of paragraph, even-spacing of words in a line to fill out to right-hand margin ('justification')
- Symmetrical arrangement of the letters in a heading in relation to the midpoint of a page ('centring')
- Tabulation of columns of predetermined width; alignment of columns of figures on a decimal point
- Provision for the addition, deletion or amendment of blocks of text of variable size, with subsequent automatic re-arrangement in context; overwriting may be used to amend characters

- The provision of bold type for headings, and of italics within text; continuous underlining can be provided automatically
- A variety of different fonts (character styles) is usually available
- In addition to the original display and printout of text, an electronic copy will automatically be held in computer memory, and any number of further printed copies may be provided
- No retyping of draft documents is ever required – the electronic data that form the template for the printed document are stored by the system, retrieved and amended as necessary on display, and then used as a new template to print the amended version.

Aids for authors

- Extensive text editing: large blocks of text can be switched from one location to another
- A change to a string of words is often made in three stages: first the point at which (or points between which) the change is to be made is identified, then the new text is entered at an area of screen temporarily cleared for the purpose (a 'window'); finally the new text is shown in its new context, highlighted by double intensity characters or characters of a different colour, and the user is invited to confirm the change
- The user may, if s/he wishes, revoke the latest command s/he made to the system
- Each word may be checked for correct spelling by comparison with a computer-held dictionary (Box 2.1) – it must be remembered, however, that the

system cannot distinguish between words such as 'there', 'their' and 'they're' unless a grammar-checking facility has also been included

- A computer-held thesaurus allows the user to look up alternative words with meanings closely associated with the one s/he has earmarked on display
- Footnotes, word counts and index construction for books are provided
- A word consistently misquoted can be changed throughout a complete text by the use of a single amended entry
- Dovetailing with computer-aided design and desktop-publishing packages allows illustrations to be constructed and incorporated in books, magazine articles or practice leaflets (compatible hardware and software are prerequisites)
- The user may assemble a complex sequence of commands to be carried out by the system, and this block of instructions ('macro') can be stored for repetitive use

Batch production of personalized letters

Letters that have a standard main body of text can have their opening remark personalized (e.g. 'Dear Mr Smith') and an address label printed by the system (*mailmerge*). This operation requires that the text of the standard letter has been prestored by the user and that a list of the names and addresses of recipients has been entered.

Names and addresses can be taken from the patient record file on the practice computer and, in this way, 'call or recall' letters can be generated for screening or immunization.

Box 2.1   The principle of word searching

- Computer inspects word letter by letter and at each step makes comparison with computer-held list
- For spelling check, whole word is compared – if no match, system warns
- For entry assistance, computer checks until sequence of letters renders word unique, then completes word
  e.g. if the letter Z is keyed in at the beginning of a word, search of the computer dictionary would show 75 possibilities
  - for ZE entered there would be 23 possibilities
  - for ZEP entered there would be 2 possibilities
  - for ZEPP entered there would be 1 possibility
  so with the entry of ZEPP the computer recognizes the word as unique and completes it as ZEPPELIN
- An alternative form of entry assistance is for the user to key in ZEP and to ask for options: the computer would then offer
  ZEPHYR
  ZEPPELIN
  from which the user would make a choice for the term s/he wishes to enter

Aids for typesetting and publishing

This facility is primarily of interest to practitioners involved in research and authorship, who may be required to construct a research paper or magazine article using word processing facilities so that it may be submitted as electronic data on a diskette. Data presented in this way allow the rapid and greatly facilitated compilation of text for magazines and books. Electronic data can also be transmitted directly from the author's computer to the compositor's computer via electronic mail.

Some word processing packages offer basic compositing facilities such as headings in different predetermined type styles and sizes, italics, chapter or book headings at the top of each page, author's name or magazine name and date at the page foot, and automatic page numbering.

The construction of illustrations requires graphical facilities not provided by elementary word processing packages. If charts and graphs are available, they can be output jointly with text to either diskette or electronic mail.

2.3 GRAPHICS PACKAGES AND COMPUTER-AIDED DESIGN

Simple monochrome graphics known as 'charting' are provided by the foremost GP systems to output line graphs, bar and pie charts, and histograms. If available, the use of colour screens enhances the differentiation of data displayed. However, the term 'graphics package' really refers to a computer application that allows the user to construct images on, or import them to, the screen, with or without colour, in preparation for printout. In the context of GP computing such an application is of very limited use, which would include the embellishment of patient advice leaflets, practice brochures or practice annual reports. Although a simple 'graphics' package to run on Windows may be purchased very cheaply, minimum hardware requirements for any 'graphics' are likely to be a fast processor, plentiful available RAM and hard disk space, a high-grade VDU and a special printer.

'Graphics packages' offer a wide range of pre-drawn outlines (*clip-art*) and assist in the construction of freehand lines and curves. Objects can be mapped from one part of the screen to another, rotated, zoomed or panned, and colours are prepared by blending on-screen in a 'palette' area from which images may then be infilled, hatched or stippled (Fig. 2.1).

'Graphics packages' can import files from other compatible software, such as word processors, and can export to desktop-publishing packages. Computer-aided design (CAD) is an offshoot of graphics that incorporates applied mathematical calculation.

Fig. 2.1 Graphics assembly of line and bar charts (Arts & Letters Apprentice, reproduced by courtesy of Roderick Manhattan Group)

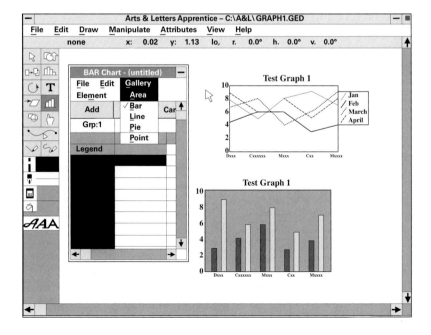

2.4 DESKTOP PUBLISHING

Practices that produce their own practice leaflets have found that the use of DTP packages halves normal printing costs. Leaflets can be printed at the practice, or a master copy may be sent to a print shop. DTP packages have taken over the compositor's job and brought to it a new versatility (Fig. 2.2).

DTP allows page presentation to be executed on screen prior to printout. This incorporates

- a wide range of print size, style spacing and colour
- page formatting – some packages allow more than one page to be planned simultaneously
- text is arranged so that it 'flows' round graphics, both text and graphical fields can be expanded or shrunk so as to fill the page exactly ('re-sizing'), and chunks of text or graphics can be transposed
- photographs can be included with graphics.

DTP packages can import files from compatible word processing, graphics, spreadsheet or database management packages. Generally, they will require at least 2 Mb RAM and not less than 5 Mb hard disk space, with a minimum of 386 processor power, a compatible printer and a VGA monitor with or without colour. Their speed of operation needs to be checked out against existing or proposed hardware specification. Packages are readily available for Macintosh and Windows, but less so for UNIX or XENIX operating systems. Prices range from £150–£750. Two of the best known are Corel Ventura and Adobe PageMaker.

If a professional print house is to be employed to replicate a master copy created by the practice, then it is essential that any images used should be made available in an electronic format that is compatible with the computer system used by the print house.

2.5 SPREADSHEETS

Spreadsheets are numerical data displays in which the data are tabulated both vertically and horizontally. This layout is one that allows crisp comparison to be made between vertical columns and horizontal rows. But there are relationships within and between rows and columns, and these relationships are known to the computer, although not routinely displayed when the spreadsheet is in use. Knowledge of the relationships allows the computer to build the spreadsheet given minimum data, or to change all affected rows and columns given a change in one subset of data (Table 2.1). When a spreadsheet has been fully labelled with its interrelationships it is sometimes referred to as a *worksheet*.

Spreadsheets may be used in practice for income and expenditure ledgers, payroll, practice accounts, claims to the health authority and subsequent payment checks, and financial audit. They allow comparison to be made, for example, between a current month's income and expenses and those of the equivalent month in the previous quarter, between values of one year and the previous year, and current values and those of an average practice. The term 'IF–THEN cal-

Fig 2.2 Desktop publishing: assembly of text and images, and assignment of font to text (Timeworks Publisher, reproduced by courtesy of GST Software)

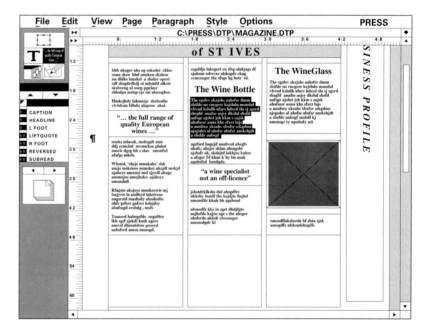

Table 2.1 The spreadsheet principle – tabulation facilitates comparison between rows and columns. Changes in hours or rate will affect both pay and tax (tax calculated at 20%)

Employee	Hours	Rate	Pay	Tax
A	1	5	5	1
B	5	6	30	6
C	4	6.5	26	5.20
D	2	7.5	15	3

culation' refers to the predictive use of a spreadsheet that will display the full effects expected if a proposed change to one piece of data were to be made.

'Off-the-shelf' spreadsheets have been dramatically successful in the commercial field, the best known being Lotus 1-2-3, Microsoft Excel, Quattro-Pro and SuperCalc (all principally DOS/Windows-based, although other versions are appearing). Spreadsheets for other operating systems are available, but are often more expensive. If the GP system supplier offers and supports a spreadsheet with the system, as most do, then this will usually be the preferred option.

2.6 ACCOUNTS AND BOOK-KEEPING

'Off-the-shelf' professional accounts packages are designed for small businesses and are not appropriate for NHS general practice, although they have an important role in private practice. Debtor files, customer statements, reminder letters, income and expenditure ledgers, overheads, profits and stock control are all provided. The most popular are Pegasus, Quickbooks Accounting, Sage, Multisoft and Tetra. NHS practice book-keeping with ledgering and balance striking may be achieved on 'off-the-shelf' spreadsheets, but all the GP suppliers now provide purpose-written book-keeping packages, many of which are of high quality and dovetail with other practice modules.

2.7 OTHER 'OFF-THE-SHELF' PACKAGES

Payroll packages may be purchased 'off-the-shelf' but do not cater for the compilation of wages reimbursement claims that need to be submitted to the health authority. Bespoke GP payroll software provides for all practice payroll requirements and is to be preferred, despite its often greater cost (see Chapter 20).

'Off-the-shelf' database management software has no place in general practice. All tailor-made GP

systems are already based on a platform of database management that basically allows storage and retrieval of data, cross-referencing, global changes to data, expansion of overall file architecture and computer searches. Database management packages have supplanted filing cabinets and card indexes.

2.8 SHAREWARE AND BULLETIN BOARDS

While subsets of software packages issued for demonstration to prospective purchasers may be obtained either inexpensively or free of charge from the makers, it is normally necessary to pay the full market price on purchase of the full package. There are two routes by which inexpensive 'off-the-shelf' software may be obtained.

Mail order

'Shareware' companies sell cut-price software with widely varying application areas, and varying quality, by mail order. There is no after-sales support.

Bulletin boards and the Internet

'Bulletin boards' usually contain files of both textual data and software programs that can be downloaded to an 'on-line' computer that has a communications card and software, a modem and a telephone line (Fig. 2.3).

In recent years the Internet has provided a cost-free milieu for the creation of a great many e-mail-based bulletin boards offering widely varying interests. Most GP system suppliers, GP user groups and the Primary Health Care Specialist Group of the British Computer Society have now developed Internet-based or direct-dial bulletin boards.

Although many bulletin boards use a computer virus filter, the medium must be regarded as a potentially infective source. (See also Chapter 18, section 18.5.)

Fig. 2.3 The Pry Marie Care bulletin board help menu screen (Courtesy of Dr Paul Bromley)

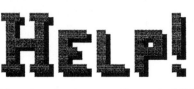

```
                    HELP!

        Press the Relevant number to access the required Help Screen.
          PLEASE LET ME KNOW IF YOU CONSIDER AN AREA NEEDS A HELP SCREEN!
  (1) Pry Marie Care Menus.              (J) Etiquette on BBs
  (2) Message Areas.                     (+)Our mailpacking facility
  (3) File Areas.                        (Q)uoting from a message in a reply.
  (4) How to Upload or Download a file.  (A)bout Archive files on PMC
  (5) All about our editors.             (D)ownload our Help File - ZIP format.
  (6) The Changing Room.                 (*)Above file, plus List, to view file.
  (7) What is Shareware.                 (#)Download our full help pack.
  (8) Combined Message Facilities.       (%)Download HELP file ASCII format.
  (X)it back from whence you came!       (H)ow to download the above Help files.
```

2.9 A BEGINNER'S GUIDE TO SYSTEM NAVIGATION

During the development of computers, some procedures that mediate the interaction between user and machine have proved so effective that they have become established practice. Although every operating system and every program is to some extent idiosyncratic, particularly with regard to the terms used to describe the procedures within it, a consensus has been arrived at with regard to the representation of data flow patterns in more advanced software. Computer literacy is now dependent upon grasping these basic concepts and becoming familiar with the terms used to describe them.

Checking the system's components

A fully assembled computer system consists of the hardware components of the individual PC you are using, the hardware components of the local area network (LAN) if you are linked to other local computers, and the electronic information contained within the system. The computer allows you to check and display the status of all hardware and software components item by item so that the integrity, connectivity and contents can be monitored.

Files and folders

Electronic information is contained within electronic *files*, each of which is named by text or acronym, and the files are arranged within larger assemblies called *folders* – terms purposely analogous to those used in paper filing cabinets. There are three types of file:

- *program files* containing motive software
- *document files* containing text

- *data files* containing other types of information such as images, charts and video.

Text-based system navigation

Early MUMPS and DOS systems were 'text based', a confusing term that simply means that they did not use a mouse, icons and the more intuitive forms of interaction of the graphical user interface. Text-based systems do have *dialogue boxes* – a rectangular space or window, superimposed upon the other screen contents, that allows question and answer interaction appropriate to the current transaction between user and system. A *prompt* by the system is a message that requires a user response which, if invalid in terms of prestored criteria, will result in the issue of an *error message* and a further prompt. Text-based systems do also have *menus* or lists of options from which a selection can be made. They also have the ability to enter data with guidance from a preprogrammed protocol, which can move the cursor on to the next 'field' of entry once a response has been validated and accepted. Other than this, cursor movement in text-based systems depends upon the use of vertical and horizontal cursor motivation keys, as a mouse is not used.

GUI system navigation

The Windows GUI operating system is so named because of its ability to embellish the concept of the subroutine window. GUI refinements include:

- *Command icons* clicking on which will invoke programs and subroutines, or open document or data files

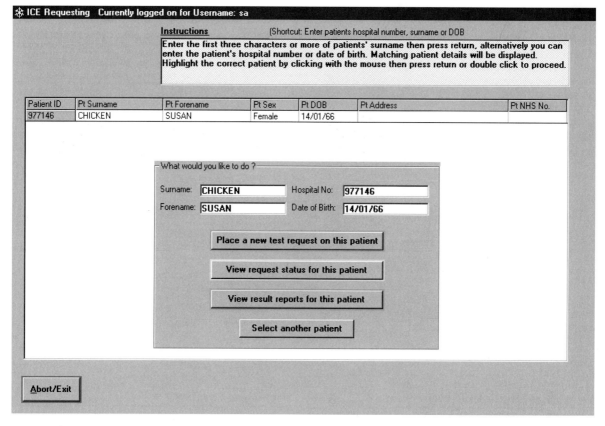

Fig. 2.4 Dialogue box and data entry window (Torex's Premiere System; Pathology and Radiology Links)

- *Bars*, strips of screen space put aside at the outer border of a Window that both enable and confirm the activation of programs and subroutines (status, task, tool, scroll and menu bars)
- *Tabs*, which mimic the titled subsection dividers in a paper card index
- The *menu* concept is also extensively used in GUIs.

The GUI employs either a mouse, trackerball or joystick to move the cursor and trigger its interaction at a given vector point on the screen. The mouse usually has left and right 'buttons' on its upper surface, and single, double, or repeated clicks on either button are all of unique significance to the system. If a mouse button is held down and the mouse moved, an operation known as *dragging* is carried out whereby a screen feature can be moved wholesale to another location. Use of a single left mouse button click often reduplicates the action of the 'return key'. The first two or three commands after 'boot-up' usually require a double click on the left mouse button, whereas subsequent commands only require one left click.

GUI primary and secondary cursors

The primary *cursor* on a GUI is a thin, upright, intermitting bar that demonstrates the point at which data entry will next take place. This is analogous to the central gap in the ribbon fork through which the letter-bearing slugs on a typewriter make their impact on the ribbon (the typing point). Mouse-based display screens also employ a secondary cursor, which typically takes the form of an arrowhead to show the point on the screen at which the user's mouse-transmitted commands will become effective. When the secondary cursor is superimposed on a *hypertext-linked* term (so denoted by being underlined, and often displayed in a different colour), its appearance changes from an arrowhead to that of a diagrammatic pointing finger. When this happens, a mouse click command will enable rapid switching to another screen defined by the term.

A commonly used convention is for the secondary cursor to be accompanied by a diagrammatic hour glass, or bee in flight, which persists while the system is in the process of activating a new routine.

Fig. 2.5 Windows 95 screen showing desktop icons (top left), main icon button bar and start button (bottom left), application menu (centre) and Microsoft Word document window available for data entry (right). Scroll bar is at right edge and task bar at lower edge of screen, with button bars overlying the Word window (Courtesy of Southampton University Computer Services)

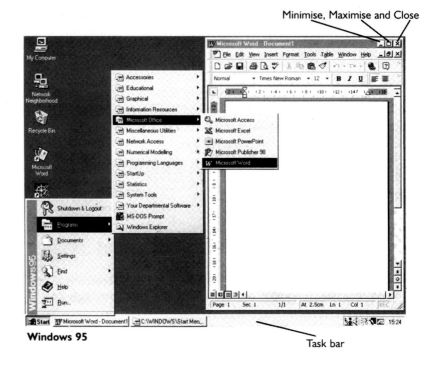

Using main programs and subprograms

Programs and data files on the computer have to be 'opened' by icon or menu selection in order to present their facilities to the user on the screen, within a circumscribed window. Programs should be closed after use by using a keyboard code, selecting the appropriate command from the menu or clicking on a small box displaying a cross, in the top right-hand corner of the window. A succession of programs can, however, be opened in series, when successive windows relating to them will be superimposed one upon the other leaving an obvious overlap (*cascade* presentation). If multiple programs are opened in parallel, then the windows for each will appear side by side (*tiled* presentation). In Microsoft Windows the names of programs currently open are also shown in the task bar located at the bottom of the screen, and clicking on these names will enable movement between open programs.

Subprograms can be selected from a list of menu options, which is unravelled downwards when the name of the subprogram category to which a particular list belongs is clicked on the *menu bar* (the latter is usually lodged just above or below the main icon button bar).

Like programs, documents must be opened before, and closed after, use.

Scrolling and paging

Vertical or horizontal extensions of the data on screen can be accessed either by *scrolling* or *paging* in the chosen direction. As with a road atlas, the presence of extensions to the data that are available are indicated by a symbol. In the case of scrolling this takes the form of a vertical or horizontal *scroll bar* – a thin strip placed at the edge of the window within which a marker mirrors the relation that the data on screen bears to the whole document. Movements to and fro are activated by clicking or holding on small icons at either end of the scroll bar or on the bar itself.

Start-up

When the system is first switched on, the process of *booting up* (a term derived from the slang expression 'pulling oneself up by one's own boot straps') begins, which copies from hard disk to memory those programs that are immediately necessary to the operation of the system.

As the Microsoft Windows convention is now the de facto standard, it is useful to quote its further routines as examplars:

• an initiating screen appears that requires the input of user name and password (the latter disguised from view), following this

- a *Start button* appears at the bottom left-hand corner of the screen, and this is accompanied elsewhere on the screen by other icons, which include:
  - '*My computer*' (which invokes an analysis of the computer's contents, listed by component)
  - the *Recycle Bin* (which enables the user to discard unwanted files)
  - the *Internet access* icon (which enables dial-up to the Internet Service Provider).

These basic command icons that appear when Windows is first started are collectively known as the *desktop*.

Activation of the start button by clicking on it summons the *Start menu*, which paradoxically includes the 'shut down' command, but which also offers access to submenu-listed programs, documents and computer settings. The Start menu also includes options to use a contents search engine to access named programs or documents (the *Run button*), and to summon *help screens*.

The documents listed will be those saved to storage by the user, and the programs will include (apart from the components of Windows 95/98/2000/NT), the subdivisions of application program packages such as Microsoft Office, plus any other software (such as the Quicken personal finance package or the Encarta encyclopedia) that has been loaded by the user.

Close down

When closing down the system, it is vital that all new data created in memory is 'saved' from memory to hard disk, otherwise these will be lost when the power is switched off. It is equally important that the system's automated shut-down procedure should be allowed to complete itself before turning off the power supply. When the procedure has been completed, a notice to this effect will appear on the screen.

Setting up new components

The term 'setup' is used to describe the process of installation and integration of new software and hardware on the system, and routines that achieve this are available for selection within the operating system.

The route through which a file is installed and can be traced is known as the *path*, and this has its own shorthand code which the computer recognizes. The relevant drive (disk) that is to contain the folder in which the file is to be placed is denoted by its drive letter, followed by a colon. The name of the folder is prefaced by a single backslash, and a shared folder on a network is prefaced by double backslashes. An individual named file within a folder will follow the folder's name, will be separated from it by a backslash, and will be followed by a dot and a three letter acronym denoting its category (e.g. *txt* for text file, *doc* for document file). A similar coding convention is used for Internet addresses.

Data processing techniques

Data stored on a system can be traced in three ways.

- A categorized index can be browsed in a manner similar to searching Yellow Pages.
- A *search engine* can be employed. Powerful programs exist for homing in by a process of pattern matching on words or phrases stored in the computer (Table 2.1).
- A *stem* or truncated word pattern match will allow the production of a short list of words, all of which begin with the same three or four specified letters, from which the user can make a final selection.

Entry of data by protocol employs a technique that first locates the cursor in the field where data are to be completed, prompts for the data required, then validates them by reference to prestored criteria. The commonest answer to a prompt may already be displayed for acceptance by default, in which case the user need only press the 'return' key.

The term *browse* refers to the perusal of a screen or sequence of screens. Text that the user wishes to process may be *selected* by highlighting it with the secondary cursor.

A document may be *reformatted* (rearranged) on screen, and text and images may be increased or reduced in size. *Print preview* allows the document's overall layout to be reviewed before printing.

The contents of screens and the findings of searches may be printed out as *hard copy* or downloaded to diskette. Help screens allow the provision of instructions on system use, and are accessed either by browsing a help index or as a context-sensitive response.

Data may be deleted *en bloc* from a document (*cut*), inserted (with rearrangement of the previous text in context), copied to another space (*copy and paste*), overwritten and so replaced, or moved from one place to another (*cut, copy and paste*).

Most modern systems allow the latest user transaction to be reversed (*undo*) or subsequently reinstated (*redo*).

Files can be deleted in their entirety by clicking on them and dragging them across to the Recycle Bin, which is emptied of its contents when the user

Fig. 2.6 Microsoft Word: Full screen window

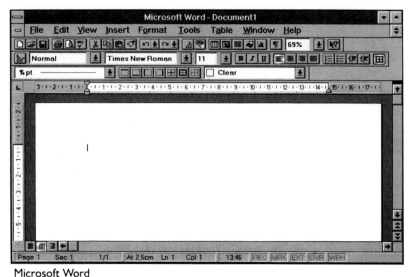

Microsoft Word

Fig. 2.7 Some special symbols used in Windows 95/98/2000

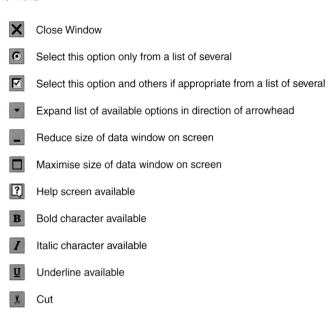

decrees. Files can also be deleted by using the appropriate submenu or keycode.

Macros are assemblies of frequently used subunits of software that are available to programmers during program construction. The facility also exists on modern systems for users to create their own macros by condensing a sequence of key depressions or mouse clicks so that these can be stored and referenced by a single code (which usually involves the depression of two keys simultaneously, or the use of Windows *shortcut* icons).

2.10 COMPRESSION

Text, and to a lesser extent images and charts, can be *compressed* on the hard disk to economize storage space. This is done by filtering out signals that record the existence and address of vacant spaces. Programs containing the acronym *zip* are used in the compression/decompression process.

2.11 WORK GROUPS

Users who jointly access the same local area network (LAN) are known as a *workgroup*. Setting up a LAN requires that each component computer is supplied with an expansion card and uses the same network protocol and *service software* to coordinate use of shared amenities. Software required by the server differs from that used on client workstations, a constraint that also applies to WAN dial-up networking, where access to the network is available through modems and telecommunication lines.

2.12 BITMAPS AND CLIP ART

A *bitmap* is the representation of an image according to the exact nature and distribution of the individual dots (*pixels*) from which it is constructed, and by which it is represented in memory. *Clip art* is an assortment of preconstructed images that can be selected from an electronic library of frames housed on the computer.

2.13 BACKUP

Backup procedures should be undertaken to replicate all user data on to security copy, such as that provided by diskette, supplementary hard disk or tape streamer. The procedure is usually automated and prevents the loss of data in the event of system failure. Programs can be reinstated by the use of the diskettes or CD-ROM from which they were originally installed.

2.14 DEFRAGMENTATION AND DISK SCANNING

Entries of data to the hard disk are constrained by the space available at each address, and fragmentation occurs with some entries occupying multiple addresses. Distribution of stored data can be rationalized by a *defragmentation* program. Hard disk storage seldom, if ever, has 100% integrity, and storage areas (*clusters*) that are faulty can be detected and circumvented by a *disk scanning* program (e.g. 'Scandisk'). Both these programs are available on modern systems.

When a system is in regular use it is helpful to have an automatic listing of average daily and monthly hard disk occupancy and corresponding spare capacity.

3 An overview of the use of computers in general practice

3.1 METAMORPHOSIS

The Babylonians used clay tablets, the Egyptians papyrus and the Greeks parchment for their records. Widespread paper-based data exchange began as primitive banknotes in ancient China, and for almost a millennium paper has remained the unchallenged vector of permanent record. Although the use of paper for books, magazines and newspapers is never likely to cease, its dominance as a medium for letters and records is being eroded by the computer. By the 1980s more than half of North American business was being conducted through electronic mail (*e-mail*), and commercial transactions are now routinely conducted by use of electronics throughout the developed world.

The medical profession is slowly but inexorably converting to computers and electronic records. In 1969 the IBM desktop pilot system initiated the use of VDUs in general practice (the IBM–Whipton Project), and first pioneered many electronic features that we now take for granted in GP computing – structured records using natural language, 'cut and paste', summary history, repeat medication and allergy records, morbidity codes, tetanus recall, audit, and telecommunication linkage with a remote computer – yet of the 400 mainly medical visitors who viewed the system, only one in four believed that their colleagues would accept the new medium or that computers would ever have a role in health care.

Attitudes were to change radically. By 1988, 20% of UK general practices had installed computers. By 1992 the proportion had risen to 70%, and by 1996 to 96%. Universality is approached as government strategies and further system development render computers virtually indispensable to modern practice. General practices elsewhere in Europe, in North America and in Australasia have also been converting to computers, although the principal application in these systems has been billing, which often involves copayments between patients and their insurance agents. Britain has been, and remains, at the forefront of development of patient management software for general practice.

3.2 INCENTIVES TO INSTALL COMPUTERS

The incentives to computerize have increased cumulatively with progressive application software development. As each of the following automated facilities (quoted in historical order) has become available, the argument for computerization has proved more compelling.

- Repeat medication control
- 'Call or recall' immunization and screening with items of service (IoS) claims
- Opportunistic screening
- Record reform, storage and retrieval (encounter forms as a transitional stage)
- Target achievement and indicative prescribing cost monitoring
- Control of delegation to practice nurse and other staff
- Acute prescribing with elimination of predictable prescribing errors
- Streamlining of practice book-keeping, payroll and accounts
- 'Personal organizer' functions
- Electronic mail to FHSA (now PPSA), pathology laboratory, hospital and bank
- Access to remote databases for a wide variety of reference material
- Checks on FHSA (now PPSA) operations – validity of register, IoS claims and other payments
- Combined referral letter, referral appointment making and referral logging
- Fundholding and Locality Commissioning

Other forms of incentive for UK practices to computerize have been

- Naked enthusiasm
- Discounts. In 1982 the 'Micros for GPs' scheme launched with Department of Industry money offered practices computers at half-price. Ciba-Geigy's subsidized software initiative of 1983 helped to launch the AMC system. In 1986 AAH Meditel and VAMP Health launched schemes to provide systems at virtually no cost, in return for practice morbidity and prescribing data. Some health authorities have negotiated bulk discount for their practices, or provided free computers
- Government policies that impose requirements on practices that can only realistically be fulfilled by the use of computers – the 1990 GP Contract, Fundholding and Locality Commissioning
- Reimbursement by HAs.

3.3 THE DIFFICULTIES OF INTRODUCING COMPUTERS INTO GENERAL PRACTICE

Daunting obstacles stood in the way of early GP system implementation, but these have slowly been overcome by improvements in design and methodology.

- At the outset, few doctors had any perception of what computers might be expected to do for them, and system designers had only the precedent of commercial applications to guide early innovations – these models proved to be totally inappropriate to general practice. The cumbersome nature of primitive equipment and software also alienated the profession.
- Early systems were prohibitively expensive, but over the past two decades both hardware and software costs have steadily fallen in real terms.
- Systems have, until recently, been unreliable. Happily, as reliance on computers has increased, so has their reliability. Hardware faults are now exceptional, and software faults can either be circumvented using hotline advice or 'patched' following remote diagnostic investigation through modems by the system supplier.
- The methodology for converting manual records to computer had not been worked out nor formalized for early systems, and disparate solutions to this problem resulted, creating barriers to later intercommunication. The cost and effort involved in record conversion constituted potent disincentives to practices. The specification of minimum data sets, the reimbursement of staff wages for the task (in some instances HAs have increased reim-

bursement levels to 100%), and the general acceptance of the need to carry out the exercise have all served to change the profession's attitude towards conversion. Processing of incoming paper reports will still be needed even after the conversion and loading of historical records, but ultimately this too will cease with the general adoption of electronic mail. The incorporation of Read morbidity codes in GP systems has had a dramatic effect on the standardization of summarization of data and on its potential for interchange.

- For many years it was alleged that doctors would refuse to type on keyboards, and that acceptance of computers would have to wait for voice recognition. 'Shoehorn' data entry techniques such as the use of the default key for the most commonly selected option, dictionary-assisted term entry, windows and menus, and 'mice' have all helped to overcome this obstacle. Encounter forms act as stepping stones to desktop computing, but most doctors and all secretaries are now happy to use keyboards.

3.4 THE COMPUTER'S ROLES IN GENERAL PRACTICE

The doctor's assistant

So many uses have been found for the computer in general practice that it becomes difficult for the uninitiated to view them in perspective. It is helpful to consider the practice computer system as having nine roles.

A: Record reformer

In contrast with most manual records, computer records are fully legible, not subject to wear and tear, may be viewed simultaneously by as many users as there are terminals, and are never misfiled nor 'missing from the rack'. They take up virtually no storage space. Computerized patient records not only log consultations but can be re-presented as summaries, preventive medicine records, chronic disease surveillance records and palliative care records. Re-presentation can be structured by episode, by problem, and by the body system affected (or by any other subdivision of the morbidity code hierarchy).

B: Administrative agent

The computer offers considerable administrative assistance in such matters as record filing and retrieval, appointment making, form filling and letter writing, monitoring transactions with the HA and PPSA, label printing for pathology samples and dispensing containers, default monitoring and automated referral.

C: Delegation controller

Criteria set by the doctor will be conveyed by the computer to control delegation of care. Activities thus regulated for practice nurses will be screening, immunization, venepuncture, prescribing, and chronic disease management clinics. Patient self-monitoring of such items as blood sugar may be controlled on the basis of results periodically downloaded on to, and analysed by, the practice computer.

D: Communicator

Computers link remote users through modems and telephone lines. This enables the practice to communicate electronically with the HA and PPSA, Primary Care Group or Trust (PCG+T), pathology laboratory, radiology department, hospitals, banks, remote databases and bulletin boards, data collection agencies, the Internet, the LMC, the Local Health Group, the Prescription Pricing Authority and the Committee on Safety of Medicines.

E: Mediator of clinical expertise

The practice computer stores comprehensive prescribing and specific case management protocols so as to be able to guide the doctor towards optimal methods of intervention.

F: Financial guardian

The computer is used to record and monitor a practice's financial affairs – HA payment checks, income maximization, private billing, book-keeping, payroll, accounts, and budgeting for Primary Care Commissioning Groups or Trusts.

G: Publisher

Practice brochures, patient advice leaflets and slips, and practice annual reports may all be produced on the practice system.

H: Auditor

The computer can be made to search its files, and analyse and re-present the results obtained for the purposes of audit and research.

I: Educator

Interactive educational packages may be loaded on the practice computer to educate and train practice personnel. Automated assessment of student prowess with national average comparison can be built in. Chart graphics, artwork and photographs may accompany these packages.

The computer will never replace the general practitioner, but it makes a very effective doctor's assistant.

3.5 THE OVERALL BENEFITS OF USING COMPUTERS IN GENERAL PRACTICE

These may be summarized as follows:

Data
- Greater accuracy
- Greater legibility
- Fewer omissions
- More control
- Faster and easier entry procedures
- Faster and easier filing
- Faster and easier retrieval
- Faster and easier analysis
- Faster and easier communication

Administration
- Greater efficiency
- Improved speed and convenience in executing practice procedures

Patient care
- Improved at all levels as a result of protocols, and greater administrative and data efficiency

Time
- Savings in doctors', receptionists', and secretaries' time

Finances
- Improved control
- Income enhanced by audit and better control

3.6 BESPOKE GP SOFTWARE

In the previous chapter we considered the merits and command structure of ready-made software packages that could be bought in the High Street. The requirements of general practice systems are so specific that 'off-the-shelf' database management software must be customized to an advanced degree if it is to achieve adequate functionality in a practice setting. Some GP software houses have preferred to construct their database software from scratch rather than modify prepackaged modules. Either way, the result is a product carefully tailored to its intended purpose – bespoke software.

By 1999, despite the demise of all but the most successful marketed systems that resulted from the introduction of accreditation, there were still around 30 on offer, and these could not intercommunicate because they used incompatible operating systems, file structures or data-terminology. In the early days of GP computer development, a golden opportunity to set functionality and data standards was ignored by NHS planners, a mistake replicated in the hospital sector. Belated efforts in the 1990s to redress this omission were more in the nature of an agonizing reappraisal than an initiative. The cost of the system reconciliation now required across the service by the NHS Executive information strategy document *Information for Health* will be many millions of pounds.

Doctors and practice staff are faced with the task of purchasing, and making the best use of, one of the many marketed systems with an eye not only on cost benefit, but also on the integration of their computer into a health service network. This entails the assimilation of knowledge of computer applications and functionality sufficient to allow an informed judgement. The remainder of this chapter is devoted to an overview of the application areas in which GP systems are employed, together with the principal services offered by suppliers. The chapters that follow will deal with each application area in greater detail, information that necessarily precedes the ultimate sections, which are devoted to computer selection and the preparation of the practice prior to its installation.

3.7 PRINCIPAL APPLICATION AREAS – AN OVERVIEW

On the basis of cumulative experience gained during the past 30 years, a consensus has been reached as to the principal features a UK general practice system should possess. As a result, most system suppliers now either market or are developing packages for the following areas of application.

- **Building the practice database** – patient record files
  - Registration
  - Consultation log – full notes in diary form but in reverse chronological order
  - Clinical summary, classified by date, body system or problem, using Read codes
  - Preventative records
  - Condition-orientated (surveillance) records and cohort clinic support
  - Medication records for acute and repeat prescribing, with use of drug databases
  - Pathology records

- Radiology records
- Hospital reports
- **Special functions**
  - GP appointments
  - Commissioning in conjunction with Primary Care Group or Trust
  - Dispensing
  - Book-keeping, payroll, accounts and banking
  - Private practice
  - Nurse triage, out-of-hours service support
  - Remote access to practice files
  - Audit and research
  - Education
  - CD-ROM reference
  - Support for near-patient testing and patient-held monitors
  - Publishing – brochures, patient instruction leaflets, business plans and practice annual reports
- **Communications** – access using EDIFACT structured messaging or e-mail to:
  - Primary Care Group or Trust
  - Health Authority and PPSA
  - Pathology Laboratory
  - Radiology Department
  - Hospital (reports, referral letters, waiting list data, service costs, appointments)
  - Telemedicine facilities
  - Remote databases, including Internet
  - Bulletin boards (news groups, conferencing, information databases, shareware)
  - Data collection for collation and analysis
  - PACT
  - CSM and REM
  - Community Health Agency
  - Mental Health Agencies
  - Social Services
  - Split-site medical centres, and remote access from portables.

3.8 WHAT THE MONEY BUYS

In contrast with the purchase of 'off-the-shelf' software modules, buying a bespoke system will result in the provision of the following facilities.

- Hardware for the practice computer configuration, which may be that suitable for a single doctor practice (with terminals for the doctor and the receptionist), a multiuser configuration with server and dumb terminals, or a fully networked configuration with server and intelligent workstations or network stations. Hybrid systems employing both dumb and intelligent terminals are also in use. Occasionally, several single-handed practices maintain segregated records on their own workstations but share a common fileserver situated at the health authority.

The system may be supplemented by portable computers for home visits, or have secondary systems where medical services are provided at split sites and are linked by land-line (a dedicated telecommunications linkage that does not require dial-up)

The choice of additional hardware such as printers or scanners, which must be fully compatible and integrated with the system, will be determined by the needs of the practice's information technology strategy

- Software with clinical, financial and communicative provisions, featuring the applications listed in the previous section
- Periodic releases of software enhancements to correct faults, and new software modules to increase functionality
- Connectivity with HealthLink and NHSnet
- Support – breakdown service, hot-line, user manual, on-site training, software-based training packages
- Morbidity, drug, and protocol dictionaries with regular upgrades
- Consumables – stationery, printer cartridges, toner or ribbons, etc.
- Maintenance contracts
- Eligibility to join a user group
- ESCROW provision (see Chapter 26)

4 The architecture of a GP system

4.1 THE NEED FOR CAREFUL PLANNING

It is said that whereas doctors bury their mistakes, those made by architects are set in stone for posterity. This is not true of some architectural howlers, following which bridges or hospitals have had to be pulled down and rebuilt from scratch. A similar process of agonizing reappraisal affects general practices that buy a system of inappropriate design, or one that underestimates their long-term requirements. A number of doctors have already changed systems once, and a few have done so twice. This is a flagrant waste of time, effort and money.

The three previous chapters dealt with the raw building materials of generic packages and of bespoke GP systems – hardware, basic computer operations, and the principal areas of application. We must now look at the way in which these elements are assembled to build a definitive general practice system. A clear understanding of the following will combine to help prevent the need for total system replacement.

- System hardware, software, dictionary and record architecture
- Those items of hardware that will tolerate system upgrades
- The applications that the practice will ultimately use
- The strategy of stepwise implementation (see Chapter 29).

The same necessity for careful planning applies to the selection of categories of data that the practice decides to store on its system. It is labour-intensive, time consuming and frustrating to have to reprocess all the manual records because a required category of data present in them was not abstracted at the first pass. Even more harrowing is the loss of data incurred by system failure or data corruption if this cannot be reinstated from backup.

It is better to learn from others' mistakes than from one's own. With careful planning, both system replacement and reduplication of data entry are avoidable. The aim must be to make the practice system as 'future-proof' as possible.

4.2 THE ARCHITECTURE OF HARDWARE, SOFTWARE, DICTIONARIES AND RECORDS

Hardware

The same basic components of hardware are now used in common by most GP computer systems, and have already been described in Chapter 1.

During the 1980s, rapid development rendered purchased hardware obsolete after four or five years of use. Currently we are witnessing progressive increases in hardware power and reliability, coupled with progressive reduction in price, so that not only has the working life of equipment been extended, but vastly increased functionality has become affordable.

The corner stone of the practice system is the fileserver, and we are fast approaching a point in development at which it should be possible to purchase a fileserver of sufficient power that system upgrades will not render it obsolete during its working lifetime.

Hard disks, although not subjected to direct mechanical degradation, have a limited life and should be replaced every 3–4 years. The degree of degradation can be assessed by using the 'Scandisk' program described in Chapter 2.

During the 1990s the introduction of Windows-based software and the prospect of requiring access to the NHSnet involved many practices in upgrading from multiuser dumb-terminal-based configurations to networked intelligent terminals and twisted pair cabling. A hardware upgrade of this magnitude is unlikely to be called for again. Printers, on-line UPS and DAT stream backup should not require upgrading during their working lifetimes.

Major software upgrades sometimes imply purchasing entirely new types of additional equipment. Remote portables, patient summoning LED displays in the waiting room, and scanners for archiving hospital reports are recent examples.

Software

Every facet of computer activity must be motivated by appropriate software, and the suite of programs that is supplied with modern systems becomes more extensive with every upgrade.

Commercial 'off-the-shelf' application packages such as Microsoft Office or Lotus SmartSuite contain modules that offer word processing, spreadsheet, database management and a variety of other features. The breadth and depth of the functionality of these suites increases with every release. GP software development is similarly expansive.

The principal hardware, software, dictionary and record components used in a GP system are listed in Table 4.1.

The architecture of computer records

Just as preventive medicine, surveillance of chronic disease, prescribing or taking a history in a new case are subsets of overall practice activity, so the records devoted to these activities are subsets of the total record system. A record policy that maintained a separate record for each function and that failed to integrate all records would either fragment data, dispersing them between the various special records, or cause the reduplication of all entries that the separate records had in common. This dilemma has never been, and cannot be, resolved using manual records.

The computer gives us an unrivalled opportunity to reshape, and use for our own purposes, each component of the general practice record in its particular context, yet at the same time to coordinate all components without the fragmentation or double entry of data.

4.3 WHY WE SHOULD CHANGE TO COMPUTER RECORDS

Other than the need to coordinate record subsets, there are many compelling reasons to change from manual to computer record systems.

- The labour-intensive and error-prone processes of pulling and refiling manual records, problems of records missing because they are in use or have been misplaced, of wear and tear, and of ever-increasing storage space, are not alleviated by a change to A4 or other improved paper record formats.

Table 4.1 Basic components of a GP system			
Hardware	**Software**	**Dictionaries**	**Records**
Fileserver	Operating system	Read codes	Registration
Distributed workstations, or network stations with VDUs, keyboards and mice	Bespoke GP software	Drug dictionary	Principal screen
Near-silent consulting room printers	Networking software	Protocol library	Prevention
Heavy duty batch printer in secretary's office	Driver software for peripheral units		Surveillance
Uninterruptible power supply	WAN communication package		Total prescribing
DAT stream backup unit	Anti-virus software		Repeat medication
CD-ROM multidrive	Backup software		Pathology
Flatbed scanner	UPS software		Archives for historical hospital reports
Modem or terminal adapter with appropriate lines out	Internet access provision		
Physical security devices	OCR software for scanner		Appointments
Twisted pair cabling			Commissioning

- Computer records are consistently legible, unlike those handwritten by most doctors.
- Record interrogation to locate a single defined item of data is always faster on computer than on paper.
- The use of 'shoehorn' techniques of data entry can make record construction by computer rapid, punctilious and accurate. Terms may also be used that are standardized for future mass searches.
- Alternative forms of record presentation, such as the ability to show a summarised or full length record, or pathology test results either as the total day's reports to the practice or as a cumulative patient record, cannot be achieved without a computer.
- New forms of patient management such as combination screening ('call or recall' complemented by opportunistic procedures) can only be undertaken if computer records are used.
- Delegation of responsibility to nursing and other staff can be controlled more effectively if records and protocols are computerized.
- The age of electronic mail has arrived. Already in many businesses, more letters are received through telephone lines and computer terminals than by conventional mail. We need computer-stored data in order to be able to automate output such as referral letters, reports and claims. In general practice, we must link with X-ray departments, laboratories, hospitals and health authorities in order to receive their communications in electronic form, which will arrive so much more promptly than paper documents. We must decide in what form we wish to receive our new electronic data. The shabby disarray of the 'Lloyd George' card wallet record shows us that we have been totally unprepared for these changes. Given a unique patient identifier between users of electronic mail, filing of the day's incoming data into the recipient computer record system can be performed automatically when the user indicates that s/he has read and accepted them.
- Computerization of patient identity details at the practice and the health authority allows the registers of the two to be reconciled rapidly and simply
- Practice research, audit and annual report preparation are exercises that proved so arduous using manual methods that they were frequently omitted. Practice activities are faithfully mirrored in a comprehensive computer record system, and their analysis can be automated.
- Other computerized procedures such as those employed during prescribing, automated decision support, commissioning, target calculations or billing, depend upon data stored in the patient record.

4.4 THE REQUIREMENTS OF THE NEW RECORD

It has been no easy matter to define those features that the general practitioner requires in the comprehensive computer record. Early in the course of development several opinion surveys were conducted, but these did little more than endorse, in a general way, the direction that prototype design was taking. In the UK it was at first hard to discover cogent reasons for computerization that would match the benefits offered by practice billing and accounting in the USA. Early system developers learned their design principles by little more than trial and error, until firmer foundations were provided by a detailed analysis of the manner in which doctors interrogated the manual record at consultation. The creation of user groups, which provide the supplier with criticisms and suggestions, now plays a highly significant part in defining and refining software, and essential design principles are later codified by incorporating them in the NHSME's Requirements for Accreditation.

Although there is individual variation between systems, the following design principles have become generally accepted.

1. There should be a screen that accommodates all details relating to the patient's registration, identity and status (sometimes referred to as demographic details).
2. There should be a log of GP consultation data ordered by date, as in the manual record, but arranged in inverse chronological order, because the most recent entries are those most frequently accessed on reattendance by the patient. There must be a link between the clinical data in the consultation log and the treatment relating to each condition.
3. A morbidity summary (summary history) should be provided, preferably structured so as to facilitate appraisal. This should combine, yet distinguish between, data from general practice, hospital and X-ray department.
4. The foremost clinical record screen should provide preferential display of the summary history, patient-drug idiosyncrasies, the names of continuously used drugs, and a list of opportunistic reminders for procedures due or overdue.
5. Special screens should be provided for data generated in consequence of the management of chronic diseases such as diabetes, hypertension or asthma – *condition-orientated displays.*
6. Screens should be provided to record preventive procedures – screening and immunization – highlighting those procedures that are due or overdue.

7. Medication records should list details of all pre-scriptions issued, and contain an identifiable sub-set for repeat medication that indicates the span of authorization and aids the monitoring of com-pliance.

8. Pathology and radiology records are required, tabulated by investigation, date and result. Abnormal results should be highlighted, and in pathology records graphs should be used to dis-play single or multiple parameter values over time.

9. When hospital reports are received through elec-tronic mail, summary statements will be redupli-cated from them to summary history before they are stored in an archival area (which must be pro-vided within the practice record).

10. Data should need to be entered once only, but should nevertheless be capable of being retrieved in context as either a consultation log entry, an item of summary, or as a component of screening or condition-orientated displays. It should be possible to retrieve data by the date they were generated, by the physiological system that is affected, by Read code, by site of consultation or by author. Data should be accessible as text, or in tabular or graphical format if appropriate. It should be possible by picking out an episode of summary history to raise the full text of that episode in the consultation log, in a condition-

orientated record, or in an archived hospital let-ter.

11. Entry of all important terms should be diction-ary-validated, and pro-formas and protocols should be used to record readings taken from commonly grouped parameters.

12. Linkage must be provided between the patient record and administrative functions such as the referral process, commissioning, claim comple-tion, billing and appointment making.

13. An audit trail must be provided to link all entries with their author, time and date, and to track all changes (the so-called 'indelible' electronic record).

4.5   BASIC ARCHITECTURE OF THE PRACTICE RECORD ON COMPUTER

There are six main clinical record screen categories – the principal screen, surveillance, preventive medi-cine, pathology and radiology, total prescribing, and repeat medication. Separate surveillance screens are required for each condition under review. All screens automatically scroll upwards in order to extend, with the exception of the consultation log on the principal screen, which scrolls downwards to allow entries to be made in reverse chronological order.

Fig. 4.1   The patient record files as the nucleus for all main practice computer activities

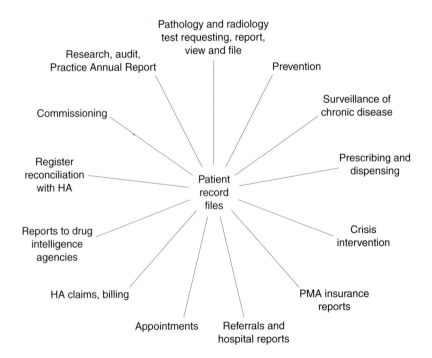

Optional scrolling as determined by the user may also take place in the reverse on all screens. Paging from one type of screen to another type for the same patient, and between screens of the same type for different patients, takes place at will. On all screens the patient identification details are shown at the top, regardless of scrolling, and prompts for action are displayed at the bottom. The principal screen should indicate by a symbol which, if any, condition-orientated screens are held for the patient. The six clinical record screens and their inter-relationships are shown diagrammatically in Figure 4.2. The following description is of a stylized system with features taken from several individual designs in order to illustrate the manner of implementation of the principles involved.

4.6 THE PRINCIPAL CLINICAL RECORD SCREEN

This screen is the master screen, and appears first when the patient's basic identification details have been entered into the system. The screen is divided into upper and lower areas. The upper area houses preferential data consisting, in order from above downwards, of opportunistic screening and other important reminders (such as default from a mammography appointment), drug and other allergies, the names of drugs authorized for repeat, and summary history. The existence of condition-orientated records that relate to chronic diseases listed in the summary history is indicated by code letters.

The lower area consists of the latest entries in the consultation log and, by scrolling, all earlier log

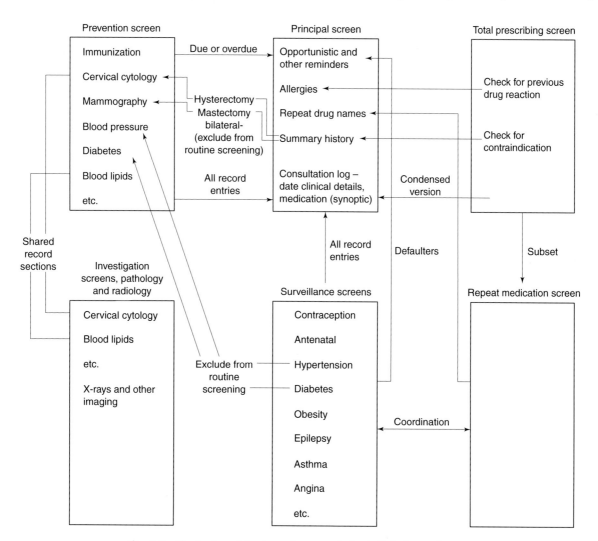

Fig. 4.2 The basic architecture of a computerized clinical record system

entries can be retrieved. Entries show the date on the left of the screen, clinical observations in the centre and a condensate of medication details on the right. As the date, clinical observations and treatment relating to the same episode of illness all occupy the same horizontal line or lines, their relationship to each other is never lost. The latest clinical log entry is the one most frequently accessed at redisplay and is therefore placed uppermost.

A summary history statement is a subset of the full clinical observations statement and, provided that the user entering data indicates the limits of the summary statement, the latter will automatically be reduplicated into the summary history area.

All important or primary terms used in the summary statement will be checked against the computer morbidity dictionary, will have Read codes allocated to them and are amenable to later search by computer. Qualifying and elaborative terms within the summary statement may also, in many cases, be coded using Read version 3. Other data that are not dictionary defined must be added freestyle. Drug allergies form another subset of the consultation log, which is preferentially reduplicated into the upper part of the principal display.

Regardless of the reduplications of subsets, the consultation log remains a complete record of all data registered at the time of patient contact. Data entered through surveillance and preventive medicine screens will also show in the consultation log, but medication will appear in it only in a condensed form. Hospital summary statements and radiology reports will be quoted in the consultation log, distinguishable from GP-originated data by appropriate flags. Pathology test data remain separate from the consultation log.

4.7 SURVEILLANCE SCREENS

The surveillance screens – one for each condition under review – show data arranged by date, parameters tested and the next review date at which the patient should be seen by the doctor and nurse. As surveillance patients are usually taking repeat medication, these two screens must correlate. Patients with hypertension or diabetes should not be called for 'call or recall' clinics for blood pressure or urine testing respectively, so there must be data correlation between the preventive medicine and surveillance screens. The condition under surveillance will appear in summary history, and the existence of surveillance screens and default from surveillance should be indicated in the preferential area of the principal screen.

Surveillance screens may show data in tabulated or graphical format.

4.8 THE PREVENTIVE MEDICINE SCREEN

This screen displays data by category, then by date, results and recall date. Preventive procedures due or overdue, or for which no records exist, are identifiable by the system and highlighted on display (allowances being made for the age and sex of the patient), and this act of recognition is the basis for 'call or recall' listing. Opportunistic reminders are also provided, which appear in the preferential area of the principal display.

4.9 PRESCRIBING SCREENS

Prescription data are entered directly on to the prescribing screen and displayed by date, drug schedule, whether authorized for repeat (and if so, duration of authorization and compliance monitoring factors) and the authorizing doctor's identity. All medication currently authorized for repeat is highlighted on the full medication screen and is also accessible as a separate subset on the repeat medication screen.

A condensed version of the prescription entry is made on the right-hand side of the consultation log. The names of repeat medication drugs are shown in the preferential area of the principal screen.

The prescribing monitor, an automated check on the doctor's choice of drug, has access to the summary history and allergies section of the principal display in order to search for contraindications, indications and previous adverse drug reactions. (When a new drug is prescribed, search is also made of the medication screen data for possible drug interactions with other concurrently prescribed medication.)

4.10 THE PATHOLOGY AND RADIOLOGY SCREENS

These screens show data displayed by category (test), date and result. Abnormal results are highlighted. Alternative presentation by 'chart' graphics is provided for pathology results quoted in series.

4.11 RELATIONSHIPS BETWEEN CLINICAL RECORDS AND ADMINISTRATIVE RECORDS

Registration

The minimum data set for patient identity and registration details is now so extensive that all GP systems house it on a special auxiliary screen of its own (see Chapter 7). Patient name, date of birth and address are taken from the patient's identity MDS and shown at the top of all clinical screens.

Appointments

The list of patient appointments for the current consultation session reciprocates with individual patient record displays. When the consulting doctor selects, by key or mouse, the next patient he wishes to see from the appointment list, the appearance of that patient's record is automatically triggered. In some systems the same trigger also displays the patient's and doctor's names on an LED display in the waiting area.

When the consulting doctor has updated the patient notes, his display will revert to the appointment list following the use of a 'toggle' key or icon.

Commissioning

Relevant identity, investigative, prescribing and referral details taken from the clinical records can be mapped to the commissioning module and save reduplication of data entry.

Other linkages

Other linkages are now being constructed between practice clinical records, MIQUEST extraction software for clinical governance and epidemiology, cooperative data systems, and social services and mental health services databases.

Dispensing practices have closely dovetailed modules for prescribing and dispensing.

4.12 BASIC DATA ARCHITECTURE

Accurate interchange of information depends upon the acceptance by all parties of a vocabulary of strictly defined terms such as that provided by the Read classification. If this is coupled with a medical dictionary providing definitions, then the manner of use and meaning of each term become unequivocal. It is equally important that the categories of data to be transmitted should be agreed between sender and recipient. Message transmission to and from general practice determines policies and actions that would be undermined by the omission of key statements.

The basic data categories used in operational communicative GP systems are jointly referred to as the minimum data set (MDS). The MDS is a conglomerate of inter-related subsets. The six principal subsets are those of the six principal patient record screens, all of which are in constant use during day-to-day patient care within the practice. These six principal MDS subsets provide the data that energize nearly all practice computer applications, with the exception of such fringe activities as practice accounts or education.

Each consultation will generate new data to be entered into one or more of the six principal subsets, and any consultation may initiate one or more derivative actions such as prescribing, referral or investigation. Each derivative action is commissioned by the creation of a message whose content is, for the most part, taken from the principal patient record subsets (Fig. 4.3).

Data used in this way are by definition shared, and must include agreed component data categories. It is mandatory that all data that may need to be shared in this way should be stored within the principal patient record subsets in the first place.

The composition of the patient record MDS is therefore determined by the requirements for the following:

- The compilation of prescriptions, adverse drug reports, referral requests and letters, pathology and radiology test requests, PMA insurance questionnaires, sickness certificates, HA claims and registration, and further appointments
- Additional patient identification categories now included in the health authority register
- Parameters that the Department of Health specifies should be tested for well person, new patient, over 74 and paediatric assessment checks, cytology and immunization programs and targets
- Commissioning
- The findings of working parties on the GP system MDS and functionality standards (the General Medical Practice Computer Systems Requirements for Accreditation, and the Bench Testing and Accreditation Project of the Standards Working Party of the Primary Health Care Specialist Group of the British Computer Society); these findings and their later amendments or substitutions will be used to shape improvements in the design of future marketed systems
- The patient record structure provided by the individual system brand used by the practice
- The practice itself.

Of these seven factors, the first four have requirements that act as absolute determinants for MDS categories. System suppliers and practices share the responsibility for specifying the remaining content of the MDS, although this is a responsibility that will

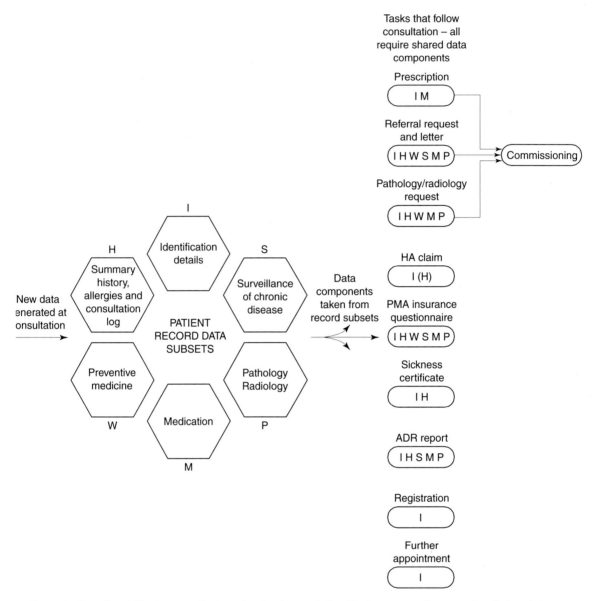

Fig. 4.3 Data flow following consultation, showing inter-relationship between patient record and shared data

diminish as the recommendations of official Standards Committees are taken up. Clearly, system design should oblige practices to enter mandatory MDS categories, but not those that are discretionary.

The cost and benefit of entering discretionary MDS categories should be assessed before these are included in computer records. Data capture takes professional and ancillary staff time and costs money. It must also be remembered that customized systems are more difficult to upgrade. Will it be worth storing data on a patient's hobbies? In what degree of detail

should exercise, diet or family history be recorded? How many previous occupations should be entered? Such decisions will be influenced not only by the needs and practicalities of immediate patient management but by a practice's special interests, including audit and research. When providing for the capture of discretionary data categories, good system design strikes a balance between consensus policy and individual flexibility.

The system designs that jointly dominate the market have coped well with the selection of minimum data categories for five of the six main clinical record screens, though the presentation of these categories is subject to considerable stylistic difference. The exception is the preventive medicine screen, which has always shown marked variation between systems, and whose design has been further unsettled by the data requirements for preventive health checks of the 1990 contract and its several amendments.

In some systems the preventive medicine record screen is called the 'At-risk' screen, but the difficulty here is that any feature in the summary medical history may be a risk factor, and there is seldom room to include summary records with full preventive records. Other designs attempt to include all opportunistic reminders or contraceptive records. Two systems allow the data categories on the preventive screen to be user-defined. These compromises are not merely uneasy, but misleading. It is to be hoped that feedback from user groups and the deliberations of the Standards Committees will, in time, iron out these anomalies.

The data categories for each of the main clinical record screens are discussed in greater detail in the following chapters.

- Identification details: Chapter 7
- Summary history and consultation log: Chapter 5
- Preventive medicine: Chapter 8
- Surveillance: Chapter 9
- Medication: Chapter 11
- Pathology/radiology: Chapter 12.

Minimum data categories will be needed both on the computer record and on the 'take-on' cards used for the summarization of manual records in preparation for loading on to computer. Not all categories of data ultimately required on the computer will be present in manual records, and these outstanding data will need to be obtained opportunistically when the patient attends the medical centre. The system should prompt accordingly.

4.13 EXTRANEOUS DATA USED IN GP SYSTEMS

The data initially required to assemble the computerized patient record, and to provide for the continuing operation of the practice system, are obtained from various extraneous sources. Some of these sources are manual and some electronic (Fig. 4.4).

Electronic data are imported either on diskettes or as telecommunication, and may incur a charge or licence fee. Data from manual sources must be keyed in to the system – a process that involves labour costs.

4.14 FURTHER DEVELOPMENTS IN GP RECORD DESIGN

Developments that are designed to produce further improvements in GP clinical record management have already reached an advanced stage. The PEN and PAD projects (acronyms for Practitioners Entering Notes and Practitioners Accessing Data) were supported respectively by the Department of Health and the Medical Research Council. The two projects were mutually complementary and were undertaken by staff centred on the Medical Informatics Group in the Department of Computer Science of the University of

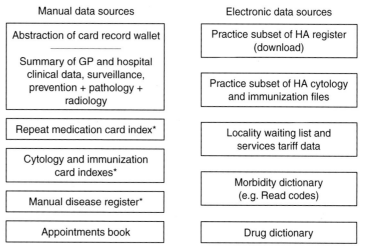

Fig. 4.4 Extraneous sources of manual and electronic data used in record building and ongoing GP system operation

Manual data sources	Electronic data sources
Abstraction of card record wallet	Practice subset of HA register (download)
Summary of GP and hospital clinical data, surveillance, prevention + pathology + radiology	Practice subset of HA cytology and immunization files
Repeat medication card index*	Locality waiting list and services tariff data
Cytology and immunization card indexes*	Morbidity dictionary (e.g. Read codes)
Manual disease register*	Drug dictionary
Appointments book	

* These data will be replicated in the card record wallet

Manchester. Data input takes place through a graphical user interface using a mouse or touch screen, with menus and graphic symbols (Fig. 4.5). Extensive 'tree-branching' protocols have been provided to assist data entry, and artificial intelligence techniques have been employed to enable the system to select lists of data entry options that the user is most likely to require in any given situation. The employment of menu choice ensures standardization of Read-coded primary morbidity terms, but the provision of anatomical diagrams and lists of grades of severity and duration of illness also allows the standardized entry of Read version 3 qualifying terms. A 'free text box' is provided for unstructured notes. PEN and PAD's data entry is not limited to clinical data but extends to treatment, investigations and referrals. Retrieval of data is offered in a variety of different formats – textual, tabular or graphical, as appropriate. The principal clinical screen contains opportunistic reminders, a summary history as a problem list, and a consultation log (encounters in reverse chronological order). As a data entry tool, the concepts that originated in the PEN project are now marketed as the 'Clinergy' system (Chapter 6).

PEN and PAD are imaginative projects whose approach is causing other system developers to review their designs.

The Good European Health Record (GEHR) is a bold scheme which has set out to be 'all things to all men' by providing a record that can be accessed by all health workers and all hospital disciplines. It purports to be compatible with all commonly used morbidity classifications and all commonly used hardware, and to produce text in most European languages using automatic translation facilities. The project's prestigious funding comes through the European Community and is backed by a large number of European commercial companies. Development is coordinated by St Bartholomew's Hospital Medical College in London.

The design and content of all records, whether medical or not, is determined uncompromisingly by the purpose for which they are used. During the 1970s an attempt at Exeter UK to develop an 'integrated medical record' for use by GPs, hospital doctors and community physicians failed for the obvious reason that the record requirements of diverse health care agencies are markedly different, and that only a very small subset of data is shared by them all. The GEHR will need to change its remit if it is to succeed.

4.15 THE ELECTRONIC HEALTH RECORD (EHR)

The UK government's 1998 strategy embodied in its policy document *Information for Health* aims to ensure that all UK general practice systems will conform to data, format and software standards so as to allow patient data to be transferred between disparate GP computer systems. In this form, such data are also scheduled to be accessible to authorized health pro-

Fig. 4.5 The 'graphical entry tool' of the PEN and PAD project

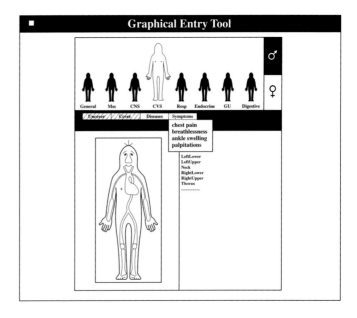

fessionals outside general practice, and to be available to health authorities for external audit.

If plans for the development of the EHR are to be realized, then the standardization of terminology, data architecture and record file structure described in this chapter will need to be fully implemented. Partisan procedures would render the whole concept of the EHR invalid.

FURTHER READING

Campbell I K 1981 Improving records in a group practice. British Medical Journal 282: 1126

Colebrook M 1982 A homemade A4 medical record system in general practice. Journal of the Royal College of General Practitioners 32: 623

Herd A 1993 Graphical user interfaces. Practice Computing, February

Kalra D 1993 The Good European Health Record. Practice Computing, February

Lippmann E O, Preece J F 1971 A pilot on-line data system for general practitioners. Computers and Biomedical Research 4: 390

McGuiness B W, Frood R A W 1981. The weaver index and register. Practitioner 225: 613

NHS Executive 1998 Information for health, an information strategy for the modern NHS 1998–2005: a national strategy for local implementation. NHSE publications, Leeds

Nowlan A 1990 PEN and PAD revolutionises record keeping. Practice Computing, September: 17

Poole N W 1980 Medical records. Update 15 February: 385

5 The principal screen

5.1 SUMMARY RECORDS – AN OVERVIEW

The patterns for the strategic deployment of goods in a supermarket so as to optimize vending have been determined with great care. Items nearest the entrance or near the till have an enhanced appeal, and a periodic reshuffle of goods forces shoppers to mull over a greater range than habit would determine.

The selection and preferential display of important items of news in newspapers is taken for granted nowadays, but the structured layout that developed this principle was given the name 'tabloid' when it was first introduced, in order to distinguish it from magazine format. Front page news has been with us ever since, with the top left-hand corner of the page usually taking precedence.

With every consultation held, every referral letter written and every PMA insurance report completed, the general practitioner realizes that there is an imperative need to introduce a working practice record that displays selected important information in a preferential and well-organized way.

The NHS general practice record is potentially one of the most important databases of its kind. It receives reports from all orthodox health agencies dealing with the patient (GP, hospital, laboratory, community health clinic, optician, midwife, deputizing service), its coverage extends from cradle to grave and it follows the patient everywhere, despite change of address or change of doctor. The total population is documented in this way.

However, access to data in the manual record wallet is made difficult. The problem is one of dilution and disorganization. There are three sections: hospital reports, pathology reports and general practice handwritten notes. Before systematic interrogation of the contents can take place, each section has to be separated, the pathology and hospital reports unfolded, all sections sorted chronologically and the pathology and hospital sections sorted by test or hospital department.

The important salient facts that are needed to summarize the patient's past medical and surgical history when determining later management are scattered throughout all three sections. These important facts are interspersed with a disproportionately large amount of obsolete and obsolescent detail in the hospital and general practice sections. Parts of the general practice section are often illegible, incomplete or otherwise unintelligible. The more bulky the record, the more self-defeating it becomes during a busy surgery. Yet, it is often in these bulky records that the past history has the greatest influence on further management.

There is nothing new about the abstraction of summary data in general practice. The original panel records of 1913 left a space for diagnosis, and the RCGP have advocated the insertion of diagnosis on the NHS manual record with a box drawn around it. Many practices summarized the contents of their bulkier manual records, or their incoming hospital reports. Some A4 records possess a sheet for summary. It is now mandatory for a training practice to have summarized at least 95% of its records, and new forms of performance-related pay are gradually pressurizing other practices to follow suit.

Although it is difficult to lay down summarizing protocols for GP notes and hospital reports that would satisfy all practices, there is a good general measure of agreement on the principles involved. One such code of rules is described in Chapter 29.

5.2 THE SELECTION OF SUMMARY DATA

The principal criterion according to which summary data should be selected is that they are relevant to further patient management months or years later.

Summary data put all a patient's risk factors in a nut-shell, and so must include not only a summary clinical history but also allergies, continuous medication, immunizations, screening procedures, and prejudicial family, occupational or addictive history, in a synoptic format. Ideally these should all be exhibited on the principal screen, although not all record designs achieve this. For simplicity, components such as immunization and screening are often displayed merely as opportunistic reminders on the principal screen when due or overdue.

Summary data must be concise, unambiguous, explicit and, though they will often be added to, should never need altering. With manual methods the creation of summary will always mean reduplication of terms already used in the conventional record. The term(s) used in summary data may reduplicate the only statement that is generated in the record at consultation, e.g. *'tonsillitis'*. When, however, summary data relate to a lengthier consultation record entry, they are a portion or subset of that lengthier statement, e.g. *'lumbar spinal pain with R sciatica – worried about possibility of losing job'* (here the summary statement is shown in italics).

Once all past records have been summarized, ongoing summary recording is accomplished at the time the clinical record is written. It is neither desirable nor necessary to perform ongoing summarization as a separate editing exercise 'out-of-hours'. In the case of both hospital and GP data, the initial summary statement can be defined at the point in time at which treatment can be rationalized, whether or not a finite diagnosis has been made. When a finite diagnosis is made this, too, becomes an essential piece of summary data, e.g. *'lumbar spinal pain with R sciatica'* (and later) *'X-ray lumbar spine: spondylolisthesis L4 on L5'*.

A surgical inpatient summary statement must include indication, operation and important sequelae, e.g. *'stress incontinence – cystocele – anterior colporrhaphy – cystitis'*.

Summarization of medical cases must also cover all salient facts, e.g. *'partial L hemiplegia due cerebral thrombosis: hypertension BP 240/130 reduced to 150/90 on lisinopril: residual L hand weakness: speech and bladder function normal'* (it should be noted that some summary data are themselves negative statements).

Abstraction of summary data side steps and omits, in both hospital and GP records, a wealth of detail which was of temporary relevance before case resolution but which, like the innocent suspects in a criminal investigation, is of little or no importance once the case is closed.

5.3 THE USES OF SUMMARY DATA

We have noted that summary data are selected on the basis of their utility to future patient management months or years later. Their important role is subsequently fulfilled in several ways.

- In case assessment as past history they indicate positive and negative predisposition to disease. A patient who has had his/her appendix removed will not experience a recurrence, whereas an attack of gout is more likely to occur in someone who has previously suffered from this complaint. Up-to-date diphtheria immunization virtually precludes a subsequent diagnosis of this disease. A patient on medication is automatically exposed to the risk of its side effects.
- In case management, summary data give positive and negative indications of the suitability of treatment. A haemorrhagic diathesis or chronic obstructive airways disease may prejudice surgery, whereas a recurrent as opposed to a single attack of tonsillitis may suggest the need for tonsillectomy. If summary data are available to the doctor for patient management, then they provide the only form of record required at one half of all GP consultations.
- The explicit nature and degree of diagnostic definition shown by summary data make them ideally suited as statements of past history for referral letters and PMA insurance reports.
- Summary data provide the best record format for teaching purposes.
- Summary data constitute the nucleus of the new computer clinical record.
- They are the data that must be accessed by automated or semiautomated checks performed during prescribing, with regard to previous drug allergies, drug–drug interactions and conditions for which drugs are indicated or contraindicated.
- They are used in the compilation of 'call or recall' clinics – sufferers from cardiorespiratory disease may be offered influenza immunization, and patients who have had previous gastrectomy or thyroid surgery may be checked for resulting deficiencies.
- Summary data are suitable for searching by computer for the purposes of practice research and practice audit, and for the extraction by MIQUEST interrogation for epidemiology and clinical governance. Together with prescribing data, and in relation to the defined population of UK general practices, they constitute a highly valued commodity for the planners of health care, epidemiologists and the pharmaceutical industry.

- Summary data are the clinical component of the computer record that is both suitable for, and requires, Read coding.
- Summary data taken together with full recent consultation data constitute the basis of the shared Electronic Health Record (EHR), which is scheduled to be available to all authorized health professionals in the NHS.

5.4 WAYS OF PRESENTING SUMMARY DATA

There are four ways of presenting summary data.

Problem-oriented records

The American physician Lawrence Weed developed a manual record system that listed clinical, investigatory and treatment details under the headings of the separate problems of which the case consisted. The problems were subdivided into active (current) and passive (concluded or past history), both of which were ranked in order of importance.

A further dimension was added to the method by the creation of a succession of versions of the record, each version showing changes in the degree of definition and resolution of each problem, and any corresponding change in the ranking order.

The method was clearly one that anticipated a switch from manual to computer storage, for on the computer the changes would show merely as amendments rather than as a replacement document.

Problem-oriented records are well suited to medical inpatient work, in which multiple problems of shifting importance are experienced, but they are of little use in most surgical cases, where there is often only one current problem and past history is past history.

In general practice, as with surgery, there is often only one current problem, but there is also the fundamental need to sift out those details relevant to future patient management and to display them all as risk factors, rather than as problems undergoing protracted investigative resolution. There is, in addition, the need to show surveillance problems in a very special way (Chapter 9).

These requirements for special record formats mean that a good deal of adaptation of the original problem-oriented concept is required if it is to be used in general practice. A compromise solution is to group summary history entries according to the physiological body system to which they refer, a procedure that will to a large extent link related problems.

Summary cards

Cards of a size and shape to fit the manual NHS wallet may be used as a summary record. The card reduplicates summary data abstracted from the wallet's contents, and it must be prepared initially by processing old records. The entries are in chronological order and the order cannot be altered. Summary cards save time when accessing the record for salient facts at consultation, when writing referral letters or completing PMA insurance reports. Summary cards make a useful transitional document upon which to prepare summary material and test it in use at consultation, prior to converting to record-driven computer systems. If summary cards are used as transitional documents, then it is of the utmost importance that all types of information available in the manual record that will subsequently be required on computer should also be contained on the card.

Such cards are available commercially and are sometimes called 'take-on' or 'transit' cards (Fig. 5.1).

More than 50 different designs of summary card are known to exist in UK general practice, and when selecting a design its user is well advised to opt for one that allows for the field expansion in summary history, medication and immunization that is likely to occur over a 1–3-year period. Most designs provide restrictive data boxes, which overflow with time and require 'continuation' cards, which tend to get lost.

Summary encounter form systems

Summary data may be printed out on computer stationery from a file of practice summary records on the computer prior to consultation. The doctor reads the summary record printout at consultation and, if further summary material is generated, he writes this in at the bottom of the form and marks the form at the point where the new material is to be inserted.

After the consultation session the practice secretary calls up the old summary records on her VDU. Using the computer keyboard, she inserts the new data that the doctor has written, to update the computer-held record. This method saves the doctor from having to use the keyboard of the display unit personally, but causes some transcription delays and errors in updating the computer record. After use, all forms have to be shredded – a wasteful procedure considering the cost of continuous computer stationery. Summary encounter documents are a useful form of record for the doctor to carry when making home visits. Encounter form systems should be regarded merely as a transitional step towards a doctor's desktop system because the doctor who uses

SYNOPSIS RECORD CARD:

{ IF ADDITIONAL CARD USED FOR SPECIAL PURPOSE, ENTER CODE P FOR PATHOLOGY H FOR HYPERTENSION – etc.

(FOR CASE ASSESSMENT – REFERRAL LETTERS PMA INSURANCE REPORT – TEACHING PRACTICE COMPUTER TAKE-ON)

Sex M/F Title	Surname – Forename(s)				Birth Date	
Previous Surname	GP No.	NHS/Private	NHS No.	Date Registered	Date NHS Record Began	Mileage Units
Address and Postcode		First Change		Second Change		
Telephone No.						
FPC Code if Practice deals with more than one FPC	Hospital Nos.				HTLV 3 Risk in lifestyle	HTLV 3 Test Date/Result

Prejudicial Family – Occupational – Social History/Tobacco Alcohol/Practice Research Data

Adverse Drug History

Clinical Details – Permanent Data Summary of Important Morbidity – Operations – Accidents – Confinements – Special Investigations Prefix H for Hospital Data – X for X-Ray Data	GP Treatment – Permanent Data Prefix £ Long Term Medication Prefix ↑ Immunisations
Date	

Urine Protein/Sugar First Abnormal if any / / =	Urine Protein/Sugar Other Recordings / / =	/ / =	/ / =
Blood Pressure First Abnormal if any / / =	Blood Pressure Other Recordings / / =	/ / =	/ / =
Prepared by	Verified by	Input by	

© Dr. J. Preece

Fig. 5.1 One type of summary card (front only shown). The card may be folded in two, and then fits the general practice record wallet, leaving the edge of the card just proud of other wallet contents. The data on this card form the nucleus of the new computer patient record, and the card can thus be used as a transfer document when records are computerized. The reverse of the card accommodates overspill from the clinical and treatment columns.

them forfeits the assistance that can be provided by interactive computer procedures.

Doctor's desktop systems

With the full implementation of the computer record by the doctor's use of a terminal at consultation, the doctor makes successive entries for successive consultations much as with the paper record, but he or she can cause automated reduplication of any or all of the statements he records into a preferential area of the record. In this way the doctor can build up summary records in the preferential record area at the same time as he makes routine consultation entries, but without extra writing.

The logistics are as follows:

The preferential area of the record is that which is read first (as with newspaper headlines); routine consultation recording is shown below this in three vertical columns that accommodate the date, clinical observations, and treatment as read from left to right ('consultation log'). Each routine consultation entry begins a new line and this line maintains a correspondence between date, clinical notes and treatment. Routine consultation entries are arranged in reverse chronological order so that the latest entry, which is most often accessed, is uppermost.

As the doctor makes his routine consultation entry, he designates that part of it which he wishes to show in summary. Systems vary in the way in which the designation can be made, but as a rule the doctor is invited to enter summary data as the first part of the routine consultation entry, and must terminate and Read code the summary statement before continuing with the rest of the entry. When the whole routine consultation entry, including the part designated for summary, has been entered on display the computer will assimilate it and redisplay the summary statement both as a part of the original full entry in the routine consultation area, and also as a reduplication into the preferential area of the record as summary.

While there is an irresistible argument for putting all risk factors in synoptic format on the principal screen as distillates from more detailed records, systems designers are sometimes deflected from doing so. The need to offer more elaborative screens for data entry, or full retrospective details with regard to procedures such as screening, immunization or surveillance of chronic disease, has sometimes resulted in all data relating to these functions being removed from the principal screen, to the detriment of its comprehensive function. It is, after all, a step backwards to make the health professional sift through the whole patient record in order to sum up an individual's health status.

If a suitable synoptic convention is used, the risk factors of nearly all patients can be accommodated on one screen, and in rare cases where this cannot be done scrolling can be employed. In this way, summary clinical history, allergies, and continuous and current acute medication can be displayed as condensed statements; detrimental family, occupational and addictive histories indicated; and screening and immunization procedures due or overdue prompted for. The date and result of first abnormal and latest blood pressure, urine and HIV tests can also be shown if available.

Well-designed synoptic presentation of summary data saves the user a considerable amount of time at consultation and reduces the chance that risk factors will be overlooked. The economical use of display space achieved means that for most patient records the latest consultation log entry or entries can be included within the lower lines of the principal display.

5.5 THE CONSULTATION LOG AND ITS RELATIONSHIP WITH SUMMARY

The day-by-day log of consultation details, which accommodates freestyle entries as well as the summary data that will be replicated in the upper part of the principal screen, is now updated and displayed in reverse chronological order in all the foremost system designs. The date referring to a consultation is shown on the left of the clinical entry, as with manual records.

Some earlier system designs used separate screens to display medication entries and clinical details, and were subsequently obliged to introduce linkages other than that provided by the date, to enable the viewer to identify the indication for which a drug had been used. It is simpler to employ the convention of displaying date, clinical details and a condensed statement of medication as three parallel columns whose horizontal relationship links them all. Fuller details of the prescription issued will, of course, appear on the medication screen.

In some system designs, all terms that are subjected to coding as they are entered in the clinical column of the consultation log are automatically replicated into summary history. The third version of the Read coding classification allows primary terms and their qualifying statements to be coded and, by using data entry protocols such as those provided by the best-known GP systems, has made the entry of rigorously defined summary data relatively straightforward. It is now possible to enter not only a general diagnosis but

Fig 5.2 The principal screen – summary: Torex Meditel's System 6000

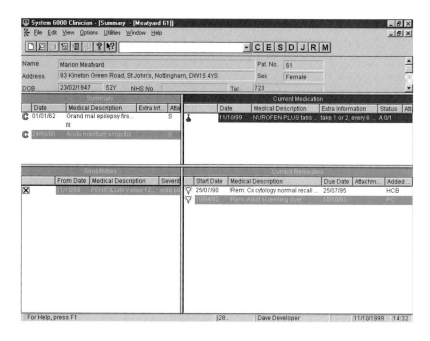

Fig 5.3 The principal screen: In-Practice Systems' Vision system's 'consultation data entry' screen

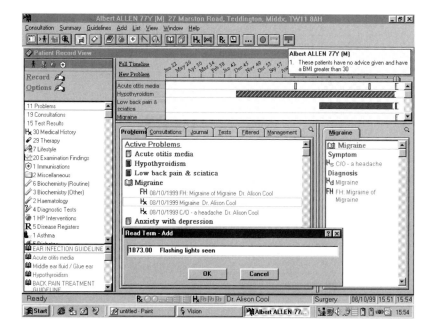

also grades of duration and severity, together with the anatomical site of a lesion (Chapter 6).

Two accessory GUI-based data entry modules have been developed for general practice, and these assist in the abstraction and coding of summary data. 'Clinergy' is a commercial development which sprang from the University of Manchester's PEN and PAD Project, and can be incorporated within most bespoke GP system software. 'Visual Read' is a Leicester-based package which can be embedded within any 32 bit Windows 95 (or above) compatible GP system. These packages are discussed in greater detail in Chapter 6.

A familiar interface

The electronic patient record looks just like a Lloyd George note. This provides staff with a familiar interface that makes learning the system very easy.

Initials of the person who entered the data (ie doctor or typist)

Shows the type of contact (ie surgery attendance)

Initials of the clinically responsible user

An ongoing problem

Diagnostic code for a cough

The numbers indicate different problems during one consultation

The drug bottle indicates a prescription

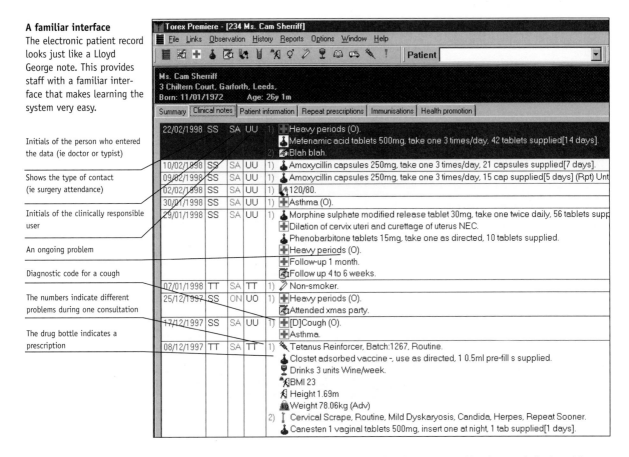

Fig 5.4 The principal screen – consultation log clinical and prescription details, integrated by date and displayed in reverse chronological order: Torex's Premiere system's 'patient record' screen

5.6 CONSULTATION LOG DATA THAT ARE NOT REPLICATED IN SUMMARY

Dictionary-derived terms and qualifying statements associated with them are the two categories of clinical data that are shared both by the routine consultation record and the summary. Other categories of data belong only in the routine consultation record. They are:

- Elaborative but obsolescent data that are recorded as part of a clinical statement but have no place in summary. A patient in the example on page 39 who had a hemiplegia might, for instance, have suffered transitory loss of consciousness, a convulsion, initial retention of urine or transitory diplopia, but after the passage of months or years these occurrences do not affect further management.

- Comprehensive medical history and physical examination records. These data, akin to those

required of hospital internists, are elicited as part of a detailed investigative procedure. Enquiry follows a standard pattern instilled at medical school and, on average, such an 'in-depth' exercise is only required once per consulting session in general practice. Protocols that act as *aides-memoire* but also facilitate fast data entry on computer have been developed for taking histories of dyspepsia, gynaecological complaints, headaches, asthma and a host of other disorders. Protocols for the examination of each physical system or for recording the salient points in a general clinical examination are also available (Chapter 23).

Unless all clinical data, whether for summary or not, can be entered on the computer, the doctor will be forced to use a double system in which some of the data are still held on manual records – a situation that has spelt doom for several systems in the past.

Fig 5.5 The principal screen: Global Clinical System (Aremis Soft Healthcare)

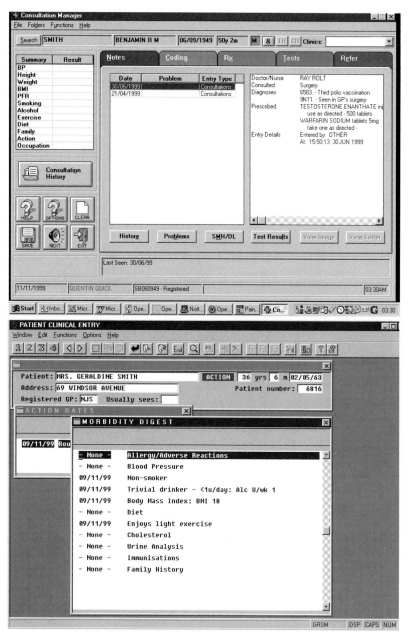

5.7 WHO SUMMARIZES DATA?

There is by now a considerable body of evidence from the UK that demonstrates that an intelligent practice records officer with adequate training, who follows strict rules, is capable of summarizing patient records. An important proviso is that this officer should be allowed and encouraged to seek professional advice when s/he requires it, and that a doctor should check and, if necessary, amend the text of all his/her work. Trained staff tend to include more detail in summary than doctors, but it is very seldom indeed that an important item is overlooked. In some parts of the UK, peripatetic teams of trained record staff offer a record summarizing service on a commercial basis.

Some general practitioners prefer to summarize all their records in person, and one prominent supplier advocated that they should do so directly through the computer terminal. The prospect is a daunting one. Often, practices compromise by requiring doctors to summarize the larger and more complex records while trained staff process the remainder.

Fig. 5.6 The principal screen: EMIS GV1 system

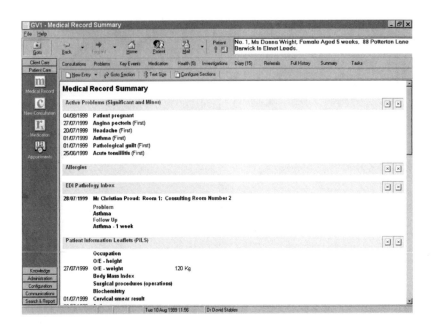

5.8 WHEN ARE RECORDS SUMMARIZED?

Summarization is a necessary preliminary to computerization, not only because it initiates the patient's computer summary record but also because it avoids loading a surfeit of obsolete data on to the computer. The summarization process is usually undertaken methodically, with notes being taken in alphabetical order and summary data written on to take-on cards. The cards are checked by the doctor and the data are then transferred to computer. Because the secretary knows how far summarization has progressed, he or she will therefore know which notes must have summaries updated from material in new hospital reports. Summarization is sometimes undertaken piecemeal, taking all notes for the next day's consultation sessions for processing and loading these summaries on to the system so that computer records can be used as soon as a system is installed. This method leads to confusion when records subsequently have to be updated from new hospital reports.

Data summarized on take-on cards and loaded on to computer are, of course, not merely a summary history but include patient identity details, immunizations, medication, allergies and all other categories of data that jointly constitute the 'minimum data set' for take-on.

After all past records have been processed and transferred to computer, further general practice notes will be entered on to the system directly at consultation, but most incoming hospital reports must still be summarized and their summary content must be entered on to the system. In practices that do not receive pathology reports electronically, test results will also still need to be keyed in. When all hospital reports are received through electronic mail, summary data will still need to be abstracted, but then, once the provisions for shared aftercare have been put in place, the full report can be relegated to archival storage. It would make good sense for hospital staff to earmark summary statements for their own and their recipients' use when they construct reports for general practitioners, and this is already established policy in some hospital departments.

5.9 STRUCTURED SUMMARIES

Viewing of summary data is greatly facilitated if it is displayed in a structured format. Systems differ in their manner of presentation, but one design uses a convention whereby the summary of past illnesses and operations is arranged in paragraphs, each paragraph representing one of seven physiological systems:

- Cardiovascular
- Alimentary
- Ears, nose and respiratory
- Obstetric
- Psychiatric
- Urogenital (other than obstetric)
- Skeletal

with an eighth paragraph to show all those conditions not accommodated in the other seven.

In this arrangement we may view a skeletal, obstetric or psychiatric history at will and in summary form. The eight paragraphs make eight roughly equal subdivisions of all summary material. The format achieved is somewhat similar to problem orientation. The appropriate positioning into paragraphs requires that the user should key in a single designating character, or use a linked Read Code, to represent the physiological system when entering a summary statement.

(The letter codes for the simple body system classification shown above may be memorized by the mnemonic *Canopus*. Canopus is a site in ancient Egypt that has given its name to clay funerary jars (canopic jars) in which the alimentary system of the deceased was stored and processed for future retrieval in the next life. Canopus is also a star in the southern hemisphere – the second brightest on display.)

Another useful convention is to distinguish summary statements based on hospital or X-ray reports from those derived from general practice. Once again, a single designating character must be entered prior to the text of the statement (e.g. H for hospital or X for X-ray).

If the month/year date of occurrence follows the diagnostic term displayed in summary, then another form of data enhancement can be achieved. For recurrent conditions such as tonsillitis, cystitis or bronchitis, the number of attacks, intervals between attacks and increase or decrease in frequency become obvious – all factors that may determine a change in management. For instance, the statement:

TONSILLITIS 12.95/ 03.96/ 09.97/ 04.98/ 08.98/ might well prompt referral for tonsillectomy.

In the past, there has been considerable variation between marketed systems in the conventions adopted for recording summary data. As we progress towards the Electronic Health Record (EHR) it becomes imperative that these differences be resolved.

SUMMARY

- The principal screen is the 'opening page' of the patient's computer record. It is divided horizontally between summary data above and the consultation log below.
- Summary data are permanently important to further patient management, and need to be separated from the excessive amount of obsolescent material within which they are embedded. They should be given a preferential position in the record.
- Summary data can be identified at consultation at the point in time when treatment is rationalized, and, although new data are continually added, old summary data should never need to be changed.
- The summary is by far the most frequently accessed area in the general practice record and it contains synoptic data that relate to all the patient's risk factors. As such it must include summary clinical history, allergies, continuous medication, due immunization and screening, and prejudicial family, occupational or addictive history. It indicates positive and negative predisposition to disease, reinforces or modifies decisions on new treatment, provides the basis for automated referral letter and PMA report construction, and assists automated checks on prescribing. It is used in preventive procedures, teaching, research and audit.
- Summary data always require Read coding and will constitute the essential basis for the Electronic Health Record (EHR).
- Methods of presenting summary data have been problem-oriented records, summary cards, summary encounter forms and the computerized record on visual display units. Only computer methods can avoid reduplicated entries or fragmentation of data between the summary section and the main body of the record.
- Summarization can be performed reliably by an intelligent practice secretary provided that s/he is trained, uses a detailed protocol and has recourse to medical opinion, and provided that the doctor verifies all the output.
- Summarization of old records to summary cards must precede take-on to computer, and this may be undertaken by working through all records in alphabetical order. Alternatively, the records for next day's consultations may be processed daily. After record computerization, incoming hospital reports will continue to require summarization.
- On the computer, the principal and many qualifying summary terms can be verified by, and entered by, dictionary-based facilities.
- Obsolescent GP data entries will be confined to the consultation log. After the extraction of summary statements, and the implementation of shared after-care, full-length hospital reports will be archived.
- Summaries can be structured so as to give enhanced viewing and to assist in management decisions.
- The consultation log should show three columns whose entries are linked horizontally to record date, clinical observations and a condensate of the

medication used. Entries are stacked in reverse chronological order because the latest is the most often accessed.

Further reading

Mould A 1982 How to improve your medical record cards. Pulse 24 April: 809

Preece J F 1988 Synopsis of record card. Update 1 Nov: 843

Tait I, Stevens J 1973 The problem orientated medical record in general practice. Journal of the Royal College of General Practitioners 23: 311

Weed L L 1969 Medical records, medical education and patient care. Cleveland Case Western Reserve University Press, Cleveland, OH

Zander L I, Beresford S A A, Thomas P 1978 Medical records in general practice. Occasional Paper 5. Royal College of General Practitioners, London

6 Read codes

6.1 OVERVIEW

On one of the many occasions during the past millennium when Anglo-French relations were under severe strain, diplomatic exchanges included a polite request from the French that used the word *demander* (meaning 'to ask'). The mistranslation prompted by the use of this word led to the brink of war. As a means of communication, language has two over-riding requirements: the same word must be used by, and must have the same meaning to, both parties.

The meaning of a word is defined by dictionaries. The use in common of a well-chosen word depends upon the general acceptance of a classification of preferred terms (which is not, it should be noted, the strict definition of a thesaurus), but until the 1990s no adequate taxonomy of medical terms was available for use in general practice. The long established International Classification of Disease, used extensively by hospitals to classify morbidity, covers diagnoses but not clinical signs, drugs or occupations. While GPs used paper-based handwritten records for private consumption within the practice, personalized and idiosyncratic use of terminology hardly mattered. The advent of computers brought to everybody's attention the fact that record keeping needed to be an exact science, and that data could not be processed and shared unless they were standardized.

Like several other embryonic coded GP classifications, the Read system was originally designed not merely to standardize but also to condense terms in order to reduce demand on the limited storage capacity of early computers. Read's structured and comprehensive approach led to his classification being accepted as the NHS standard, and his concept, the original purpose of which was to provide a mechanism for the preparation of GP record summaries, subsequently became the victim of its own success. Burgeoning demand from a user base that by now spread across the whole medical spectrum, caused expansion of the number of coded terms from an original 250 to 500 000. This explosive growth in turn necessitated drastic revisions, both of the degree of detail stored in each code and of the structure of the underlying database architecture. Progressive upgrading refinements have tended to dislocate exact correspondence between successive releases of the codes, and some practices have been using systems that put them in the invidious position of having logged codes from more than one release, with consequent incompatibility. Mapping programs that attempt to convert codes from one release to another can only cope with terms for which exact correspondence still exists, with the result that labour-intensive adjustments to achieve reconciliation have to be made at practice level. Although implementation of the Read codes is now a Department of Health requirement for system accreditation, and most practices use them, the Department of Health has been careful not to specify a particular release in its requirements, and the organization responsible for propagating the codes has been careful to assure users that all releases will continue to be supported, at least in the short term.

6.2 STRUCTURE

The four byte set

Read's original plan was to produce a system of codes based on tree-branching architecture in which each of four successive characters in the code, read from left to right, represented a finer degree of detail. The leftmost character was either a numeral signifying a 'process of care' (such as a symptom, sign or test), an upper-case character signifying a 'diagnosis', or a lower-case character signifying a 'drug' (Table 6.1). Having thus defined the term's primary grouping, the three remaining characters, which might be numbers or letters, were used to add increasing degrees of specificity.

Table 6.1 An example of the original Read code system

Term	Read code	ICD-9-CM equivalent
Circulatory system disease	G	390–459
Ischaemic heart disease	G3	410–414
Acute myocardial infarction	G30	410
Anterior myocardial infarct	G301	410.1

The version 2 (five-byte) set

In response to the need for a further degree of definition, which was not always available in the ICD, Read added a fifth character to his code structure. In the above example, 'anterior myocardial infarct' could now be defined more specifically as 'acute anteroseptal infarct' with a Read code of G 3011, although the ICD code could achieve no further layer of definition and remained 410.1.

The introduction of the fifth character brought with it the additional advantage of increasing the possible number of code permutations from 58^4 to 58^5, and the opportunity was now taken to rationalize the presentation of exact synonyms as 'extensions' to their preferred term.

Versions 3 and 3.1

The adoption of Read codes as an NHS standard led to their infiltration throughout secondary care, pathology, nursing, the dental profession, other allied professions and patient administration. Not only did this further expansion multiply the number of codes manyfold, but it exposed a fundamental defect in the database architecture of previous releases. Using tree-branch scaffolding, a node can give rise to multiple subdivisions but have only one antecedent – the branch from which the twigs sprang. Paper-based morbidity classifications, when faced with duplicating a term such as asthma in order to place it within more than one category (in this case to exhibit it as both a respiratory and an allergic disease), must either use two different codes or one that is replicated out of sequence. Computer-based classifications can store not only the target code for a term but also the addresses and identities of all other codes with which the target code has a relationship. The computer storage architecture that enables this is called a relational database, a structure that allowed Read to link a term with both multiple subclasses and multiple antecedents. In this way, not only could synonyms that had been appended in version 2 (5-byte) be related, but qualifying statements ('qualifiers') could also be coded in their own right, and could be linked in, with the nature of the relationship being recorded.

It is now possible to code complex statements such as 'pulmonary embolism, secondary to thrombosis of the right long saphenous vein, secondary to Mercilon therapy for contraception'.

The massive and intricate new database required that access be provided by an innovative, high-calibre 'sort engine'.

6.3 DERIVATION AND RELATIONSHIPS WITH OTHER CODING CLASSIFICATIONS

Read codes are a superset of the other classifications from which they were originally derived, to which has been added unique new sections. Where there is correspondence with other classifications, this can be exposed by cross-reference. Thus demonstrable linkages exist between the Read classification and ICD 9, ICD 10, OPCS 4.2, BNF, OPCS and SOC occupations, DSM-III, SNOMED, CPT-4, ICPC, OXMIS, SOC and PPA, and the RCGP 'Classification and Analysis of GP Data'.

The Read classification is an attempt for the first time to include all the terms needed throughout medicine and its administration. It covers:

- Diseases
- History/symptoms
- Examination/signs
- Occupations
- Diagnostic procedures
- Pathology tests
- Radiology/diagnostic imaging
- Preventive procedures
- Operative procedures
- Other therapeutic procedures
- Administration
- Drugs/appliances
- Health status
- Social factors
- The field of dentistry
- The field of nursing

- The fields of other allied professions
- Diagnosis-Related-Groupings.

6.4 DEVELOPMENT, DISTRIBUTION AND SUPPORT

The Read Clinical Classification (RCC) is developed on a continuing basis by the NHS Centre for Coding and Classification (NHSCCC), which was originally headed by James Read himself. In 1990 the copyright of the RCC was purchased on behalf of the NHS, and since that date no royalty payment has been due from NHS users.

Between 1990 and 1999 distribution, updating and support had to be paid for by purchasing a licence granted by Dr Read's private company, Computer Aided Medical Systems (CAMS). In April 1999 these functions also became the responsibility of the NHS when the NHSCCC became a component of the NHS Information Authority. Although licences must still be obtained from the authority by NHS users, no licence fees are now charged to them. GPs normally obtain their RCC licences through their clinical system suppliers, who are responsible for providing accessing software and for installing and upgrading the RCC database on client systems.

CAMS still provides component technology and training to suppliers when required and distributes the RCC elsewhere in the world.

6.5 SELECTION OF CODED TERMS DURING BESPOKE GP SYSTEM USE

The convention was originally adopted throughout most GP systems to display coded terms together with their codes during the selection process, though it is now usual to reveal the term and conceal the code from display. Unfettered use of synonyms has been allowed so as not to prejudice uptake of the Read system. Coded terms may be selected at data entry in several ways.

- The first three or four letters of the term required may be entered, following which a picking list can be displayed of all terms that begin with those letters, from which ultimate selection is made. Some systems have introduced the principle of allowing the user to specify a general category of code in order to reduce the size of the picking list.
- Data entry protocols offer pathways that are already paved with preferred coded terms, each of which can be selected by a single key depression.

- Some systems allow a short picking list to be produced that is ranked in the order of frequency of use made by an individual health professional.
- Display of a patient's pre-existing coded problem list can be used as the basis for reselection of a term by the doctor or nurse.
- Shortened picking lists of terms describing commonly occurring conditions can be displayed to facilitate rapid selection.
- Regional anatomical diagrams can be presented, in relation to which commonly associated symptoms, signs and morbidity can be summoned by mouse-based selection.
- A user can browse the overall RCC database by category and subcategory, or by access to the synonym dictionary.

6.6 SELECTION OF CODED TERMS FROM GUI-BASED IMPORTED PROGRAMS

When originally introduced on 'text-based' systems, Read-coded term selection involved progression through a succession of submenus with repetitive use of the return and cursor keys before the point of definition was reached. The tedium and delay involved in this process prompted developers to seek less fatiguing ways of reaching the Read endpoint, and the introduction of GUI technology spawned two innovative packages in the late 1990s. Both relied on the use of anatomical diagrams from which the user could initiate the selection process, and further refinement of definition was obtained by using the mouse to pinpoint options from carefully tailored, context-sensitive submenus. Such methods not only select via the body system route but would allow representation of summary data classed by body systems – a format that is not very far removed from problem orientation.

Clinergy™ GP and Visual Read are data entry programs that require compatibility with Windows 95 or above, need to be embedded within host GP practice management systems and cannot be used with dumb terminal configurations. The two packages, which both use Read version 3, are closely similar in approach but differ in the fine detail of their pathways. The anatomical drawings they use make them suitable for demonstration to patients.

Clinergy™ GP is the commercial package derived from the data input component of the University of Manchester's PEN and PAD project. Two pathways are offered, one for quick data entry (QDE) of common straightforward topics, and the other, the graphical topic selector (GTS), providing a more finely detailed protocol for data selection (Figs 6.1, 6.2).

Fig. 6.1 Clinergy™ GUI data entry screen

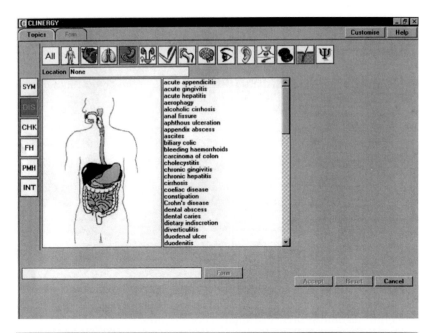

Fig. 6.2 Clinergy™ data entry of fine details

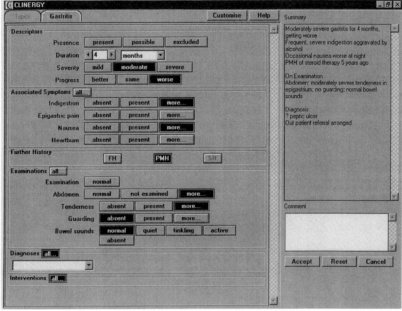

The QDE screen does not possess anatomical drawings but shows two parallel columns. The left column lists common topics, selection from which fills the right-hand column with a list of possible associated symptoms, signs and disposals, from which choices are to be made.

The GTS protocol is initiated by selection from a button bar offering access to anatomical drawings of alternative body systems – in particular those relating to cardiovascular, respiratory, gastrointestinal, genito-

urinary, muscular, skeletal, central nervous, ocular, aural, endocrine and dermatological categories. Drawings are shown on the left of the screen and, when an organ within a body system is selected by the user, a picking list of possible diagnoses relating to it is triggered on the screen's right-hand side. Subsidiary details are then captured through another data entry screen, which offers multiple choice values to parameters such as associated symptoms and examination. There is also scope for logging the results of a comprehensive physical examination, system by system.

Clinergy's minimum requirements are a Pentium PC with 16 Mb of RAM, Windows 95 and compatible GP bespoke software. It can be obtained from Semantic Technologies Limited, Enterprise House, Lloyd Street North, Manchester M15 6SE, tel: 0161 226 3859.

Visual Read was developed by Leicester GPs Paul Roper and Andrew Sharp. Its inaugural button bar offers access to drawings of general areas of the body such as thorax or abdomen, from which body systems or individual organs can be selected. In relation to any of the diagram's components, provision is made for recording a history, examination, investigation, diagnosis, plan or procedure. Results can be tiled under the patient's identity details as previous findings, as a current consultation or encounter, or as a summary. Fine details are selected from successive submenus, and free text can be added. The completed data entry protocol can then be filed away in the patient record.

Visual Read has some attractive additional features. Successive submenu choices are represented by a cascade of subsidiary windows. If the cursor rests in a space immediately adjacent to the organ on display, a list box of all non-specific terms likely to be related to it appears. A list can be obtained for all generalized conditions that may affect or be associated with a specified organ, and ill-defined symptom complexes are also allowed for. Multimedia tutorials on topics

such as ECG interpretation are provided as part of the package (Fig. 6.3).

Minimum requirements for Visual Read are a 32-bit configuration, Windows 95/NT and compatible GP bespoke software. The package is supplied by Visual Read Ltd, 82 London Road, Leicester LE2 0QR, tel: 0116 255 7348.

GUI-facilitated Read coding has such obvious visual appeal that it is destined to be incorporated in the designs of all major GP system suppliers. The facility is already offered as standard by MediDesk and the Safe Clinical System. The EMIS system's protocol engine MENTOR also offers data access through anatomical diagrams.

6.7 READ ONCE, WRITE MANY TIMES

Read coding is now applied either overtly or by computer protocol to all areas of GP clinical data activity. Once selected and stored, a coded term can be accessed unequivocally and repeatedly for a host of subsequent purposes. Importantly, these include the following:

- Sharing clinical data with other health professionals – referral letters, pathology and radiology requests, commissioning, PMA insurance reports, requests to social services, transferring GP records to other practices

Fig. 6.3 Visual Read data entry tool (with acknowledgements to Novartis)

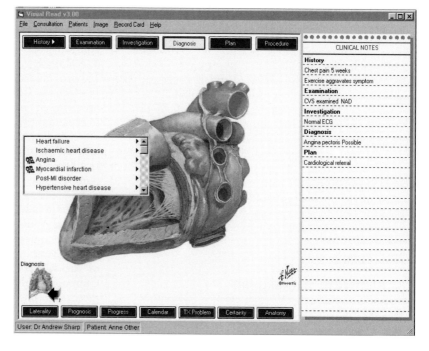

Fig. 6.4 The Read code dictionary: full listing of Read codes (Practice Made Perfect GP system)

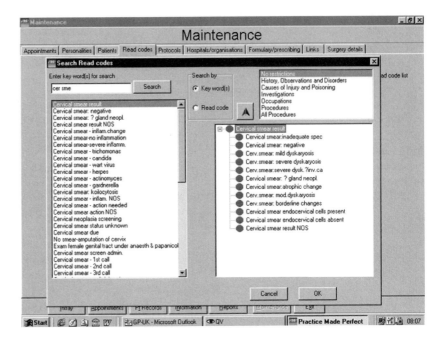

- Computerized cross-checks for prescribing, expert clinical systems, nurse triage systems
- Computerized searches for 'call and recall', defaulter identification, opportunistic reminders, audit, research and statistics
- Computerized clinical protocols are activated by, and extensively use, Read codes – the uptake of evidence based medicine will depend heavily upon the use of preferred defined terms
- Claims formulated for budgets, prescribing and services
- Resource management at practice, PCG+T and national level
- Some printout will be related to coded terms, e.g. prescriptions and patient instruction leaflets
- Coded data entered within one record field or format can be replicated automatically to all other record fields or formats to which those data also belong, so that rekeying should never be necessary.

Searches on GP system patient files that contain a mixture of RCC releases should either specify search criteria for each release separately or else be limited to the core term that all releases have in common.

6.8 HISTORICAL BACKGROUND

- In 1982 Dr James Read was a general practitioner in Loughborough and cooperated with Tim Benson in the development of the Abies GP system for which the first set of codes were designed.
- In 1988 the RCC was recommended by the Joint Computing Group of the RCGP and GMSC (BMA) for adoption as a national standard classification.
- In 1990 the RCC copyright was bought by the NHSE for use throughout the NHS. The NHS Centre for Coding and Classification (NHSCCC) was set up to develop the system further, with Dr Read as executive director, while Dr Read's private company Computer Aided Medical Systems (CAMS) was given the sole rights to market, license and provide technical support for the product.
- In 1993 the Clinical Terms Projects were set up, involving 55 working groups and 2000 clinicians, to expand the codes so as to cover the requirements of secondary care, pathology, dentistry, nursing, other allied professions and administration.
- In 1994 incorporation of the RCC within GP computer systems became a requirement for accreditation.
- In 1995/6 adverse reports were lodged by the National Audit Office and Silicon Bridge Research over the contractual arrangements between NHSE and Dr Read for financing the further development of the RCC. A later report by the House of Commons Public Accounts Committee endorsed these criticisms.
- In 1997 the number of coded terms exceeded a quarter of a million.

- In 1999 the NHSCCC became a component of the NHS Information Agency, and distribution and support responsibilities passed to the NHS.

6.9 OTHER MORBIDITY CLASSIFICATIONS USED IN GENERAL PRACTICE

- ICHPPC (International Classification of Health Problems in Primary Care) – published on behalf of WONCA in 1975 and 1979, and redefined as ICHPPC 2 in 1983
- ICPC (International Classification in Primary Care) – used by the rest of Europe and adopted by the World Organization of National Colleges and Academies; first published in 1987 by WONCA
- ICD (the International Classification of Disease), versions 9 and 10 – also used widely throughout Europe and other continents
- RCGP Classification and Analysis of GP Data 1984
- OXMIS (Oxford Medical Information Systems) Problem Codes 1978
- SNOMED (Systematized Nomenclature of Medicine; American College of Pathologists)

A joint initiative to combine the advantages of the two classifications is being undertaken by the NHSCCC and SNOMED. The resulting database is scheduled for release in 2001.

SUMMARY

- Accurate intercommunication requires that all parties use mutually preferred terms whose meanings are unequivocally understood. In the context of clinical record keeping and medical messaging, this calls for a comprehensive classification of available terms matched to meanings which are defined by authoritative medical dictionaries.
- James Read pioneered a taxonomy that classified terms in medical use and allowed for exact synonyms and qualifying statements related to the primary term. The terms are lodged, together with the alphanumeric codes allocated to them, in a relational database that requires access from a high calibre search engine.
- Read's classification (RCC) has been adopted for standardized use throughout the NHS, and maintenance and further development is now the responsibility of the NHSE. RCC codes are in widespread use throughout general practice,

secondary care, nursing, dentistry and NHS administration.

- GPs obtain their version of the RCC database and regular updates to it through their clinical GP system supplier on licence. The RCC integrates closely with the clinical system, and the use of coded terms is essential to computer-based clinical messaging, automated cross-checks, computerized searches, protocol use, the submission of electronic claims and resource management, at all levels of the NHS. Use of the RCC is a requirement for GP system accreditation.
- The early development of the RCC introduced successive releases with increasing refinement of detail so that later releases could not always be mapped to earlier ones except at root level.
- The RCC is a superset of 12 other coding systems, but also includes new unique material.
- Read-coded terms can be entered on practice systems by a number of different methods, which accelerate the selection process. GUI-based anatomical diagrams are being adopted as an initial method by which an accurately targeted short picking list of relevant terms may be triggered.

FURTHER READING

Department of Health 1990 New clinical classification will streamline computerised medical records. Press release, 29 March

Department of Health 1994 CMO Update Communication 4. New National Thesaurus, November: 1

Doctor Magazine 1998 NHSE faces code rap. Doctor 12 March: 2

Doctor Magazine 1998 Health chiefs slated in spending probe. Doctor 13 August: 15

Herd A, 1994 Are Read codes good for GPs? GP 12 March: 2

GP Magazine 1994 GP friendly Read codes due next year. GP 16 September: 55

NHSE 1996 NHS centre for coding and classification announces staff changes. Press Release 39/96: 2–3

Practice Computing Magazine 1997 Editorial comment. Practice Computing, February

Read 1990 The Read clinical classification. Computer Aided Medical Systems: 1–17

The Read Clinical Classification 1987, 1989, 1991, 1992 Technical overview, Read Codes Enquiry Pack and Incorporation of Read Codes into Hospital Systems. Computer Aided Medical Systems text published by permission of HMSA

Technology Monitor 1990 Technology Monitor, September: 50

7 Registration, download and list match

7.1 PRACTICE REGISTERS

The Oxford dictionary defines the term 'register' as an official or authoritative list. An entry in the appropriate register can legitimize acts as diverse as matrimony and the right to practise medicine. In the general practice context, manual age–sex and disease registers have been used for a number of years – the former as a means of checking capitation payments and initiating 'call' clinics for certain preventive procedures, the latter as a tool for epidemiological research within the practice and as a list of those with chronic morbidity who should be offered influenza immunization. Both these manual registers were usually housed on card indexes, and both have been ousted by computer searches of electronic practice records. Although the term 'age–sex register' is still sometimes applied to a search routine involving these two attributes, there is no longer a discrete register as such, nor the need for one. The computer can search on these, or any other acceptable attributes defined by the user, with impressive flexibility.

The most important register from the practice's point of view is, of course, the practice patient register, which is held on the practice computer – a list of the identification details of all patients who have contracted to receive primary care. This register is now replicated as closely related subsets, both in the responsible PPSA and in the National Central Registry at Southport. (In Scotland, Health Boards have similar functions to PPSAs and HAs in England and Wales. Future to references to all PPSAs and HAs will be understood to refer also to Health Boards.)

Only one manual register can justify its further existence after the introduction of the practice computer record. This is the Deskbook for change of patient status, a running list of all changes to patient identity details, which is kept in the reception area and is updated by all staff members to whom such infor-

mation is periodically given. At regular intervals, batches of amendments are loaded on to the practice computer records, and transmitted to the PPSA using Registration Links software.

7.2 MANUAL AGE–SEX REGISTERS

It is worth reviewing the severe limitations of the manual age–sex register (ASR), if only to explain the success of one of the GP computer's early applications.

The manual ASR ranked patients by sex and in date of birth order, and was promoted by enthusiasts as a practice management and research tool. It was used to check total and age-related capitation payments and to invite patients in selected age bands to attend for preventive procedures. The limitations were as follows:

- The register was a separate entity from the medical record and had to be updated individually as shifts in practice population and changes in name and address occurred. This meant locating cards by date of birth within the index, and thus required information that first had to be obtained from the record card wallet.
- Only a few of the applications claimed for the manual ASR could be run entirely from it – MMR immunization, and paediatric and geriatric screening. For most preventive procedures, further recall depends upon the date and nature of the previous recall procedure. For instance, a patient's date of recall for cytology will be dictated by the date and result of her previous test, as well as by her age.
- The target population for 'call or recall' may not be limited to a particular age band. Thus influenza immunization should be offered to patients with ongoing cardiac or pulmonary morbidity, regardless of age.

- Some patients in the age band under review should be excluded from 'call or recall' – hypertension screening need not be offered to someone who has had a recent blood pressure check.
- The task of maintaining the manual ASR index and the clerical procedures associated with its application in practice ('call or recall' letters and claims) commonly absorbed 20 or more hours of clerical time each week.

7.3   MANUAL DISEASE REGISTERS

Manual disease registers were subdivided into sections, each of which catalogued all practice patients suffering from one particular disease, and therefore omitted those patients with no morbidity. *Incidence* measures the first episode of a disease in a given population per unit of time, whereas *prevalence* measures the number of patients suffering from a disease at any one time (whether as a first episode or not). If the distinction between first episode and continuing or recurrent disease was made in the register, then calculations of incidence and prevalence could be made, given knowledge of the total number of practice patients as denominator. Clearly, these are tasks better undertaken by the computer.

7.4   PATIENT REGISTRATION WITH A PRACTICE

The tripartite contract between patient, doctor and state paymaster in the UK begins with registration. All citizens are so registered with a locality GP throughout their lives, and the cumulative record created as a result of every encounter between patient and health professional follows the patient from practice to practice on re-registration.

The signed GMS 1 contract, which records details of the identities of the applicant patient and accepting doctor, together with the services to be provided, is required to be made available to the PPSA. (In some cases GMS 1 forms may be retained at the practice when electronic registration takes place.) If the transfer is from its own area of responsibility, the PPSA checks the registration details against those held on its own computer, making any necessary changes, and re-registers the patient in the new doctor's name. The PPSA confirms the fact and the date of registration to the new GP and initiates per capita payments, with special rates applying to patients aged 65–74 years and those over 75 years. The manual record is obtained from the relinquishing practice and forwarded to the accepting practice. The PPSA also recalls records of deceased, emigrating or enlisting patients.

If patient transfer involves two different PPSAs, if the patient has been abroad, in the armed forces or in a long stay institution, or if the registration involves a newborn or immigrant, then the NHS Central Registry must ratify the change, allocating a new NHS number if appropriate. The Central Registry maintains a national database of the identities and NHS numbers of all UK citizens.

7.5   REGISTRATION PROBLEMS

For the first 40 years of the NHS, registration and re-registration depended upon the use of an array of alternative paper forms and postal or courier services. The defects of the paper based procedure were as follows:

- Verification of PPSA registration could only occur when the manual NHS record was received in the practice, stamped with the registration date. The clerical processes involved in each stage were subject to delay and some degree of inaccuracy. The accepting GP might only realize that the registration process had failed when, a considerable time later, the patient's NHS record could not be found in the practice files.
- In every practice there were a number of NHS records (cumulative with time, and up to 10% in city practices) for patients no longer attending the practice. Some of these were de-registered but their records had escaped recall. Some had re-registered elsewhere, unknown to the PPSA whose area they had left ('ghost patients'). Ghost patients played havoc with the denominator in target achievement calculations and often meant that the NHS was paying two capitation fees for the same patient.
- New babies might not be registered by their parents with the practice for many months. Elderly patients who wintered abroad for more than 3 months might be removed automatically from a doctor's list and fail to re-register on return, as did prison inmates on release.
- A cross-check on whether an individual patient was registered required a phone call to the PPSA. A cross-check with the PPSA for all patients registered against all manual records held by the practice was a formidable and rarely undertaken procedure. A numerical count of practice-held NHS records could give, at best, only an approximation to the number registered with the PPSA, and practices relied heavily on the accuracy of PPSA clerical procedures for the calculation of their capitation fees. When PPSA and practice registers were eventually reconciled nationwide prior to comput-

erization of the registration process, extensive surveys showed that discrepancies of detail of one sort or another had lain dormant in the records of between 25% and 50% of all patients.

Computerization solves all the problems of the manual process, and Registration Links has proved to be one of the outstanding early achievements of the government's IM and T strategy.

Fig. 7.1 Registration details screen: Torex Meditel System 5

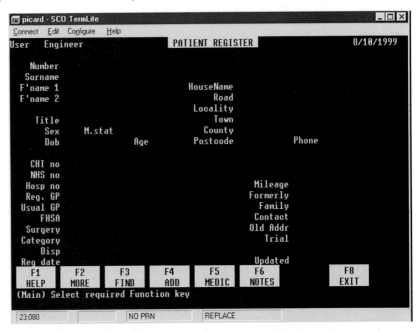

Fig. 7.2 Registration details screen: new GPASS system

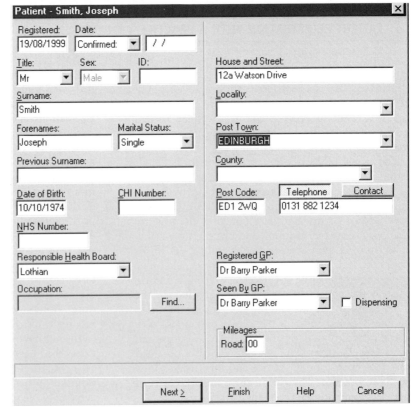

7.6   REGISTRATION LINKS

The radical changes that were applied to the registration process in the 1990s began with the first linkages between FHSAs and the NHS Central Registry in the autumn of 1990. The reforms that took place in the data traffic between FHSAs and GPs were brought about in two stages.

- In July 1996 a suite of four new, simplified and streamlined paper forms (GMS 1–4) was introduced to regulate GP–FHSA data traffic. These replaced the array of 19 heterogeneous and clumsy documents that had previously been used. The new forms, which incorporated the new 10-numeric-digit NHS patient number, recorded registration (GMS 1), maternity services (GMS 2), temporary services (GMS 3) and GMS items of service (GMS 4).
- Electronification of interchanges between GPs and FHSAs, using their respective computer systems via the Racal HealthLink, enabled data structured in keeping with the new GMS 1–4 format to be transmitted and, to a large extent, processed automatically.

GP–FHSA Links were first piloted by the FHS Computer Unit in September 1992. In December 1994, the NHSE relaunched its IM and T strategy with amendments that included provisions for Links and the new NHS number. FHSAs prioritized the adoption of GP–FHSA Links, manipulating preferential reimbursement in an effort to achieve NHSE uptake targets. (The introduction of e-registration to all computerized practices by April 1997 was attempted but not realized.) In November 1996 the HealthLink network buckled under the rapidly increasing demand placed upon it by e-registration and had to be upgraded as a matter of urgency. Ultimately, by the end of the 1990s, conversion was more or less complete.

The conversion process had called for a significant effort from practices. A considerable amount of staff time had been spent in training and in reconciling registers, while the main beneficiaries were seen to be the FHSAs, whose clerical procedures could now be automated. Inevitably, the fact that 'ghost' patients had at last been exorcized meant that capitation fees were correspondingly reduced in most practices. However, the overall advantages of e-registration were indisputable, and benefited GPs, FHSAs and patients:

- GP, FHSA and Central Registry registers became much more accurate, and tallied with each other.

- Patient record transfer was accelerated.
- Paperwork was considerably reduced, both in practices and, more especially, in FHSAs.

7.7   GMS AND OTHER PRACTICE PATIENT REGISTERS

So far, we have spoken of registration as if it were a single procedure. Strictly speaking, each practice maintains six separate concurrent patient registers – GMS, CHS, maternity, contraception, emergency treatment, and temporary residents, and, although most patients will attend the same practice for the first five of these services, the population of all registers can vary from one another.

Temporary residents are, of course, a case apart, but some practices do not undertake maternity or child health development work, in which event their patients must register elsewhere for these services. Form GMS 1 accommodates registration for both GMS and CHS, as the two services are rarely separated, and form GMS 4 details Item of Service claims for one or more GMS registered patients. Form GMS 2 registers patients for maternity services (and claims for them), and GMS 3 registers and claims for temporary residents, emergency treatment and contraception.

There are four categories of applicant who complete the GMS 1 registration/re-registration form:

- those transferring from another doctor
- the newborn. Although parents of a newborn child will obtain from FP 58 from the Registrar of Births and Deaths to whom they report the birth (a form that allocates a new NHS number and invites registration with a GP), a practice's best interest is served by asking parents to complete a GMS 1 form during the puerperium, since this will pre-empt potential delay in registering the infant. As a consequence of registration, parents are provided with the child's record of immunizations and screening procedures (a folder colloquially known as 'the Red Book'), and an appointment should be made by the practice for the initial screening consultation, noting the date and time in the folder. Ironically, although the child's name appears preprinted on the folder, the NHS number does not.
- immigrants. If not already allocated, a new NHS number will subsequently be issued by the Central Registry.
- patients leaving long stay institutions or the armed forces, or having temporarily resided abroad.

With the introduction of electronic registration, the use of the pre-existing patient-held 'medical card' (FP 4, originally derived from the wartime identity card), fell into abeyance.

7.8 SETTING UP REGISTRATION LINKS

Registration Links software, which must of necessity be compatible with the practice management software and accredited by the NHS Computer Agency, is provided and supported by the GP system supplier.

The program prompts for, and validates field by field, the data otherwise recorded on the GMS 1 paper form:

- the patient's title, surname, first names, previous surnames
- date of birth, sex, NHS number
- home address, post code, telephone number
- town and country of birth
- if relocated, details of the previous domicile and previous UK GP, with relevant dates
- conjoint registration for CHS, practice dispensing and NHS organ donation (rural payment claim details are added by the practice)
- source and date of application for registration
- doctor's acceptance and date of registration with the practice.

The system must record the date it uploads these details to the PPSA and the date of confirmation of receipt by the PPSA. Amendments to registration details must also log dates of transmission to, and receipt by, the PPSA.

7.9 LOGISTICS

In order to implement Registration Links, the following steps must be taken:

- The GP system supplier must commission an electronic mailbox for the practice from Racal or BT Syntegra.
- Hardware should be reviewed. The GP system supplier's advice on the status of all pre-existing and proposed hardware should be obtained. Basic connective hardware requirements are a modem, communications card, and dedicated telephone socket and line. For most practices, 15 Mb available hard disk space on the server will suffice.
- The supplier's Links software must be installed, and should include a tuition program with dummy records.

- A Links maintenance contract should be obtained from the supplier.
- Training, preferably provided over two days, should be arranged by the supplier in conjunction with the PPSA.
- Target dates should be set for all inauguration milestones.
- The Deskbook for Change of Patient Status should be initiated.
- Reconciliation must be provided between the GP and PPSA registers. Initially, the practice is asked to provide the PPSA with a diskette listing registered patients by sex and in age order. Crosschecks by the PPSA, using the practice diskette and its own electronic register, allow the production of a printed exception list, which the practice must work through manually. When adjustments have been incorporated, a further practice diskette is downloaded and sent to the PPSA for comparison. This cycle of readjustments must be repeated until full reconciliation is achieved. For a practice of 10 000 patients the process of reconciliation is likely to take a minimum of one working week.
  Patients who do not appear on the PPSA register but whose manual records are held by the practice should be asked to complete form GMS 1 forthwith, unless they have left the practice, in which case their records should be returned to the PPSA. When patients appear on the PPSA register but not in the practice files, their records should be traced or replaced.
- The PPSA must now test both ends of the GP–PPSA linkage using dummy records.
- A security copy of the practice files must be taken, and the system will then be able to 'go live'. Daily changes of patient data will be stored on the practice server as they are loaded by practice staff, and two-way autodial-up and transfer to the PPSA will take place each night.
- New patients will have new records raised on the practice computer, which must include the date on which acceptance was acknowledged by the PPSA. Changes in status will be transferred regularly to the computer from the manual Deskbook.
- A list will be printed out for patients leaving the practice, in order to facilitate the selection of wallets from the manual files.
- When transferring manual record wallets between practice and PPSA, the fact of receipt or dispatch should be noted in the patient's computer record. An audit trail of all steps in the registration procedure must be kept by the practice management system, and must be available for inspection by proper authority.

- The PPSA prompts the practice each quarter for the production of an electronic or printed practice list size, which must show age-related subgroups, to be used as the basis for calculating capitation and target payments. Paper GMS 1s are submitted to the PPSA quarterly.
- Extra registration data were recorded during the days of fundholding, and these included previous name, aliases, place of birth, ethnic origin and patient's hospital number. It may be advantageous to retain these details for practice or commissioning purposes and, if so, arrangements should be made with the system supplier for their transfer to the practice management system database.
- The act of patient registration should automatically trigger the practice system to prompt for the initiation of other new patient procedures such as the issue of health questionnaires and practice leaflets, an appointment for new patient checks and the monitoring of claims in association with those checks, and the inauguration of the new patient computer record. Screening procedures, immunization, and contraception will be offered if the response to the questionnaire shows these to be appropriate.

7.10 LISTMATCH SOFTWARE

The NHS Central Registry at Southport, which is in electronic communication with all 98 PPSAs, not only acts as a coordinating source of reference for NHS numbers and patient identity details, but is well placed to provide accurate statistics on population distribution. Given the fact that practice populations and medical responsibilities are accurately defined at local level by the UK registration process, the potential for the development of more sophisticated statistical investigation is impressive and almost unique to this country.

The data categories that are jointly used to identify patients uniquely throughout the NHS are the NHS number, date of birth and surname. The primary task of the Central Registry is to ensure that all patients are registered and that no entries are reduplicated. It therefore has absolute power to determine the NHS number, exerts this power through PPSAs, and, when discrepancies between PPSA and GP registers involve the NHS number, the PPSA version will be held to be correct by definition.

The registration details held in respect of each patient on the PPSA computer are:

- title, surname and first names
- previous surnames
- NHS number (both former and new)
- date of birth

- sex
- home address, arranged in five lines – house name, street number and name, district, town, county. In the computer's dictionary the latter three of these items are jointly represented by a unique code, which can be used to check their validity, and which will also generate the identity of the local health authority
- post code, which may also be checked for validity and which is used to generate the deprivation index
- telephone number
- town and country of birth
- the GP with whom registered
- rural mileage weighting
- CHS status
- dispensing status
- organ donation status
- if relocated, details of previous domicile and previous UK GP, with relevant dates
- date and source of request for registration
- date entered on PPSA register.

If discrepancies between PPSA and GP registers occur with regard to the patient's surname, forenames, date of birth, sex, address or post code, then it is highly probable that the version in the GP register is correct. Discrepancies are most often caused by failure to update changed details, although typographical errors and mis-spelling also occur. Discrepancies in the identity of the registered GP can only be changed in the PPSA register by completion of a GMS 1 form.

'Listmatch' software loads the GP and PPSA registers and displays them side by side on the screen or as printout. Discrepancies between the two are highlighted, and the highlight is applied to the detail on the register that is most likely to be at fault – the practice in the case of the NHS number, and the PPSA in the case of names, date of birth, sex, address or post code. The two main types of discrepancy are:

- whole record mismatch, where a record appears on one register but not on the other. A list of these discrepancies is printed out by the system.
- field mismatches, in which one or more fields are discrepant. Field mismatches result in a side-by-side printout or screen display with the discrepancies highlighted. Discrepancies may be corrected on-screen, and developments are under way to allow automatic correction to take place, subject to safeguards. Error assignment to one or other register can be over-ridden by the user.

Listmatch software was the brainchild of David Jehring, a Worcestershire GP, and was extensively tested by the Wycombe Primary Care Computing Project using predominantly Update Systems. Its suc-

```
              H A Entry              Practice Entry
              -  -                   -  -
              Mr. Andrew Other       Mr. Andrew Other
              Male                   Male
              09 02 1929             09 02 1929
              NHS 1234560789         NHS 1234560189
              Inglenook              Inglenook
              14 Any Street          14 Any Street
              Troytown               Troytown
              Blandshire             Blandshire
              BL22 9NT               BL22 9NT
              Dr. Haver              Dr. Haver



              H A Entry              Practice Entry
              -  -                   -  -
              Miss Peta Grimes       Mr. Peter Grimes
              Female                 Male
              10 03 1942             10 03 1942
              NHS 1234056789         NHS 1234056789
              Inglenook              Inglenook
              140 Any Street         14 Any Street
              Mans Estate            Mans Estate
              Troytown               Troytown
              Blandshire             Blandshire
              BL22 9NT               BL22 9NT
              Dr. Haver              Dr. Leech
```

Fig. 7.3 Examples of reports of field-mismatches – entries underlined are those the system considers likely to be in error (Courtesy of Listmatch Software)

cess has spawned a number of imitations, and the principles it established formed the basis for the production of the PPSA exception list.

7.11 THE DESKBOOK FOR CHANGE OF PATIENT STATUS

The only manual register that can justifiably be retained once a practice computer system becomes operational is the Deskbook for change of patient status. The book is used to record identification details of all patients signing on with the practice, new births, patients temporarily removed from the list, all records recalled, and changes of names and address. This allows a check of patients who have signed on but whose registration has not been endorsed by the PPSA, or whose records have not been received, and

helps to distinguish between manual records recalled and those missing for any other reason. The book's main use, however, is as a central source of corrected patient identity details from which computer records will be updated, whence amendments will subsequently be replicated and transmitted to the PPSA by GP-PPSA Links. Those responsible for updates should confirm that they have fulfilled their duties by recording their action, together with their signature and the appropriate date, in the Deskbook.

NHSE system accreditation requirements now include provision for recording the date and the source of the request for registration or de-registration, so provision for recording these details should also be made in the Deskbook.

Computer systems must provide evidence of change and date of change of registration details, whether and when these have been notified to the

PPSA, and whether and when the PPSA confirmed registration.

Registration status and dates are searched during the process of defining populations for capitation and target payments.

The Deskbook is usually kept in the practice reception area, but must be assiduously maintained by all practice staff when notified of changes by patients.

Since the introduction of the 1990 contract, new patient registration has been linked to practice obligations to perform, and claim for, new patient checks and to issue practice leaflets. To this end it is wise to set up new patient computer records at the time of registration whenever possible. (Initial data for the record may be obtained from patient questionnaires.) This will enable all linked procedures, including

---

Box 7.1   Augmented patient identity details

The basic details required for the entry of a patient to the HA register suffice to provide for unique identification and for the needs of PPSA administration, but are insufficient for comprehensive GP system use. This augmented list of details associated with patient identity will be needed as a minimum data subset in a comprehensively formatted GP record.

1. Details recommended by the Primary Health Care Specialist Group of the British Computer Society (November 1991)

Surname	Telephone number (work)	Registering PPSA
Previous surname (e.g. maiden)	Occupation	Medical insurance
Forename (s)	Registered GP	Rural mileage etc
NHS number	Usual GP	Last update
Title	Next of kin/emergency contact	Last data check date, and scrutinizer
Date of birth	Date registered	
Sex	Registered status (e.g. current ...	Exempt status (script fees)
Marital status	Date of transfer/leaving	Type of exemption
Address	Reason for transfer	Source and date of request for registration)
Post code	Location for manual notes (multisurgery practices)	
Health district of residence		
Telephone number (home)	Dispensing status	

As a minimum data set for comprehensive identity details, the above list is incomplete and should include the following

2. Ethnic origin Hospitals attended and patient's hospital numbers	Required for commissioning
3. Patient status: NHS or private	Required for practices with private patients
4. Aliases Place of birth	Required for augmented PPSA register
5. At least one previous or alternative address Date and source of request for registration or de-registration	Requirements for NHS Management Executive system accreditation

The PPSA register's preferred format for the patient's address is that it should be recorded in a five line format – house name, street number and name, district, town, county. The last three of these items can be checked using a coordinating computer directory.

Postcodes will already have been added to the details received in the exceptions list from PPSAs, but they may otherwise be obtained from local post offices.

Many of the above items will not be available on the record card wallet and will need to be prompted for when the patient attends the medical centre. Highlighted omissions should then be rectified by the receptionist where possible.

PPSA registration, to be monitored (see also Chapter 8).

SUMMARY

- Manual age–sex and disease registers have been superseded by computers, which can search the patient record files by age, sex, disease, or any other standardized parameters, on demand.
- Patient registration with a practice is a contract for the primary care responsibility for each patient. Separate practice registers exist for GMS, CHS, maternity, contraception, emergency treatment, and temporary resident care, although, as a rule, the first five of these types of service will be provided by the same practice.
- Registration is initiated by the practice and subsequently notified to and confirmed by the PPSA, but these processes are subject to errors and delays if manual methods are used. Electronic linkage between the practice and the PPSA will allow simultaneous and accurate registration details to be recorded at both sites.
- Patient registration by the practice should initiate other new patient procedures, such as the issue of health questionnaires and practice leaflets, the offer of checks and the monitoring of claims associated with these checks, the offer of screening, immunization, or contraception if appropriate, and the inauguration of the computer medical record.
- When a computer system is installed in a practice, the registration details of all patients must be recorded. If the computer system communicates with the PPSA through Links, then these details must include surname, first names, title, previous surnames, date of birth, sex, NHS number, address and post code, telephone number, town and country of birth; if relocated, details of previous domicile and UK GP with dates, CHS, practice dispensing and NHS organ donation details, doctor's acceptance with date, and source and date of registration request. These details must be logged on the practice computer and uploaded to the PPSA nightly. The dates that the source provided the information, the date of uploading and the date of confirmation of the receipt by the PPSA must be logged – data that must also be kept with regard to all subsequent amendments.
- A total reconciliation between practice and PPSA computer registers must be effected, and this can be done by submitting a practice-originated diskette for PPSA checking, following which discrepancies can be processed at the practice. Discrepancies between the two sources are common and, as the Central Registry has absolute discretion in determining NHS numbers, the PPSA version of the latter will be deemed correct by definition. Discrepancies in patient name, date of birth, sex or address will lead to the assumption that the practice version is correct. Software is now available to provide for the rapid resolution of these problems.
- The Deskbook for change of patient status is used to record all changes in patient registration details as they are reported to the practice. Periodically, these amendments must be recorded in the practice computer records and notified to the PPSA.

FURTHER READING

Information Management Group, NHS Management Executive 1993 General medical practice computer systems requirements for accreditation (applicable from 1 April 1994)

Jehring D 1992 Patient registration and Listmatch software. Practice Computing, July: 11

8 Preventive medicine and item of service claims

8.1 INTRODUCTION

Prevention is better than cure, cure is better than the stalemate of long-term therapeutic control, which in turn is better than progressive disease. Absolute prevention is the unattainable ideal, which, if realized, would remove the need for all other forms of medicine and the doctors who practise them.

The general practitioner's three main roles – crisis intervention in acute disease, preventive medicine, and the maintenance control of chronic disease – are all materially assisted by the computer. For dealing with new acute problems in their role as interveners in crisis, doctors may use the whole past record on computer, or subsets of it structured so as to provide rapid access to important positive and negative evidence. For preventive medicine, the computer provides total administrative support for 'call or recall' clinics, a reminder facility for opportunistic procedures, and sophisticated performance enhancement routines. For the maintenance control of chronic disease, the doctor can summon special displays of sequential information, purposely selected from the patient's computer record, each display dedicated to the control of a specific condition.

There is a fundamental distinction to be made between the search of an apparently healthy population for signs of impending disease, and maintaining control once that disease has become established. The clinic administration, and therefore the data-processing requirements of the two, are in direct contrast. In the former, the total practice population or, more probably, a subset defined by age, sex, occupation or family history, is invited by letter to attend a 'call' clinic for the performance of a test. Only if the test is abnormal will they be redirected for treatment. In the control of established disease a batch of patients, defined jointly by the condition for which they are being treated, are reappointed from check to check

('cohort' clinics). The continuing health of such cohorts of patients usually depends upon continuing medication, and default requires prompt action. The relationship between 'call' and cohort clinics, and their contrasting computer requirements, is shown in Figures 8.1 and 8.2.

8.2 'CALL OR RECALL' AND OPPORTUNISTIC SCREENING

Call clinic management becomes more complex after the first record search. Although defaulters will be re-identified at subsequent searches, there will be the need to re-appoint some patients for procedures that are in effect repeats – a second dose of tetanus immunization, for instance, or a repeated cervical smear where the first proved inadequate. As such re-appointments are usually tacked on to further 'call' clinics, the composite term 'call or recall' is often used. Opportunistic screening is complementary to 'call or recall' and is provided by computer-generated timely reminders placed prominently in the consultation record. These reminders prompt the doctor to suggest a due preventive procedure when the patient attends the medical centre for an unassociated reason.

'Call or recall' clinics require the expenditure of time, effort and resources such as postage and stationery in the production of summoning letters. They have the logistical advantage of mass production, which makes the most effective use of staff. Their main drawback is their disappointing take-up rate, which may be as low as 40–50% for some screening procedures – a measure of the low priority accorded to them by patients in the absence of adequate publicity. In order to improve uptake, counter-measures such as scheduling clinics outside normal working hours, offering creche facilities at the medical centre, performing cytology at the patient's

Fig. 8.1 Relationship between 'call' and 'cohort' clinic populations

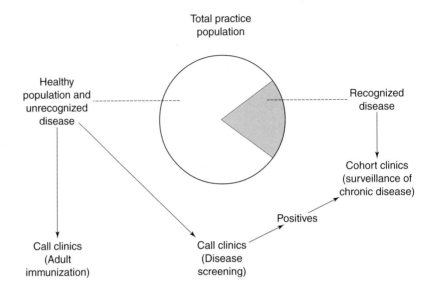

Fig. 8.2 Uses of computer by 'call' and 'cohort' clinics

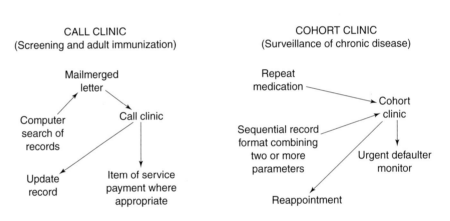

home, and coercion on the part of the health visitor have all been tried. A personalized summoning letter signed by the patient's own doctor seems to contribute to greater compliance.

Opportunistic screening secures a much better patient response – partly because of the direct and personal recommendation which the doctor has made, and partly because the patient may not need to make a separate journey to the medical centre. The procedure, if carried out by the doctor, extends the time taken over the consultation but does not involve the cost of summoning letters. However, it fails to provide for patients who have no other cause to consult their doctor.

'Call or recall' requires a clearly defined practice population and is, therefore, well suited to use under National Health Service conditions in the UK, where every patient must be registered with a doctor. It is difficult or impossible to implement under health systems in which doctors are paid purely by item of service and patients are given an open choice of doctor with each new illness, because under these conditions summoning letters may be taken to imply solicitation. Without a defined practice population, opportunistic screening can be used, but patient mobility between practices poses problems of record continuity. This can be overcome by the use of the patient-held record, and the introduction of the 'smart card' (a credit-card-style innovation that stores electronic data and can be carried in the patient's wallet) has been successful in the medical context in the USA.

A combination of 'call or recall' and opportunistic procedures gives the best results – the non-responder to one method being identified and encouraged to

Fig. 8.3 Opportunistic screening: Seetec's GP Professional System

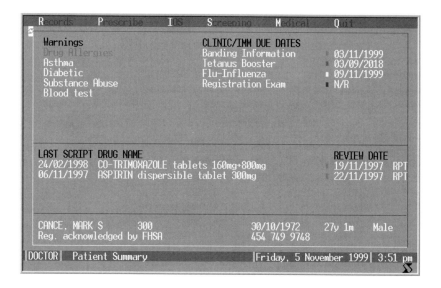

cooperate by the other. Even the fact that an invitation is issued twice (by whatever method) seems to increase the response rate.

Many preventive procedures, whether immunization or screening for incipient disease, when sanctioned by authority are paid for individually (in most developed countries), or by target achievement (in the UK), and as such contribute significantly to practice income. Most of the procedures practised in both immunization and screening can be delegated to ancillary staff under supervision. Immunization, testing of blood pressure and urine, height and weight, visual acuity, hearing, and all venepunctures can be performed by trained nurses. The sparing use of medical manpower serves to make this lucrative means of improving health standards additionally attractive.

Preventive medicine as a whole may be divided into communal hygiene, and personalized screening and immunization. The latter two are now, save for mammography, predominantly the responsibility of general practice. It is significant that this responsibility cannot be discharged without the use of computers.

8.3 THE 1990 CONTRACT

Health service reforms as they affected general practice in 1990 placed increased emphasis on information interchange, accountability and prevention. Coupled with these reforms, and in open recognition of the fact that they could scarcely be introduced without computers, partial direct system reimbursement was instituted.

There were five initial categories of reform, to which the fundholding and indicative drug amount initiatives would be added later:

A. preventive policies – 3-yearly checks, elderly checks, paediatric development checks, new patient checks, target payments and authorized preventive clinic assembly
B. practice publications – practice leaflets (brochures) and practice annual reports
C. minor surgery
D. provision to the FHSA of basic practice details
E. changes in the methods of GP payment.

The first and last of these reform categories rendered the administration of prevention considerably more complex. All GP system suppliers had to provide major upgrades to meet the requirements of the new contract.

Modifications made to the contract in 1993 abolished routine 3-yearly checks and introduced 'triple-band' screening in their place. Clinic assembly claims and fees were also phased out, being replaced by payments linked directly with protocol-based triple-band screening, and diabetes and asthma supervision.

By the end of the 1990s further modifications were introduced that abolished the 'triple-band' framework and merely required practices to submit their own proposals for preventive policies for approval by the Local Health Promotion Committee.

From 1999 onwards, evidence-based justification for intervention promulgated by the National Institute for Clinical Excellence (NICE), and locally determined Health Improvement Plans, have exerted steadily increasing influence over practices' preventive policies.

8.4 SCREENING

It must be clearly understood that only a limited number of diseases can be pre-empted by presymptomatic detection. The prerequisites for an effective screening procedure are:

- a straightforward test that has a high degree of reliability
- a long latent interval between the development of a positive test and the development of the disease against which the test warns
- a significant improvement in the outcome of the disease if detected and treated during the latent interval, as opposed to the outcome of treatment after the disease has become established.

Screening procedures are more acceptable to policy makers if they can be shown to save money in terms of the ultimate cost of care. For this purpose it is necessary to calculate the cost of preventing one case of the disease in question and compare this with the cost of treating an unscreened case. In this context the argument for preventing chronic disability such as stroke illness is a compelling one.

The viability of screening policies has come under intense scrutiny in recent years. The National Screening Committee (NSC) was set up in 1996 to advise UK ministers on the introduction, review, modification or cessation of national population screening programmes, and determined criteria for appraising the viability, effectiveness and appropriateness of individual policies. The Cochrane Collaboration uses in-depth investigation of existing reports (meta-analysis) as the basis for providing a framework for evidence-based practice, and includes screening in its remit.

Although responsible authority has now endorsed the effectiveness of the cervical cytology and mammography screening programs, there has been considerable controversy over its decisions to reject non-specialized breast examination by palpation, and screening for prostatic cancer. The NSC has over 300 discrete pilot programmes on its register, the detailed appraisal of which will take many years. The 1990 GP contract attempted to introduce an all-patient life-span monitoring policy, with stipulated minimum test parameters selected so as to ensure that the population would be checked for child development, cervical cytology, hypertension, diabetes, hyperlipidaemia, obesity and other known cardiac risk factors, but the

rationale and methodology for scrutinizing the last five of these variables nationally are still under dispute.

General practice cannot stand idly by while the pundits argue and, although routine 3-yearly checks and banding have been abandoned, must still discharge its basic responsibilities with regard to the early detection of diabetes and hypertension, because to await symptoms in these conditions worsens their prognosis. Whereas screening for both these maladies involves examination of the total population, screening for some other disorders will only be required within subgroups determined by age, sex, race, family history or associated morbidity. If the practice computer is to be able to search for selected subgroups, it is essential that the pertinent criteria used when defining such searches should be stored in the patient record in the first place.

Litigation further complicates the debate on the selection of diseases to be screened. Stroke illness is no longer regarded as an act of God but as a failure on the part of the doctor to act. In the USA, GPs who fail to put cases of atrial fibrillation on anticoagulants risk being sued. Where conflicting advice exists (as for instance between the CMO and the manufacturers of HRT and oral contraceptives over the value of breast palpation in cancer detection) the GP must decide not only what is in the patient's best interest but what action will avoid accusations of negligence.

Each practice needs to be *au fait* with the current thinking on prevention, to be prepared to search its patient record database periodically using those criteria that identify subsets at risk, and record in the patient notes what action has been taken, even if this is limited to giving lifestyle advice. Box 8.1 is an attempt to codify current thinking on screening policy in line with existing published reports, but every practice has its own responsibility for compiling such a table and keeping it up to date.

8.5 THE COMPUTER'S ROLE

Manual records can no longer provide for the data processing requirements of modern preventive medicine. If unstructured record wallets were to be used, then those for the whole practice would need to be sifted through every time a screening operation was planned. Age–sex registers facilitate compilations of 'call' lists but cannot cope with recall or opportunistic screening, and make the recording of change of patient identity details difficult. The recall index, in which patients' cards are ranked by the date when their next recall is due, cannot be used for a 'call'

Box 8.1 List of suggested screening procedures

(Each practice should prepare and update its own suite of screening policies in line with NSC guidelines)

Well-established screening procedures
- *Cervical cytology*. Cervical cancer incidence is 24 cases per 100 000 population p.a. HPV testing gives a 70% positive prediction rate
- *Mammography* (augmented by electropotential). Breast cancer incidence is 54 cases per 100 000 population p.a.
- *Child health surveillance*
- *Antenatal care*
- *The elderly* (over 74 years)

Prejudicial family history
- *Colorectal cancer FH*. ?Faecal occult blood tests combined with either barium enema or colonoscopy, or else flexible sigmoidoscopy ?every 2 years between ages 50 and 69
- *High risk breast or ovarian cancer* (two first- or second-degree relations with B. or O. cancer). ?Genetic testing and tertiary specialist care. ?6-monthly GP checks and 3-yearly mammography
- *Diabetes FH*. Take IA2 blood test in childhood. Take gestational GTT

High risk of osteoporosis
(Early natural or surgical menopause, vertebral deformity, osteopenia on X-ray, long-term corticosteroids, anorexia nervosa, alcohol abuse, hyperparathyroidism, thyrotoxicosis, malabsorption syndrome, partial gastrectomy, myeloma, hypogonadism in males, FH osteoporosis or multiple low trauma fractures)
- Dual energy X-ray absorbiometry

Sexually-active females
(Contraception clinic attendees, termination cases, GUM referrals, partners of positives)
- Swab or urine test for *Chlamydia trachomatis*

Known CVS risk factors
(Hypertension, hypercholesterolaemia, cigarette smoking, diabetes, marked obesity)
- Carotid or femoral artery bifurcation scan for atherosclerosis

Antenatal care
- Syphilis, hepatitis B, anaemia, rubella status, ?GTT, ?endomysial antibodies for coeliac disease

Race
- Haemoglobinopathies, thalassaemia, sickle-cell disorder

New immigrants
- Heaf test for tuberculosis

Patients on OCT or HRT
- ?6-monthly GP checks and triennial mammograms

The ageing myocardium
(All aged 65–75 years, in order to assist in stroke prevention)
- ?ECG to detect atrial fibrillation

Established or incipient myocardial degeneration
(Post-myocardial-infarction, elderly hypertension, angina, diabetes, auricular fibrillation)
- Echocardiography to quantify LV dysfunction and prevent heart failure

Under active NSC consideration
- Cystic fibrosis
- Down's syndrome
- Fragile X syndrome
- Haemoglobinopathies
- Ovarian carcinoma
- Child health surveillance
- Genetic testing

Pending consideration
- *BC10* ageing gene, which can mutate to become carcinogenic (discovered in 1999)

search based on age and sex, and do not cope with opportunistic screening or lend themselves readily to the updating of patient identity details. Structured preventive record cards included with the record wallet provide for opportunistic reminders but do not allow 'call or recall'. Features such as target calculations, and automated letters and claims are, of course, only possible if computers are used.

8.6 INTEGRATION WITH NATIONAL SCREENING PROGRAMMES

The first 'call or recall' systems on computer were community-based in the UK. Following the success of mass miniature radiography in helping to eradicate tuberculosis, attention turned to the early detection of cancer, and mass screening programmes for cervical cytology and mammography were inaugurated. It was considered essential to set up a cohesive national administration to eliminate variation between practices and provide for rapid processing in cases of abnormality. In taking primary responsibility for cancer 'call or recall', Local Health Authorities used an FHSA register as a source for the call process, and names and results were then transferred to a computerized recall register.

Use of the FHSA register, correlated with the Central National Registry at Southport, ensured that patients who had moved area but failed to re-register were not missed, and that patients were not registered simultaneously in two different areas. Individual patient details for those whose status or address had changed had to be brought up to date before summoning letters were sent out, and this was achieved by sending a draft list of patients to each practice for correction. Following this, patients were summoned for screening, results were forwarded and abnormal cases were processed.

Although the practice was not primarily responsible for the administration of cancer screening under these arrangements, it had to carry out the following procedures:

- The prior notification list had to be checked to ensure that all practice patients in the given age band had been listed for screening. The practice had also to amend all individual patient details that required updating, and remove from the list the names of those who should not be summoned. If the practice computer housed the patient's clinical and preventive records, then the process of checking the prior notification list was made easy. A list of patients in the relevant age band was produced by the computer, then each of these records was

accessed by computer through the list to allow the necessary comparison to be made. Manual checks took an average 5 minutes per record; computerized checks took 30–40 seconds.
- Persistent defaulters to cancer screening appointments had to be followed up by the general practitioner. It was important that the fact of default should appear in a prominent place in the computerized consultation record, so as to prompt the doctor to give opportunistic counselling when the patient next attended the medical centre. Periodic searches of the records by computer to give lists of persistent defaulters could be provided for health visitors, so that follow-up by home visits could be considered.
- In the case of cervical cytology screening, the practice was already involved in the screening process and was in any case responsible for the collation of results from all screening sources. It was also responsible for the rapid referral of abnormalities. A recall register was essential, run in parallel with the local health authority listings, and, if computerized, could be taken simply as a search function on the preventive medicine or pathology file of the patient record. A computer-maintained list of all urgent cases could be kept in a prominent place in the system in order to ensure that none were overlooked.

With the more widespread use of practice computers and the added incentive to meet targets, many practices have now taken primary responsibility for their own cytology 'call or recall' operation, although both cytology and mammography continue to be supported by central processing. With increasing electronic communication between the practice and the health authority computer, regular reconciliation of patient registers between the two have become the norm, and there is no reason why a facility for sharing data should not extend to cytology and mammography files.

8.7 COMPUTER SUPPORT FOR OTHER SCREENING PROCEDURES

New patient checks

New patients must be offered a consultation in writing within 28 days of registration with the practice.

Logistical requirements
1. Complete registration form GMS 1 – for the whole family, if applicable.
2. Replicate GMS 1 details on computer for e-registration and transmit to PPSA.
3. Issue practice leaflet (brochure).

4. Allocate appointment for new patient check. Generate invitation letter on computer, giving it or posting it to the patient and recording the fact of issue (not applicable to patients under 5 years of age). Appointments must be for a date within 3 months of registration.

5. Record patients' response to invitation letter on computer.

6. Issue new-patient questionnaire: try to obtain replies at the time of registration. Enter results on to computer.

7. Enter new-patient check results on to computer – *minimum data set*: patient identity details (registration); previous illnesses, operations or serious injuries; immunizations, allergies, current medication, previous tests for breast and cervical cancer; adverse family, social or occupational history; life style (diet, exercise, smoking, alcohol, drug abuse, solvents) and current health. The assessor must offer an examination to include height, weight, BP, and urine for albumin and sugar. Body mass index and cardiac risk index will be calculated by the computer.

8. Generate new-patient check claim on computer for submission to PPSA within 6 months.

9. Plan and discuss health policy with patient, and record recommendations on computer. Update immunization, screening and contraception provision if required, and claim.

10. Record date and source of application for registration, and dates of submission to, and confirmation of acceptance of registration by, the PPSA.

Screening for patients already on practice list

Geriatric, paediatric and well-person checks all employ 'call or recall', with complementary opportunistic screening schedules. The logistical requirements are:

1. All practice patient records on computer: registration details, appropriate screening files and subset selection criteria as a minimum.

2. Periodic search of patient files by date of birth and other subset selection criteria for those who are due for, but who have not received, the appropriate screening procedure. Although much geriatric and well-person screening is carried out opportunistically, those not attending surgery will still need to be called. The Paediatric Assessment Register will not necessarily be a subset of the general practice register, and a copy of it has to be made available quarterly to the HA as the basis for CHS capitation payments.

3. Send mail-merged letters offering appointments. Geriatric patients have the right to require a home visit when replying, and this must be scheduled separately.

4. Enter screening results on computer, using protocol to ensure compliance with minimum data set. Home visits to the over-74s may be accompanied by a minimum data-set printout, whose completed details may later be keyed in to the computer record by the practice secretary.

5. The records of defaulters should be flagged with opportunistic reminders. Health visitors should be involved in encouraging compliance where default has occurred in paediatric or geriatric assessment.

6. Plan and discuss resulting health policy with patient, and record recommendations on computer. Schedule any immunizations needed, and print out diet sheets or other instruction leaflets. Arrange referrals, pathology tests, or reappointment at surgery or condition-orientated clinic as necessary.

7. Audit performance annually to assess efficiency. Include results in practice annual report and reports to PCG+T.

Geriatric screening protocols and well-person health promotion procedures must be approved by the Local Health Promotion Committee on behalf of the HA (Figs 8.4 and 8.5). The minimum data sets for paediatric assessment are laid down in the official protocols for the Child Health Surveillance Programme. For the logistics of cohort clinics, see Chapter 9.

8.8 TARGET ACHIEVEMENT

Cervical cytology, and infant and preschool immunization, have been singled out for a special type of incentive payment – target-related fees. Lower and higher performance targets have been set for both cytology and childhood immunization, the achievement of which, when the relative contributions made by hospital and community health agencies have been taken into account, determine the GP's fee. Failure to achieve the lower target results in no fee being paid. The schedule for cervical cytology will illustrate the principles involved in the arrangements made for both these programmes.

8.9 CERVICAL CYTOLOGY TARGETS

Payments are made in relation to lower and higher percentages of eligible women on the practice list who

```
MINIMUM DATA SET

SMOKING:
Cigarettes [    ] day  Cigars [    ] day  Pipe tobacco [    ] oz/wk  Inhale [ Y/N ]

DIET:
Unrestricted / High fat / High calorie / Low fibre / Low fruit + veg

Health conscious / Low fat / Low calorie / High fibre / High fruit + veg

Vegetarian / With fish / With eggs / Supplemental iron tablets

Medical diet for (state condition) ...........................

EXERCISE:
At least 30 mins sustained vigorous exercise [ 3 / 2 / 1 ] times per wk

Failing which at least 30 mins intermittently vigorous exercise

                                            [ 3 / 2 / 1 ] times per wk

Failing which at least 30 mins walking [ 3 / 2 / 1 ] times per wk

Less than above [    ]

ALCOHOL INTAKE:
Units per week [ 1-5 / 6-10 / 11-15 / 16-20 / over 20 / nil ]

B.P. [    ]     URINE ALBUMIN [ + ] [ - ]   URINE GLUCOSE [ + ] [ - ]

HEIGHT [    ] cm.        WEIGHT [    ] kg.          B.M.I [    ]

SIGNIFICANT FAMILY HISTORY:
Cardiovascular, obesity, diabetes, hyperlipidaemia, carcinoma breast /

ovary / bowel, others
```

Fig. 8.4 Specimen data entry protocol and minimum data set for well-person screening

have received adequate smears during the previous 5½ years. Eligible women are those in the age range 25 to 64 (21 to 60 in Scotland) who have not undergone total hysterectomy. Assessment of target achievement is carried out by the PPSA on the first day of each quarter. Computerized 'call or recall' programmes may be run by the HA, but, because target achievement is at stake, it makes better sense for the GP system to assume full control.

Logistical requirements
1. Patient records on computer: registration and cytology files as minimum.
2. Record all previous tests – date, whether performed by GP, hospital or HA clinic, results as Read codes to include whether smear was adequate. Record dates of all further tests taken the results of which are awaited.
3. Record all total hysterectomies, including date.
4. *Call*: Search records quarterly of all registered women 25–64 (21–60 in Scotland), for those who have not had an adequate smear during the past

5½ years. Exclude those who have had a total hysterectomy and those whose results are pending.
5. *Recall*: Patients whose previously abnormal smear results have prompted trigger dates for retesting (if the HA is initiating 'call or recall', check that its list of patients to be summoned corresponds with the list produced by the practice system).
6. Mailmerge letters of invitation.
7. Update records with new procedure and result using Read codes, including adequacy criteria. Set trigger dates for retesting abnormals.
8. Opportunistic reminders for defaulters, to receive 'ad hoc' testing or reappointment.
9. The computer will provide a list of defaulting patients who need to be coerced into accepting smears, either at the medical centre or at home, for the practice to attain targets.
10. *Audit*: calculate percentage of eligible women who have had adequate smears during the past 5½ years and check against PPSA printout statement each quarter.

Fig. 8.5 Draft letter to patients over 74 offering a domiciliary visit and consultation, and recording the minimum history data set (Courtesy of BMA GMSC survival guide to the new contractual arrangements, March 1990)

Dear

I am writing to offer you the opportunity to come and have your health assessed and to have a home visit from a member of our practice team.

There are a number of questions we would like you to answer before we see you. But I must stress there is no obligation on you to either answer these questions or accept a home visit.

Surname: Forenames:
Address:

Postcode:
Telephone number:
Do you live on your own?
If not, who else lives with you?
How is your eyesight?
How is your hearing?
How far are you able to walk?
Can you get around your home alright?
Can you walk upstairs?
How is your memory?
Do you have any problems controlling your bowels or bladder?
Are you receiving any tablets, medicines or other treatments?
Please list:

Are you taking any tablets or medicines that you have bought from a chemist?
Please list:

Are you receiving any special help at home (for example home help, meals on wheels)?

Are there any matters you would like to discuss with us?

Can you come to the surgery for your health check?

Do you want to have a home visit?

If you would like your health assessed and can come to the surgery, please make an appointment. If you cannot come to the surgery but would like a home visit, please ask for one. If you do not wamt to take up this offer at the present time please let us know so that we can avoid troubling you further.

Yours sincerely

8.10 IMMUNIZATION TARGETS

The principle of attaining lower and higher performance targets also applies to childhood immunization. Once again, HA computer programs have been the norm, but target and payment achievement by the practice will tend to suffer if patients are given the impression that they are expected to attend the HA clinic. Many practices prefer not to computerize 'call or recall' for infant injections but to reappoint manually at each medical centre attendance, starting with the mother's postnatal attendance (when claims for maternity, contraception services and child health surveillance at 6 weeks of age will have been completed, and the parent-held folder that records checks and immunizations will have been initiated). Protection against diphtheria, tetanus, poliomyelitis, pertussis, measles, mumps, rubella, *Haemophilus influenzae* B and meningitis will have been catered for in this way. The preschool booster will need to be the subject of recall (dovetailing with a child development check), either from the practice or the HA.

Separate targets, each with higher and lower levels of attainment, are set for infant immunizations fully completed by the age of 2 years, and for preschool boosters for children aged 5 years, on the first day of the quarter to which the target applies.

Second doses of adult immunization schedules are also more appropriately handled manually for such diseases as tetanus or hepatitis A and B, where the second attendance will be by reappointment at the time of the first attendance, although the first dose may have resulted from a 'call' search. Subsequent boosting doses are then initiated by recall, supported by opportunistic reminder. Immunizations, other than those that attract target payments, are paid for as item of service claims if so authorized by the HA. In addition to details of the vaccine, patient and doctor, practices must specify whether an immunization given constitutes an initial or reinforcing dose, as the corresponding fees differ.

The act of infant immunization must necessarily be logged on the computer record so that, in future, defaulters may be identified by opportunistic reminders or summoned by recall. Lists of such defaulters should be generated at the beginning of the third month of each quarter, so that target achievement may be enhanced. Audit of target achievement will take place as for cytology at the beginning of each quarter to allow comparison with the PPSA statement.

8.11 PREVENTIVE RECORD ARCHITECTURE

Display screens

Crisis intervention in primary care is patient-motivated, but the onus for prevention has been placed squarely on the doctor's shoulders by the 1990 contract. Efficient record data processing is therefore a legal as well as an ethical necessity. Preventive procedures generate a discrete subset of patient data, which is displayed in three ways:

- As sequential comprehensive historical recordings arranged by date for each parameter and quoting results, action required if any, and next due dates. A series of screens is often required to accommodate voluminous preventive data; access to them may be scrolled or paged. Parameters such as blood pressure may be displayed as graphical output, and cardiac risk or body mass index will require access to arithmetical functions.

- As a single preventive master screen, which summarizes the current status of all preventive parameters to include date of latest procedure, latest result, action required if any, date claimed if appropriate, and next due date.
- As opportunistic reminders for procedures due or overdue, posted to the principal clinical record screen (see also Chapter 5).

Some systems replicate cervical cytology results with dates in pathology records, and data included in the minimum data set for geriatric or other well-person screening will be replicated in other appropriate areas of the clinical record.

Data entry screens

Display screens derive their data from data entry screens and dialogue boxes which act as *aides-memoire* for prevention, prompting for all outstanding data categories and for the completion of claims at patient attendance. Data entry protocols for procedures such as paediatric surveillance or geriatric screening are highly specific and require HA approval.

Preventive audit screen

This supporting screen enables computer search, statistical computation and graphical display to demonstrate preventive performance, both as numbers and percentages, in relation to the total practice population. Results can be expressed per practice or per partner.

Target achievement, screening and immunization response and yield, item-of-service workload and claims (which may be extended to include temporary residents, night visits, maternity, contraception, minor surgery, emergencies, immediately necessary

Fig. 8.6 Entry of preventive medicine data: flu vaccination details logged through Torex Medical's Premiere system using an ISIS template

Header

Observation

Restricts the value of the observation (ie to influenza)

Allows you to further refine the observation

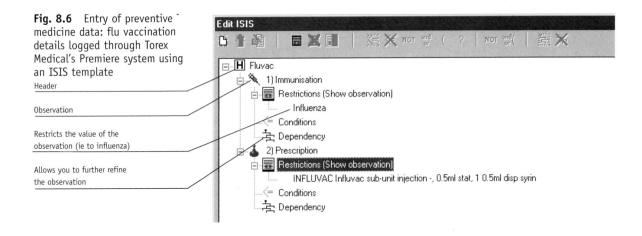

> **Box 8.2** Preventive master screen details
>
> **Name   Sex   Address   Date of birth   NHS number**
> Immunization type – last given date – batch, dose & site – claimed date – next due date
> Cervical cytology – last smear date – result and code – action and code – next due date
> Mammography – last test date – result – action and code – next due date
> Contraception – last check date – method – side effect code – claimed date – RM till date – next due date
> Blood pressure – test date – result – action if any – next due date
> Height – weight last test date and result – BMI† – next due date
> Urine albumen – last test date – result – next due date
> Urine sugar – last test date – result – next due date
> Occupation*   Social class*   Hereditary taint
> Diet – exercise – smoking – alcohol – addictive drug codes
> Cardiac risk grading†
> Current health symptom codes
> Details checked by – date checked – last consultation date
>
> Tests due or overdue are highlighted with flashes
> Data missing are highlighted
> * Data entry validated by dictionary. All codes are Read and therefore also validated on entry
> † Data calculated by program
> Protocol is trimmed for use in accordance with sex and age
> All records show author's identity

treatment, anaesthetics and dental haemorrhage), and new patient checks may all be audited and compared with past years, or local and national averages. The results may be included in the practice annual report.

8.12   ITEM OF SERVICE CLAIMS

The original concept of the NHS was that it should be based purely on capitation payments to doctors. However, the inequity of not rewarding maternity services with dedicated fees rapidly became apparent, and for many years these were the only items of service that could be claimed. During latter decades, the profession's representatives negotiated a series of further segregated payments for specific aspects of the doctor's workload, and these diversified the claim procedure to an extent that by 1996 no fewer than 19 different claim forms were in circulation. At this point the need for reform became imperative, and the forms GMS 1–4 were introduced, not only to simplify matters but as a prelude to computerization. At the same time, the procedure for claiming reimbursement for personally administered drugs was streamlined.

Form GMS 1, which initiates capitation for all GMS and CHS services, has been described in Chapter 7. Forms GMS 2, 3 and 4 are used to claim for piecemeal services that are paid for in addition to capitation,

and each GMS 4 form can accommodate up to 10 claims relating to one or more patients for services of the same type. The function of the forms can be replicated by, and is rapidly being displaced by, computerization, a change that is facilitated by the fact that only GMS 1 and 2 now have to be signed by the patient.

IoS Links were first piloted in 1993 using Racal HealthLink, and software from the GP system suppliers. An NHSE target for uptake by 80% of computerized practices was set for April 1997, although not realized. IoS Links uses the same modem, telephone line, carrier, and mailbox facilities as e-registration, and it is an NHSE prerequisite that the latter shall have been operational in a practice for at least 3 months before e-IoS is implemented.

- E-IoS software is supplied and maintained by the GP system supplier.
- After installation, the system is tested by the PPSA which also arranges training and hotline support, and provides a reconciliation diskette each quarter.
- It is necessary to appoint and train at least one responsible staff member as an e-Links operator.
- Details of previous contraceptive and CHS services and claims, and hysterectomy records, must be available to the system.
- For the first 6 months of e-IoS, parallel paper claims should be used as backup.

Fig. 8.7 Item of service claims: In-Practice Systems' Vision system.
Screens showing (a) Picking list for access to claim type (b) Completion of
individual claim (c) Claims status report

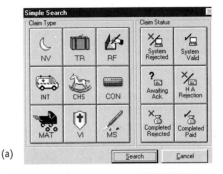

(a)

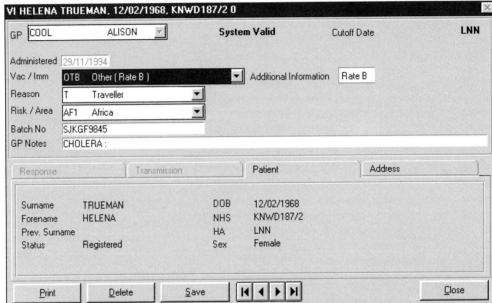

(b)

(c)

- IoS software is invoked automatically on the practice system when relevant Read-coded procedures are recorded in the patient's computer record. The system compiles each claim by replicating data to which it already has access (patient, practice and PPSA identities, date and procedure) and, through dialogue boxes, invites the user to add further details such as the reason for immunization, or the pack size and batch number of a vaccine. Completed claims are then stored on the practice server pending auto-transmission to the PPSA, which occurs each night. The system detects incomplete or erroneously completed claims and stores them, together with claims rejected by the PPSA, so that all can be accessed under the categories of individual doctor or type of procedure, and can subsequently be reprocessed.
- The system also prepares claims for personally administered drugs (PADs), which should include medications, vaccines, suture strips, dressings, pessaries and local anaesthetics. For most preparations, individual prescriptions must be printed and accompany the computerized claim, but monthly multiclaim procedures now apply to vaccines against influenza, typhoid, cholera, hepatitis A, hepatitis B, and meningococcal and pneumococcal infections. Multiclaim details must include vaccine type, brand or maker, formulation and pack size, dose and doctor. In due course all these procedures will become fully electronic.
- The system must also be capable of providing a listing of all patients by date and procedure for whom a particular service has been carried out, so that cross-checks can be performed by the health authority.
- Although the reforms of 1996 greatly simplified the mechanism for claims, there are never the less still eight logistically different types of claim procedure in operation:
  - Individually reimbursable immunizations, which require additional claims for reimbursement of PADs
  - Target-related payments
  - Registration examination, contraception (advice only or IUCD), anaesthetic, arrest of dental haemorrhage – all claimed individually
  - Maternity, requiring patient's signature, with claim completed in stages
  - Minor surgery sessions, claimed in batch
  - Night visits, claimed in batch following cooperative fax or e-mail download
  - Temporary resident (two types; telephone advice qualifies), plus or minus additional services
  - Private travel immunizations, e.g. yellow fever.

Fig. 8.8 Torex Meditel System 5 capitation statistics audit

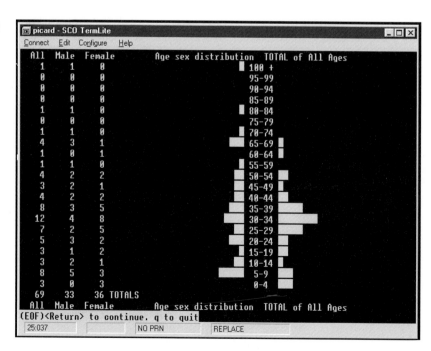

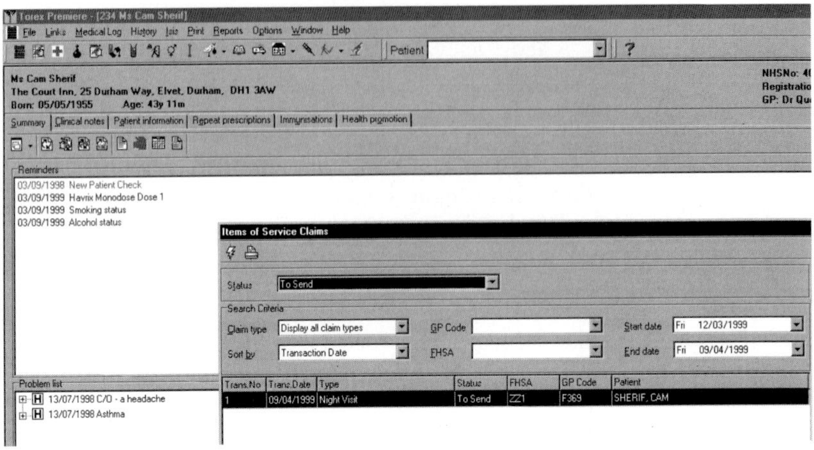

Fig. 8.9 Semiautomated assembly of Item of Service claims: Torex Medical's Premiere system

8.13 TARGET-RELATED PAYMENTS

In order to calculate target-related payments, the practice system must search the practice files for all patients treated and all at risk. Childhood immunization, preschool boosters and cervical cytology are the procedures involved. Performance targets are pegged at two levels, the upper of which attracts correspondingly greater financial reward. If the lower target is not attained, no payment is made. The actual amount of payment will be calculated in relation to treatment carried out in practice as opposed to other venues, to list size and to national norms.

The formulae used to calculate target-related payments are shown in Figure 8.10.

Criteria for the inclusion of patients and procedures within target calculations are of necessity highly specific. Patients must be registered with the

Fig. 8.10 The formulae used to calculate target-related payments

1. Target achievement calculation

$$\text{Target achieved} \quad \text{if} \quad \frac{\text{Number receiving procedure}}{\substack{\text{Total number in at-risk group} \\ \text{(colpectomies excluded)}}} \times 100 \quad \substack{= \text{ not} <70 \text{ or not} <90 \quad \text{immunization} \\ = \text{ not} <50 \text{ or not} <80 \quad \text{cytology}}$$

(for lower and upper targets respectively)

2. 'Maximum per annum sum payable' calculation for practice

$$\frac{\substack{\text{Total number in at-risk group} \\ \text{(colpectomies excluded)}}}{22 \text{ (imms) or } 430 \text{ (cytology)}} \times \substack{\text{Tariff determined by upper or lower target} \\ \text{for procedure per 'national average doctor'}}$$

3. 'Actual payment' calculation for practice

$$\star \quad \frac{\substack{\text{Number procedures carried out by} \\ \text{practice as opposed to HA or hospital}}}{\text{Number procedures needed to reach target}} \times \substack{\text{Maximum per annum} \\ \text{sum payable for practice}}$$

* If number of procedures carried out exceeds number required to reach target in question it will be automatically scaled back to target level

practice. Only full courses of infant and reinforcing immunization, and adequate smears count. Colpectomies are excluded from the at-risk population. The final immunizing dose is regarded as the point of calculation if patients move to another practice. Age bands assessed are those children aged 2 or 5 on the first day of the payment quarter, or women of 25–64 (in Scotland 21–60) smeared within 5½ years of the payment quarter.

The data relating to all these criteria must be recorded in the patient's immunization and cytology files and selected by a fresh search for each new calculation, since the populations and their data are constantly changing.

Definitive target calculation on the part of the practice necessarily requires that data held on the health authority central database shall be accessible to the practice computer system. A pioneer project entitled GP Key, set up by the South East Thames RHA, has provided local GPs with the facility to interrogate the authority's mainframe from a Windows workstation in the practice, and download weekly data relating to practice patients who have been immunized in schools or community clinics. Uptake levels, target achievement, defaulter identification, payment checks and comparable national statistics have all been built in. GP Key has set the standard that is likely to be adopted nationally.

8.14 AUDIT

GP supplier software must provide an audit trail so that each link in the chain of data transfer from originator to payment can be identified. For purposes of cross-checking, a quarterly report should be prepared by the practice system which lists PPSA payments and IoS procedures by type, patient and doctor. This should also provide comparisons with previous and subsequent quarters, and with the equivalent quarter of the previous year. Where discrepancies are revealed, rogue categories must be checked item by item. Target-related payments must be similarly checked.

The HA is entitled to make spot checks on practice computer records after payments have been made, in order to monitor the integrity of the e-IoS system and its users. The practice may be required to list all patients for whom IoS services have been provided.

Fig. 8.11 Target achievement audit: Torex Medical's Premiere system

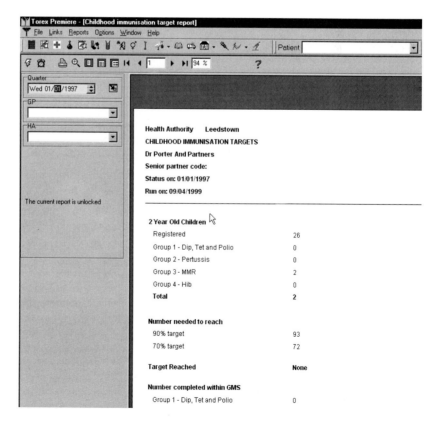

8.15 THE ADVANTAGES OF IOS LINKS

In contrast with Registration Links, which is primarily of benefit to the PPSA, IoS Links brings significant benefits to both PPSAs and practices:

• Staff time is saved because claim and payment procedures are accelerated. E-IoS claim completion takes approximately one-seventh of the time required to find and fill in an equivalent paper form.
• Claim and payment procedures are more accurate.
• Most practices find that their income has been increased by electronification, because fewer claims are overlooked by practice staff. (Contraceptive claims have been found to increase by 25% in some practices.)
• Prompt submission of registration data and all claims often enhances target achievement.
• Electronic claims are considerably more convenient than their paper-based counterparts because:
  – the patient's signature is not required for most claims
  – the electronic form is produced automatically
  – most of the data for the claim are preloaded.
• The extensive photocopying that many practices used in order to monitor their manual procedures is abolished.

Problems encountered in using IoS links

Although some practices record IoS claims on the paper GMS forms, which are then passed to clerical staff to key into the system, IoS Links software is so easy to use that many doctors and nurses now enter claims directly on to the computer as and when services are provided. This sometimes results in claims being overlooked when two health professionals are jointly involved in the provision of services – the cooperative and the practice, the doctor and the practice nurse, or the doctor and the midwife. Claims may also be missed when more than one service is provided at a time, such as during home visits or when giving telephone advice. These problems were also, to some extent, inherent in the manual claim procedures,

Table 8.1 The eight logistically different types of service claim procedure used in UK general practice

Type of service	System requirements
1. Straightforward IoS claim Contraceptive services Anaesthetic Dental haemorrhage	Log procedure on patient record: Individual claim is triggered as per GMS 4
Registration check	As above, but issue New Patient Questionnaire, practice brochure, etc.
2. Maternity	First and subsequent attendance data logged on patient record Practice maternity documents pack issued to patient. Patient's signature obtained. System prompts for and autocompletes claim when due as per GMS 2
3. Night consultation	E-mail download from cooperative 'dawn report' with autofile in patient record and autoclaim as per GMS 4
4. Temporary services	Complete paper GMS 3 form for return of clinical notes to own doctor Log patient identity and 'services rendered' details on system for autoclaim and payment checking purposes
5. Minor surgery	Session details already logged on minor surgery database. Batch autoclaims as per GMS 4
6. Target-related payments	Incorporate community health and national statistical data to calculate target achievements and check payments
7. Immunizations reimbursable individually under NHS	Log procedure and drug on patient record and autoclaim as per GMS 4 Autoclaim reimbursement for personally administered drug, either individually or in batch if the latter applies
8. Private practice	Private practice database of patients, procedures, and debtors (patients, insurance companies, or solicitors), billing and accounts

and can be overcome by adopting a well disciplined practice protocol.

SUMMARY

- 'Call' clinics are constructed from those patients at risk in the general practice population, who are apparently healthy but who will include some cases of incipient disease. Once assessed, the results obtained will determine subsequent attendance at 'recall' clinics. In both cases, mailmerged letters may invite attendance, the computer record will be updated and semiautomated claims will be completed. Those patients who do not attend 'call or recall' clinics can be contacted opportunistically when they next consult. Those found to be suffering from incipient disease are referred to dedicated 'cohort' clinics.
- Screening and immunization by 'call or recall' contrast with cohort clinics for chronic disease management, in which the same group of patients is recurrently reappointed, monitored, usually takes continuous medication and must swiftly be followed up in the event of default.
- Prevention may for the most part be delegated and significantly increases practice income. The 1990 NHS contract, and its 1993 and 1998 amendments, made GPs responsible for new patient, paediatric, geriatric and well-person screening, and introduced target-related payments. Recognizing that these measures required practice systems, the government also inaugurated computer reimbursement.
- Prevention by screening is only viable for a few diseases, several of which were catered for by the contract's proposals, but future practice preventive policies will be determined by NICE guidelines and local Health Improvement Plans. Meanwhile, GPs should at least consider screening their practice population for diabetes and hypertension.
- Cervical cytology and mammography both require synergy between the practice and the Local Health Authority.
- The logistical requirements of new patient, paediatric, geriatric and well-person screening, cervical cytology and immunization are precise and well catered for by the practice computer.
- Preventive record architecture displays data in three ways – as a comprehensive historical record, as a summary of current preventive status, and as opportunistic reminders posted to the principal clinical record screen. Data entry screens feed the display screens and ensure that no data required for record completion, patient management or claims are omitted.
- Audit of preventive procedures is required for both practice, PCGT and national statistical purposes.
- Item of service claims procedures were subjected to reform in two stages. First, the pre-existing array of 19 separate heterogeneous forms used for GP returns to the FHSA was replaced by a much simplified set of four. Subsequently, practices that had converted to e-registration were upgraded to electronic transfer of IoS claim procedures whose data replicated those contained on the revised paper forms.
- E-IoS claims have saved time and effort, increased practice income, and proved to be more accurate and convenient than manual procedures.

FURTHER READING

Akerman F M 1982 Prevention and screening. Update 1 July: 52

Brimblecombe F S W 1978 Implementation of vaccination programmes. Journal of the Royal College of Physicians 12: 246

British Medical Association 1986 Cervical cancer and screening in Britain: Professional Division report. British Medical Association, London

Department of Health 1998 Clinical examination of the breast. Circular PL/CMO/98/1, PL/CNO/98/1. Department of Health, London

Draper G J 1982 Screening for cervical cancer: revised policy. The recommendations of the DHSS Committee on Gynaecological Cytology. Health Trends 14: 37

European Research Organisation on Genital Infection and Neoplasia 1998 Eurogin Conference Report

GP Magazine 1998 GP Chlamydia screen to be 'opportunistic'. GP 15 May: 4

Gregory R, Swinn R A, Wareham N et al 1998 An audit of a comprehensive screening programme for diabetes in pregnancy. Practical Diabetes International 15: 2.45–2.48

Illingworth R S 1982 Basic developmental screening 0–5 years, 3rd edn. Blackwell Scientific Publications, Oxford

Kirby R 1998 Early detection – should we screen for prostate cancer? Geriatric Medicine, October: 21–22

Macleod J et al 1999 Postal urine specimens: are they a feasible method for genital chlamydial infection screening? British Journal of General Practice 44: 455–458

McPherson A 1985 Cervical screening, a practical guide. Oxford University Press, Oxford

Meadow R 1982 Routine developmental assessment – is it worthwhile? Update 1 January: 57

National Screening Committee 1998 First report. http://www.open.gov.uk/doh/nsc/nsch.htm

Preece J F, Lippmann E O 1971 Record design for the computer file in general practice. Practitioner (Suppl), August: 3

Royal College of General Practitioners 1981 Health and prevention in primary care. Report from General Practice 18. Royal College of General Practitioners, London

Royal College of General Practitioners 1982. Healthier children – thinking prevention. Report from General Practice 22. Royal College of General Practitioners, London

Roberts A, 1982 Cervical cytology in England and Wales 1965–80. Health Trends 14: 41

Ross E M 1985 Immunisation against diphtheria, tetanus, pertussis and polio. Practitioner 227: 795

Rowlands S, Bethal R G H 1981 Rubella vaccination: screening all women at risk. British Medical Journal 283: 827

Sampson M 1998 Screening for diabetes and impaired glucose tolerance in the elderly. Geriatric Medicine, March: 51–54

Secretary of State for Health 1998 Our healthier nation. Government Green Paper. http://www.open.gov.uk/doh/ohn/ohnhome.htm

Shepherd S G 1985 Opportunistic screening using the computer. Update 15 July: 145

Tudor Hart J 1980 Hypertension. Churchill Livingstone, Edinburgh

9 Supervision of chronic disease

9.1 OVERVIEW

The increasing longevity of the population of developed countries brings with it a disproportionately high prevalence of chronic morbidity. In addition to his roles in crisis intervention during illness and in preventive medicine, the general practitioner must shoulder a steadily increasing burden of responsibility for the treatment and supervision of continuing chronic disease.

Some idea of the size of the surveillance problem can be gained by considering hypertension, with a prevalence estimated at 10%. If we assume that most patients with raised blood pressure should be reviewed periodically, with or without active treatment, surveillance of this condition alone represents a massive increase in practice workload. If to this we add the need for surveillance of diabetes, asthma, epilepsy, thyroid disease, gross obesity, the dependent elderly and a host of other problems, then adequate control can scarcely be achieved by the doctor acting alone.

At this point it becomes imperative to enlist ancillary help. Just as doctors can delegate the writing of

Table 9.1 Surveillance problems

Chronic disease	Blood tests related to drug control	Other tasks
Hypertension	For:	The elderly infirm
Angina	anticoagulants	Contraceptive pill
Diabetes	penicillamine	Antenatal care
Asthma	azathioprine	Other conditions of special practice interest (for research purposes)
Gross obesity	cytotoxics	
Thyroid disorders	Levels of:	
Rheumatoid arthritis	phenytoin	
Pernicious anaemia	digoxin	
Anaemia from:	lithium	
gastrectomy		
menorrhagia		
peptic ulcer		
poor iron absorption		
Hypercholesterolaemia		
Hyperuricaemia		
Epilepsy		
AIDS		
Selected chronic psychoses		

repeat prescriptions to secretaries, subject to stringent preconditions and an efficient system, so, in a similar manner, they can preset the criteria for the maintenance of control of certain chronic diseases and share the responsibility for care with the practice nurse. As the majority of cases under surveillance require long-term medication, the repeat prescription routine will need to dovetail with the surveillance procedure. As most cases needing surveillance will undergo progressive deterioration if uncontrolled, defaulters must be detected and encouraged to comply. Some chronic diseases require continuing attendance at hospital, because specialist expertise, investigation or treatment are necessary. These cases call for accurate apportionment of responsibility and information interchange between primary and secondary care.

9.2 AN INCREASINGLY ELABORATE AND CENTRALLY CONTROLLED PROCESS

Since the introduction of the 1990 NHS reforms, the Department of Health has steadily increased its control over the methodology of the care of chronic disease in general practice. The 'carrot' of dedicated funding for asthma and diabetes clinics has been counterbalanced by the 'stick' of requiring that formal protocols for the conduct of surveillance clinics are submitted by practices for approval by health authorities, adhered to, and checked by audit.

New emphasis on chronic disease management within the NHS has prompted a number of elaborative developments at practice level.

- GPs are devoting more time to postgraduate medical education, which centres on those diseases requiring surveillance.
- Nurses are being trained and accredited by specialist educational centres dedicated to the surveillance care of chronic disease (especially those dealing with asthma, diabetes, epilepsy and mental health).
- The apportionment of responsibility for care between consultant, GP, nurse and patient is now much more clearly defined.
- Cooperational clinical and administrative records, shared variously between consultant, GP, nurse and patient, are being developed and used. (Increasingly, these adopt electronic formats.)
- Practices now keep a register of all patients suffering from each surveillance condition, run 'cohort' clinics to manage these conditions, and identify and follow-up defaulters.
- Arrangements are made for the continuing education of surveillance patients and for the inductive education of new patients.

- The guidelines provided and updated by national organizations such as the British Thoracic Society, the British Diabetic Association and the National Institute for Clinical Excellence (NICE) for the control of surveillance are implemented by protocol. Some NICE guidelines are passed to general practice using the PRODIGY electronic vehicle.
- Criteria for diagnosis are becoming standardized, and scoring systems are being introduced to enable the grading of risk factors and gravity status.
- Individual care plans are formulated for each patient and incorporate:
  – detailed patient management policies taken from protocol and individual circumstances
  – instructions in self-help
  – provision for obtaining repeat medication
  – schedules for review.
- Policies for referral to consultants, dieticians, chiropodists and eye care professionals are agreed at PCG+T level.
- Clinical parameters for initial examination and reviews are agreed at PCG+T level.
- Self-treatment techniques and patient compliance are monitored.
- Audit of process and outcome are implemented, using MIQUEST and other extraction software, and the results are made available to the PCG+T. Progress made towards targets set by government NHS strategy and the St Vincent Declaration is noted.

Quantitative health care performance indicators, specified in April 1999 by the UK government as they affect general practice, are shown in Box 9.1. The effectiveness of practice surveillance policies will be a major factor in determining how well a practice's performance compares with its peers as measured by the indicators.

Practices will not only be graded by the use of the indicators, but 'league tables' of performance will be released, and qualification for performance-related pay in the form of 'quality payments' will to some extent depend upon them.

When first introduced in 1999, quality payments were determined by standards of clinical and medication record keeping, prescribing, immunization, chronic disease management, the maintenance of chronic disease and other registers, and ease of access to a GP. Details are subject to review.

GP systems must ultimately cope with the massive increase in data processing requirements ushered in by these elaborative surveillance developments. Progress towards a comprehensive NHS electronic surveillance system will necessarily be piecemeal.

Box 9.1   Healthcare performance indicators relevant to general practice (suggested for England by the government 1999, data based on a report in Doctor magazine 15 April 1999)

Health improvement
- Deaths from all causes – patients aged 15–64
- Deaths from all causes – patients aged 65–74
- Cancer registrations
- Deaths from malignant neoplasms
- Deaths from circulatory diseases
- Suicide rates
- Deaths from accidents

Fair access
- Early detection of cancer

Effective delivery of appropriate health care
- Disease prevention and health promotion – percentage of target population vaccinated
- Early detection of cancer – percentage of target population screened for breast and cervical cancer
- Asthma, diabetes and epilepsy management
- Mental health in primary care – volume of benzodiazepines prescribed
- Cost-effective prescribing – cost per patient of: combination products; modified-release products; drugs of limited clinical value and cost per dose of inhaled corticosteroids
- Discharge from hospital
- Management of severe ENT infection, UTI, heart failure

Efficiency
- Length of stay in hospital – casemix adjusted
- Generic prescribing
- Unit cost of maternity – adjusted

Patient and carer experiences of NHS
- Delayed discharge for those aged 75 or over

NHS health outcomes
- Conceptions in under-16s
- Adverse events or complications in treatment
- Emergency admission for people aged 75 and over
- Infant deaths
- Survival rate for breast and cervical cancer
- Avoidable deaths

9.3   REVENUE FROM SURVEILLANCE

Item of service fees are payable for maternity and contraception services under the NHS, and specific payments are made per doctor for asthma and diabetes supervision, provided that the protocols used by the practice for the management of these conditions have received prior HA approval. The practice computer must be programmed to prompt for these claims. The increased capitation rate for elderly patients, revenue from influenza immunization and the official reimbursement of practice nurse pay at 70% all help to offset the cost of surveillance clinics.

Some practices have succeeded in negotiating the payment of special fees from their HAs for conducting prothrombin time assay and special cancer management procedures, on the grounds that these are devolved forms of secondary care.

9.4   MANUAL PROCEDURE FOR SHARED RESPONSIBILITY IN SURVEILLANCE

After initial diagnosis, the doctor manages the case until s/he is satisfied that therapeutic control has been achieved. S/he then sets the criteria by which the nurse is to measure continuing case control. S/he determines the length of the review cycles (measured in weeks) to schedule both the treatment and nurse supervision until the doctor's own next assessment of the patient. S/he authorizes repeat medication with a supply that synchronizes with the nurse review cycles, and directs the patient to reappoint for the appropriate future surveillance clinic. The nurse holds clinics at suitable intervals. For each clinic s/he raises a list of patients who should attend, and who have already been given appointments. S/he selects the NHS records for these patients (records that will include surveillance records sheets) and constructs, and arranges for signature, the repeat prescriptions appropriate to the condition under review. At the clinic the nurse checks each patient for the preset criteria s/he has been given, and updates the record. If the criteria are met s/he issues the prescription and re-appoints the patient. If the criteria are not met, s/he reappoints the patient to see the doctor forthwith. S/he identifies and follows up defaulters. Figure 9.1 shows the inter-relationship of the doctor and nurse review cycles.

Problems inherent in the manual process

Every step in the process is undertaken manually; this is labour-intensive. Coordination of all data and activities must be the responsibility of one member of staff – the surveillance nurse. In order to ensure that all patients under surveillance remain accounted for, especially those referred back to the doctor, and defaulters who have escaped the nurse's immediate control, s/he must keep a detailed manual surveillance register for each type of cohort clinic. The register

must be checked regularly against the patient NHS records to ensure that the two tally, because some patients will have attended the doctor or been seen at home for intercurrent problems, renewing their medication at the same time. When s/he identifies defaulters, the nurse sends a handwritten letter to encourage compliance and to offer a further appointment.

9.5 PRINCIPLES OF COMPUTERIZATION

The computer acts as coordinator of the surveillance activities, and it stores and retrieves the special format surveillance records. The computerized surveillance records dovetail with computerized repeat medication. The computer helps to keep track of patients who need review by the doctor or who have defaulted.

A description of two contrasting systems will serve to illustrate the potential of the computer in surveillance applications.

Encounter form system

This term has been used to describe a computer system where the doctor amends a paper record that is later transcribed on to a computer record by a secretary, thus sparing the doctor the need to key in data. The paper document may or may not contain preprinted past record material. The method is prone to transcription delay and errors. If the encounter form is a computer record printout, much shredding of expensive continuous computer stationery may follow each session.

Fig. 9.1 Inter-relationship of the doctor and nurse review cycles

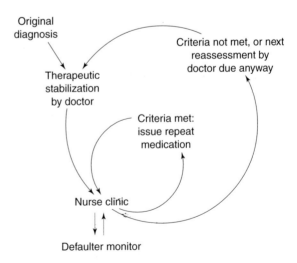

Probably the most successful application of encounter form systems lies in the use of a combined repeat medication and surveillance encounter form. The continuous stationery supplied free for practice use by the HA for printing repeat medication shows the preprinted empty prescription form on the left-hand side of a wide sheet. To the right of this lies a totally blank page, separated from the prescription by perforations to allow separation after printing. The blank page can be used to print out a surveillance encounter record with details taken from the surveillance file held on computer store. This can be linked to the production of a repeat prescription taken from the computer's repeat medication file (Fig. 9.2).

The two forms are printed out in parallel and used in the nurse-operated surveillance clinic. Armed with the pile of twinned forms, the nurse assesses the patients and updates the surveillance encounter forms. Where criteria for control are met, s/he issues the repeat prescription and the secretary transcribes the encounter record on to computer. The pile of residual twinned forms will constitute documents upon which further action must be taken, either by reference to the doctor or as defaulters. The nurse is thus spared the need to keep a manual surveillance clinic list. As a double check, the computer can search the surveillance records for those patients who have not attended within a defined interval.

The doctor is responsible for the initiation of entries in both surveillance and repeat medication files on computer, s/he must sign the repeat prescriptions and may also use an encounter form when subsequently consulted by the patient. In addition, the encounter form may be used by the nurse when making home visits, such as to the dependent elderly.

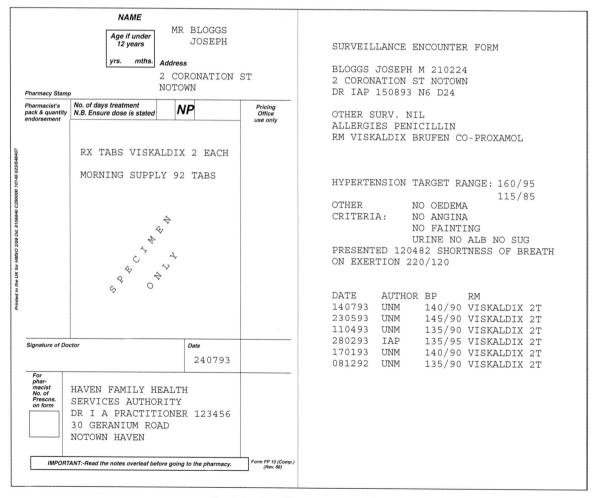

Fig. 9.2 Surveillance encounter form

Encounter surveillance records have the disadvantage that, while used in this form, they are segregated from the main manual clinical record. This fragmentation is overcome in record driven systems, where the whole clinical record is housed on computer.

Record driven systems

When all consultation data are made on a computer record, the computer has the power to represent them on display in alternative ways. Thus, although all entries on the record are initially made in chronological order, regardless of category, selected material may be retrieved from the computer memory and reassembled according to need. In this way, the doctor may call for all immunization data, a summary clinical history or all data relating to hypertension. In the case of surveillance screens, the data will all relate to the condition under review and there will be a separate screen for each condition.

With the power to call forward a surveillance record at will from the general medical record, the doctor and nurse can operate surveillance clinics directly from the visual display unit. Interactive procedures assist the user in making data entries. The patient record is never fragmented nor missing, and the same record can be viewed by as many users as there are terminals. Repeat prescriptions are written directly from the medication screen of the clinical record. The record driven system monitors non-controlled and defaulting patients by producing cumulative lists of both automatically. Integration of all functions is achieved by the record driven system and transcription delays and errors are avoided.

The records of patients supervised for asthma and diabetes in accordance with HA criteria for chronic disease management should be flagged so that periodic computer search for lists and numbers of these patients may be used in support of the practice's claims for payment.

The computer checks payments from the HA/PPSA for asthma and diabetes care alongside other quarterly payments.

The details required on computer surveillance records shared by doctor and nurse are shown in Box 9.2.

9.6 SURVEILLANCE RECORDS SHARED WITH THE HOSPITAL

In the healthcare systems of several developed countries surveillance is shared between primary care and the hospital, and a patient-held record then becomes a useful method of centralizing and sharing clinical and medication data. Records that reduplicate the entries made on the patient-held record must also be kept by both physicians, otherwise all evidence will perish if the patient loses the record.

Successful manual records using this principle have been applied to antenatal care (the 'cooperation card' of the UK), and to diabetes surveillance in which patient urine test results are incorporated in the multiuser record. Parent-held records have been employed satisfactorily in multiuser paediatric screening. In all these applications, the patient's motivation to guard the record has been assisted by his/her involvement in the process of care.

9.7 SHARED ELECTRONIC RECORDS

Smart cards

In the USA, where patients may select at will a different physician as appears appropriate to each new complaint, clinical data are necessarily fragmented

---

Box 9.2 Details required on computer surveillance records shared by doctor and nurse

Patient identification details

Drs name/doctor and nurse review cycle/date of next appointment with doctor

Codes of other surveillance screens/patient allergies/all repeat medication (names only)

Condition reviewed/criteria to be met

Comments as to onset and major landmarks of disease

Nurse entries	Date	Author code	Special measurements (e.g. blood pressure, weight)	Repeat medication of condition under review
Doctor entries	Date	Author code	Free style clinical observations including special measurements	Changes in repeat medication of condition under review

between users. To overcome this difficulty, a patient-held document similar to a credit card has been introduced in some areas – the so-called 'smart card'. The smart card carries electronic data with details of patient identity, important medical problems, long-term medication and drug idiosyncrasies, and insurance status. The cards and the equipment for recording and reading them are surprisingly inexpensive, and access to them can be limited by a system password.

In the UK, with its defined practice populations, there is no problem of data fragmentation between practices, but the smart card principle might be used as a shared record between general practice and hospital. UK pilot trials have led to the conclusion that a record in whose upkeep the patient is not involved, that the patient cannot read, and that carries no financial implications for the patient is frequently forgotten by the patient. A smart card that carried details of chronic pathology, continuous medication and drug allergies could conceivably be used by a doctor's or pharmacist's computer system to cross-check the suitability of new medication. As a vehicle of basic permanent patient-held details, such as blood group or the need for antibiotic cover during dental extraction, it would have limited use because it cannot be read visually.

The electronic personal organizer

One of the most interesting developments in patient-held electronic records has occurred in relation to diabetic care. The simple enzyme urine test strip for glucose has been adapted as a means of assaying blood glucose, for which one drop of blood from a finger prick suffices.

Because of the vagaries of artificial lighting, human colour vision and diabetic visual acuity, a simple pocket-sized reflectance meter was developed with its own light source, wavelength selection and intensity sensor. A digital read-out of blood glucose is achieved with a considerable measure of accuracy. The addition of a clock-calendar and an electronic memory enables patients to store, automatically, several hundred test results, which the machine can display serially. Moreover, by using an extension lead, these results can be tabulated, analysed and displayed graphically on an on-site computer, or fed through the telephone to a remote computer in hospital. It takes little imagination to see that by increasing the memory, the display and the key input of the reflectance meter, a sophisticated 'personal organizer' for diabetics could be developed, which would not only guide them in control, with reference to their individual care plans,

but could be used to maintain their medical records in hospital and general practice, and link both. The reflectance meter has already been shown to reduce complications in that most critical of all diabetic care areas – antenatal management.

This type of patient-held electronic record has implications for the management of other chronic conditions such as asthma (linked to a peak flow monitor), epilepsy (with a seizure log), angina pectoris or cardiac arrhythmias, in which careful monitoring of attacks by the patient is the key to improved control, and in which more detailed records are required both at hospital outpatients and in general practice. Where it is safe to do so, advice on better control could be programmed into the 'personal organizer' and, if the situation demanded it, the patient's recorded log could be fed to the practice or hospital computer through the telephone line, for medical advice to be given by telephone.

9.8 DIRECT TELECOMMUNICATION RECORD ACCESS

In future, telecommunication links will allow GPs and hospital doctors to view relevant sections of each other's records for patients under shared surveillance. A secure 'shuttle' record, which can be viewed and updated by both GP and consultant, will be an ideal solution and needs to use the same basic principles as those established for record sharing between GP and nurse.

9.9 SURVEILLANCE PROTOCOLS

Local and national protocols for the surveillance of chronic diseases are now used extensively in general practice and are of two types. Administrative protocols determine the logistics of running clinics, and patient management protocols guide the supervision of individual cases (see Chapter 23). Increasingly, it is becoming necessary to obtain local hospital and HA approval for protocol use, without which, for instance, specific fees for asthma and diabetes care will not be authorized.

The National Institute for Clinical Excellence is tasked with encapsulating evidence-based intervention within national guidelines for use by health professionals. Some of these guidelines will be incorporated within electronic protocols and supplied to practices and PCG+Ts using the PRODIGY protocol engine.

Expert protocols that accurately define the boundary of responsibility between primary and secondary care, and offer referral decision-making assistance, have been developed by the Wolfson Computer Laboratory.

9.10 GRAPHIC ENHANCEMENT OF SURVEILLANCE RECORDS

All forms of surveillance measure the same parameters repeatedly over time, and these measurements are visually enhanced by being represented as graphs on the visual display unit. The graphs may travel from left to right, as on paper, or, because visual displays usually scroll upwards and downwards, the direction of flow of the graph may be from above downwards, thus enabling successive pages to be viewed in continuity. (Some displays do scroll both vertically and horizontally.)

Most surveillance is also concerned with two variables other than time, and requires the titration of one variable against the other – blood pressure and drug dosage, blood glucose and insulin dosage, prothrombin time and anticoagulant dosage, or body weight and dietary calories (Fig. 9.3).

Some conditions require more than two parameters to be recorded, such as the incidence of convulsions and the oral dosage and blood level of phenytoin in epilepsy. Such representation is markedly enhanced by the use of colour screens.

The computer has the additional advantage that it can perform statistical analyses on data before representing them. In this way, an average blood pressure, a mean 24-hour distribution of blood glucose (the 'modal day') or a mean 24-hour distribution of anginal attacks may be shown.

Special software is needed for graphic representation. Bar charts, pie charts and histograms are facilities that are usually included with 'charting' graphics, a feature of most spreadsheet packages. Colour graphics not only need purpose-built software but also have special equipment requirements – processor, hard disk and display.

9.11 SPECIFIC SURVEILLANCE PROGRAMMES

In addition to the measures outlined on page 84 for surveillance programmes in general, the following considerations apply to individual conditions.

9.12 ASTHMA SURVEILLANCE

Overview

In the UK, asthma causes around 1500 deaths each year and now affects 1 in 7 children. No satisfactory explanation has been offered for the fact that its incidence has doubled during the past 20 years, nor as to why it is less prevalent in some East German cities, where the air is considerably more polluted than it is in comparable urban areas in the West.

Throughout the UK, the efficacy of treatment for asthma varies considerably, and in 1996 a National

Fig. 9.3 The graphical representation of multiple parameters in a surveillance record (Nowlan 1990)

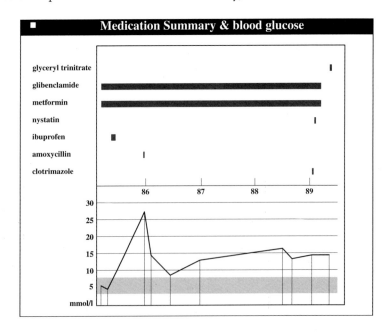

Asthma Campaign survey identified a high proportion of patients who were dissatisfied with their treatment. The suggestion that some practices underdiagnose the condition is supported by surveys, which show that overall control is poorer in practices whose spending on preventive inhaler prescribing falls below average.

Against this background, the Department of Health has introduced its general practice chronic disease management initiatives, the National Asthma Campaign has been launched, and a battery of different sets of guidelines has been released from sources such as the British Thoracic Society (BTS; 1990), the International Paediatric Asthma Consensus Group (1992) and the RCGP. As judged by fewer admissions, fewer days off work and fewer courses of oral steroids and antibiotics, improved control of asthma has been achieved by combining adequate patient education with self-management of anti-inflammatory therapy guided by peak flow measurements.

It is useful to base the assessment of patients at consultation on scoring systems such as that produced by the Midland Thoracic Society (Table 9.2), and to base the construction of patient self-management plans on the BTS 'step' charts (Fig. 9.4).

Referral policy should be agreed with local consultants. Patient education can be assisted by use of the National Asthma Campaign leaflets on self-management and peak flow techniques.

Asthma records on computer

The condition-orientated patient record for asthma should accommodate the following data:

- Current and past history
  - Past medical history
  - Past asthma history
  - Past asthma medication
  - Current asthma medication
  - Other concurrent medication
  - Symptoms (scored)
  - Trigger factors and allergies
  - Family history of allergy
  - Occupational and smoking history
- - General physical examination
  - Height, weight, peak flow (predicted and actual)
  - Device technique
- Chest X-ray
- Confirmation of diagnosis
  - Exercise test
  - Reversibility test
  - Steroid trial
  - Home peak flow monitoring

- Initial education including peak flow and inhaler technique
- Self-management plan
- Follow up appointment date
- Influenza immunization where appropriate.

Peak flow meters and spirometers are now available with built-in memory to record times, dates and results, with the additional provision that they can be

Table 9.2 Asthma scoring scale (Courtesy of Midland Thoracic Society)

	Score
FEV_1	
> 90% of predicted	0
> 80% of predicted	1
> 70% of predicted	2
> 60% of predicted	3
> 50% of predicted	4
> 40% of predicted	5
> 30% of predicted	6
> 20% of predicted	7
Extra bronchodilator usage	
Less than once daily	0
Once daily	1
Two to four times daily	2
More than four times daily	3
Nocturnal asthma in last 7 days	
No waking at night	0
Any early morning asthma	1
Early morning asthma > 2 hours	2
Waking at night once a week	3
Waking at night two to three times	4
Waking at night > three times a week	6
Waking at night every night	7
Effect on lifestyle	
No wheezing, cough or breathlessness	0
Mild wheeze or cough not needing extra treatment	1
Any time off work or activities due to asthma	2
Loss of 5 days or more in a month	3
Emergency visit to GP or A&E	4
Hospital admission	5
Extra drugs since last visit	
No extra drugs	0
Any more treatment	1
Course of antibiotics	2
Increase in inhaled steroids	3
Increased oral steroids	4

Management of chronic asthma in adults and school children | Outcomes

STEP 1

Occasional use of relief bronchodilators

Inhaled short-acting beta agonists as required for symptom relief are acceptable. If they are needed more than once daily move to Step 2. Before altering a treatment step ensure that the patient is having the treatment and has a good inhaler technique. Address any fears.

STEP 2

Regular inhaled anti-inflammatory agents

Inhaled short-acting beta agonists as required *plus* beclomethasone or budesonide 100–400mcg twice daily, or fluticasone 50–200mcg twice daily. Alternatively, use cromoglycate or nedocromil sodium, but if control is not achieved start inhaled steroids.

STEP 3

High-dose inhaled steroids or low-dose inhaled steroids plus long-acting inhaled beta agonist bronchodilators

Inhaled short-acting beta agonists as required plus *either* beclomethasone or budesonide increased to 800–2,000mcg daily, or fluticasone 400–1,000mcg daily via a large volume spacer *or* beclomethasone or budesonide 100–400mcg twice daily, or fluticasone 50–200mcg twice daily plus salmeterol 50mcg twice daily.
In a very small number of patients who experience side-effects with high-dose inhaled steroids, either the long-acting inhaled beta agonist option is used or a sustained-release theophylline may be added to Step 2 medication. Cromoglycate or nedocromil may also be tried.

STEP 4

High-dose inhaled steroids and regular bronchodilators

Inhaled short-acting beta agonists as required with inhaled beclomethasone or budesonide 800–2,000mcg daily, or fluticasone 400–1,000mcg daily via a large volume spacer *plus* a sequential therapeutic trial of one or more of:
☐ Inhaled long-acting beta agonists
☐ Sustained-release theophylline
☐ Inhaled ipratropium or oxitropium
☐ Long-acting beta agonist tablets
☐ High-dose inhaled bronchodilators
☐ Cromoglycate or nedocromil

STEP 5

Addition of regular steroid tablets

Inhaled short-acting beta agonists as required with inhaled beclomethasone or budesonide 800–2,000mcg daily or fluticasone 400–1,000mcg daily via a large volume spacer and one or more of the long-acting bronchodilators *plus* regular prednisolone tablets in a single daily dose.

STEPPING DOWN

Review treatment every three to six months. If control is achieved a stepwise reduction in treatment may be possible.

In patients whose treatment was recently started at Step 4 or 5 or included steroid tablets for gaining control of asthma, this reduction may take place after a short interval.

In other patients with chronic asthma a three- to six-month period of stability should be shown before slow stepwise reduction is undertaken.

Steps 1–3

☐ Minimal (ideally no) chronic symptoms, including nocturnal symptoms
☐ Minimal (infrequent) exacerbations
☐ Minimal need for relieving bronchodilators
☐ No limitations on activities, including exercise
☐ In adults and school children, circadian variation in peak expiratory flow (PEF)<20%
☐ In adults and school children, PEF ≥80% of predicted or best
☐ Minimal or no adverse effects from medicine

Step 4 (and Step 5 in adults and school children)

☐ Least possible symptoms
☐ Least possible need for relieving bronchodilators
☐ Least possible limitation of activity
☐ In adults and school children, least possible variation in PEF
☐ In adults and school children, best PEF
☐ Least adverse effects from medicine

Management of asthma in children under five years old | Notes

STEP 1

Occasional use of relief bronchodilators

Short-acting beta agonists as required for symptom relief but not more than once daily. Before altering a treatment step ensure that the patient is taking the treatment, the inhaler is appropriate and inhaler technique is good. Address any concerns or fears. Mildest cases may respond to oral beta agonist.

STEP 2

Regular inhaled preventer therapy

Inhaled short-acting beta agonists as required *plus* cromoglycate as powder (20mg three to four times daily) or via metered dose inhaler and large volume spacer (10mg three times daily) or beclomethasone or budesonide up to 400mcg, or fluticasone up to 200mcg daily. Consider a five-day course of soluble prednisolone (see Notes for dosage) or temporarily double inhaled steroids to gain rapid control.

STEP 3

Increased-dose inhaled steroids

Inhaled short-acting beta agonists as required *plus* beclomethasone or budesonide increased to 800mcg or fluticasone 500mcg daily via a large volume spacer. Consider short prednisolone course. Consider adding regular twice-daily long-acting beta agonists or a slow-release xanthine.

STEP 4

High-dose inhaled steroids and bronchodilators

Inhaled steroids (up to 2mg/day) and other treatment as in Step 3. Slow-release xanthines or nebulised beta agonists.

STEPPING DOWN

Regularly review the need to decrease treatment and step down as indicated.

Monitor all changes in treatment by clinical review.

Notes

Patients should start treatment at the step most appropriate to the initial severity.

A rescue course of prednisolone may be needed at any step or any time (for children under one, 1–2mg/kg/day; for those aged one to five years, 20 mg/day. Maximum daily dose is 20mg).

The aim is to achieve early control of the condition and then reduce treatment. Until growth is complete, any child requiring beclomethasone or budesonide >800mcg daily or fluticasone >500mcg daily should be referred to a paediatrician with an interest in asthma.

Fig. 9.4 British guidelines on asthma management

made to 'flag' readings to show whether these were taken before or after use of a reliever inhaler. Results can be downloaded by cable to a PC, represented graphically and analysed statistically. Further development should allow these assaying devices to be furnished with a small screen so that output of test readings can be accompanied by textual advice taken from the appropriate 'step' of the self-management plan.

Computer support for asthma clinics

• The foremost GP systems now provide modules that support the appropriate data input, record for-

mats and follow-up monitoring of the more important chronic diseases such as asthma.
• Two different protocols are required: one for clinic administration and one for patient management. Both protocols must be approved by the HA if the relevant management allowance is to be claimed.
• As failure of disease control has implications for secondary care, patient management protocols must be formulated in conjunction with the local provider trust.
• The clinic administration protocol, like the asthma surveillance record, must provide for the accurate delegation of responsibility to the practice nurse (specialized training with the issue of a diploma for nurses is available from the National

Fig. 9.5 Asthma management screen: new GPASS system

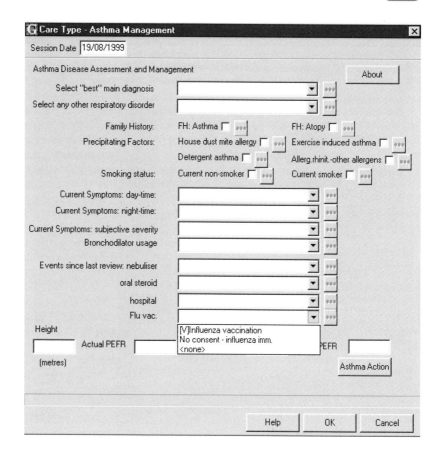

Asthma Training Centre at Stratford-upon-Avon).

- Protocols must be stored in electronic folders in the protocol library database, and must be capable of amendment. Patient management protocols must be available for viewing at the time that the patient record is on screen, and will constitute the basis upon which the patient's individual management plan is constructed.
- Close links must be provided between the surveillance record and the repeat medication record.
- Links with the practice appointments module will allow appropriate reappointment and the monitoring of missed appointments to be carried out.
- Opportunistic reminders for procedures associated with asthma management, such as smoking cessation and influenza immunization, are built in.
- Patient education screens are provided, and patient instruction leaflets can be printed.
- Audit of the process and outcome of care is required for PCG+T/HA use and will employ

MIQUEST, or equivalent, extraction software and performance indicators.

Computer-aided investigation of asthma in the community

During the past two decades, computer correlation has been employed by several large-scale projects investigating asthma in the community. Data on inhaler consumption have been used as a means of identifying poorly controlled patients, history questionnaires have been distributed to detect undiagnosed asthmatics, and the collation and analysis of a large number of asthmatic case records has enabled the construction of a model that can be used to predict the risk of acute attacks and hospital admissions.

Perhaps the most innovative of these projects was that fielded by the Queen Elizabeth Hospital at Welwyn Garden City in 1992. This linked GPs and hospital clinicians by telecommunicated terminals in order to record all asthmatic morbidity and treatment.

Box. 9.3 Guidelines suggested by the British Diabetic Association for annual review of diabetes

This is a suggested protocol. The tasks performed, and those responsible, will vary. However, it is the responsibility of the GP to ensure that all the recommended procedures are undertaken annually.
The data accumulated at the annual review can be collated for the purposes of clinical audit and service evaluation.

Initial discussion
1. General health and wellbeing and life with diabetes, including driving.
2. Glycaemic control:
   - self-monitoring results
   - symptoms of hypoglycaemia and hyperglycaemia.
3. Knowledge of diabetes and self-management skills, including importance of good metabolic control and a healthy lifestyle.
4. Specific enquiry about tobacco and alcohol consumption and level of physical activity.
5. Specific enquiry about symptoms of diabetic complications, including
   - problems with vision
   - chest pain and shortness of breath
   - claudication
   - symptoms of neuropathy, including impotence.

Examination
1. Weight and body mass index.
2. Blood pressure.
3. Eye examination:
   - distant visual acuity (with glasses, if worn – use pinhole if acuity reduced)
   - fundoscopy through dilated pupils (using tropicamide).
   Alternatively, fundoscopy may be performed by a specially trained and accredited optometrist, or, where a formal retinal photography screening programme has been organized, fundal photographs taken.
4. Foot examination:
   - footwear and general condition of skin and nails
   - deformity and ulceration
   - peripheral pulses
   - vibration and pin-prick sensation.
5. Inspection of injection sites in insulin-treated patients.
6. Further clinical examination, as indicated.

Investigations
1. Urinalysis for proteinuria.
   If protein detected, an MSU should be arranged and consideration given to measuring the albumin excretion rate.
   Arrange microalbuminuria screening in:
   - all patients with type 1 diabetes
   - patients with type 2 diabetes who do not have documented ischaemic heart disease (IHD) – the presence of microalbuminaemia in these patients is a very strong risk factor for IHD.
2. Blood test (ideally 2 weeks before so that results are available at annual review), for:
   - HbA_{1c}
   - serum creatinine
   - serum cholesterol.
   In the presence of ischaemic heart disease, a fasting lipoprotein analysis is also recommended.
3. Further investigations, as indicated.

Management
1. Glycaemic control:
   - dietary management – consider referral to state-registered dietician
   - treatment regimen – oral hypoglycaemic or insulin
   - understanding of the relationship between blood glucose, dietary intake and physical activity.
2. Management of identified cardiovascular risk factors.
3. Management of long-term complications.
4. Individual management targets.
5. Management plan for next 12 months:
   - referral to state-registered dietician, state-registered podiatrist, specialist diabetes clinic or other specialist, as indicated
   - contraception and plans for future pregnancies, where appropriate
   - future reviews.

Recording of annual review findings
1. Written and/or computerized medical record.
2. Patient-held record.
3. Practice diabetes register.
4. District diabetes register, where this exists.

The network data were also used to support nurse-run hospital-based asthma clinics.

9.13 DIABETES SURVEILLANCE

Diabetes is suffered by 1–2% of the population, and 2–3% of those with impaired glucose tolerance (IGT) become fully fledged diabetics each year. New criteria for diagnosis were proposed by the American Diabetic Association in 1998 (subsequently endorsed by the WHO), according to which patients with IGT demonstrated fasting glucose levels between 5.8 and 6.9 mmol/l, whereas overt diabetes was diagnosed in those whose levels equalled or exceeded 7.0 mmol/l. The new criteria bring improved correlation with subsequent morbidity. IGT does not predispose to retinopathy but carries similar risks to diabetes in its ability to cause atherosclerosis and early death.

As with asthma care, the 1993 amendments to the 1990 NHS reforms introduced diabetes management guidelines, and flat payment rates per principal per year for carrying them out. The general principles for surveillance quoted on page 84 obtain, but must be augmented by factors particular to diabetes.

The St Vincent Declaration of 1990, agreed by the World Health Organization and European diabetes organizations, called on member governments to implement policies that would reduce new diabetic blindness by a third, end-stage renal failure by a third, limb amputation for gangrene by a half, significantly reduce mortality and morbidity from coronary heart disease, and make pregnancy as safe for diabetics as for non-diabetics. In response, patient management protocols were issued by the British Diabetic Association (BDA), the British Geriatric Special Interest Group in Diabetes, and the Clinical Standards Advisory Group. In 1990 the Eurodiabeta Project, part-funded by the European Commission, was established to pool and standardize specialist views on the management of diabetes and enshrine these views in a computerized protocol that could be used Europe-wide by hospitals and GPs. Local Diabetes Services Advisory Groups advise health authorities on the implementation of suitable local policies.

The BDA protocol for case management is reproduced in Box 9.3, and the computerized record must accommodate data relating to it.

Quantifiable parameters are blood sugar, fructosamine/HBA-1, BMI, urinary protein, blood urea/creatinine, blood pressure and visual acuity, and these can be represented graphically. The practice must keep a register of diabetic patients, submissible to the HA in support of its claim for dedicated clinics,

and a strong case has been made for the compilation of district-wide registers. Defaulters to review must be identified and followed up.

Practice nurses can subscribe to the Roehampton Training Programme in Diabetes Care for which a certificate with credit rating is obtainable. Liaison should be established with the District Specialist Diabetic Nurse, who can be used to educate new patients, and with the Hospital Diabetes Liaison Sister. Further nurse education is obtainable through the Federation of European Nurses in Diabetes (FEND).

Individual patient management plans, review schedules and arrangements for repeat medication and education must be provided, and new patients should be referred to a registered dietician within 4 weeks of diagnosis. Other referral policies involving a diabetologist, ophthalmologist, chiropodist and nephrologist must be agreed with local providers. Self-care techniques and injection sites should monitored. The condition-orientated record for diabetes must accommodate details of all the above activities (Box 9.4). The memory glucose meter (e.g. Glucometer, Medisense) is now in common use, and is described more fully in Chapter 21.

Audit should identify the percentage of diabetic patients who are being catered for through protocols, and should list patients with pre-existing and new complications. Quantifiable parameters can be employed to measure the effectiveness of care.

There is increasing pressure on practices to screen, on a regular basis, close relatives of diabetics, elderly and grossly obese patients, and those who have had gestational diabetes.

Marketed computer systems that support diabetes care

Prototype computer systems for use in general practice which record diabetic patient data, manage protocols and produce reports, were fielded by Invicta (the NIDDMS system), and by Dr Colin Kenny of Dromore, Co. Down (the DiabSys system). These have now been superseded by surveillance modules produced by the main GP practice management system suppliers.

Computerized diabetes databases

The DIP-IN database provides information on diabetes for multiprofessional use.

The DIABCARE database sited at Bogenhausen in Germany has collated data from 45 diabetes centres in 21 countries in order to compare care performance.

Box 9.4 Diabetes review minimum data set (based on Financial Pulse Management Clinic 23 June 92)

Name	Address	NHS number	Date of birth		

History		**Examination**			
Smoking, alcohol		Height, weight, BMI			
Self medication		Blood pressure standing, lying			
Prescribed medication		Visual acuity (? + pinhole)			
Diet		– corrected		R	L
Exercise		– uncorrected		R	L
Self monitoring		Retinopathy		R	L
		Injection sites			
Known complications					
Symptomatic hypoglycaemia		Lower limbs			
Symptomatic hyperglycaemia		Ulcers		R	L
Retinopathy		Peripheral vascular disease		R	L
Cataract		Ankle jerks		R	L
Peripheral vascular disease		Vibration sense (seconds)		R	L
Ischaemic heart disease		Posterior tibial pulse		R	L
Stroke		Dorsalis pedis pulse		R	L
Peripheral neuropathy					
Sexual dysfunction		**Memory glucose meter download**			
Raised creatinine					
Proteinuria		**Education**			
Infections					
		Referral?			
Investigations		Dietician			
Urine		Diabetologist			
– Glucose		Ophthalmologist			
– Proteinuria		Chiropodist			
– Microalbuminuria		Nephrologist			
		District specialist diabetic nurse			
Blood					
– Glucose-random fasting		**Represcription**			
– Creatinine					
– HBA_1, fructosamine		**Reappointment**			
– Lipids		Practice nurse			
		GP			

9.14 CARDIOVASCULAR SURVEILLANCE – HYPERTENSION

Computer-aided diagnosis

10% of the British population has a raised blood pressure. If ignored, hypertensives have markedly increased risks of stroke, myocardial infarction, peripheral vascular disease, renal failure, retinal degeneration and heart failure. Even if efficiently treated, hypertension and its sequelae constitute the greatest drain on medical, nursing and pharmaceutical resources of any single disease.

British Hypertension Society guidelines (1998) specify that levels over 140/90, (140/80 in diabetics), using Korotkoff sounds 1–5, should be regarded as hypertensive and, if persistent, liable to cause premature end-organ damage.

For many years discrepancies between sphygmomanometers and assay techniques bedevilled the accurate monitoring of low-grade hypertension, but recent refinements in equipment engineering have

Fig. 9.6 Data entry screens for assessment of a diabetic case (Chronic disease management. NEMAS clinical audit software, courtesy of Dr Murray Lough)

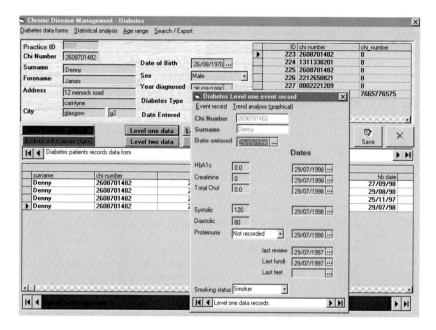

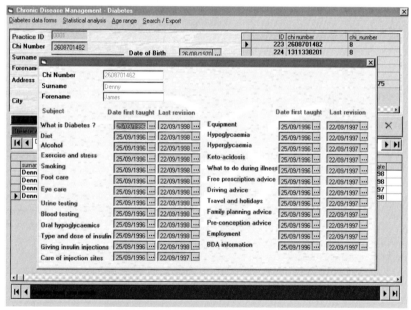

improved matters. Moreover, devices that the patient can use at home, whose operations are almost all automated, and whose results can be stored and downloaded to practice computers, mean that a cluster of recordings that obviate 'white coat hypertension' can be obtained.

The Omron 1C blood pressure monitor uses the oscillometric method of assay, is battery operated, has an automatically inflatable cuff, and is shock-resistant and simple to use. With the cuff in place, the patient has only to press the On/Start/Off button successively to prime the cuff and monitor, to record in memory, and to shut down the system. A second button logs a symbol on the time-scale to record the position of an 'event' whose identity is defined by the user. An LCD screen displays values for systolic and diastolic pressures, and pulse rate. The device memorizes up to 350 separate readings, taken over a timespan of up to

Box 9.5 Diabetes clinic support: system requirements

- Care strategy statement and process of care protocol, agreed with HA and local providers, must be stored on system (objectives, targets and criteria must be defined)
- Construct practice register of diabetic patients
- Prompted and validated data input routines must be used for diabetic minimum data set recording
- Prompts must be provided for procedures required by the process of care protocol
- Use condition-orientated shared care record architecture to accommodate nurse and GP input, delegation of responsibility, and contributions from dietician, diabetologist, ophthalmologist and chiropodist
- Dovetail with acute and repeat medication routines
- Implement decision support modules
- Formulate management plans for individual patients
- Input readings from blood glucose meter memory, and other pathology test results
- Use patient education screens, and provide for printing of patient instruction leaflets
- Dovetail with appointment system for re-appointment and monitoring of failed appointments. Print standard reminder letter and display opportunistic reminders on screen for procedures due or overdue.
- Compile list of all diabetic patients with quoted values of parameters required by process audit. Submit patient list with copy of the protocol of care to the HA in support of claim for the diabetic care fee. Include process audit in report to the PCG+T
- Provide search routines to identify and list relatives of diabetics, the grossly obese, and elderly patients so that opportunistic prompts and standard 'call' letters may be issued for screening purposes

Fig. 9.7 Condition orientated record: In-Practice Systems' Vision system's cardiovascular data entry screen

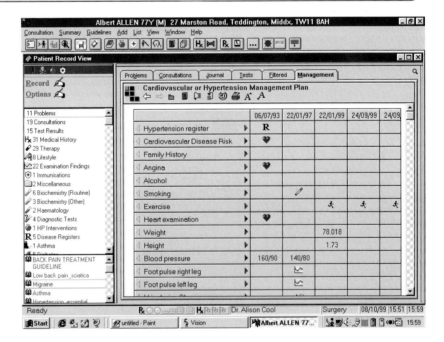

64 days, and an integral date/time clock labels each reading.

When the next assessment of the patient occurs, readings are downloaded through a cable to the doctor's PC and can be displayed on the computer screen as tables, trend graphs, or bar charts over time. Results can be demonstrated as actual, mean, maximum, minimum, or SD values.

The Profilomat 2 is an alternative model of automated blood pressure monitor that downloads results to a PC.

Graphical computer records

However obtained, systolic and diastolic blood pressure readings should be entered in the hypertensive

Fig. 9.8 Graphical representation of blood pressure: Global Clinical System, Aremis Soft Healthcare

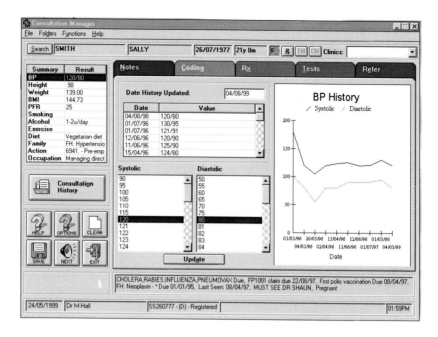

patient's computer record and can then with advantage be redisplayed graphically in conjunction with medication dosage over a time base. Ideally, these records will also show normal range values and provide for the superimposition of one week's readings on the next, so as to represent a typical (or 'modal') week's output. Effects produced by particular weekday or weekend activities are highlighted by these methods. Where repetitive readings are taken within successive 24 hour periods, a 'modal' day's readings may be constructed by superimposition and will help to identify circadian variations.

Risk assessment by computer

Hypertensive blood pressure readings are at once diagnostic, prognostic, and portray the effectiveness or ineffectiveness of therapy. They must be accompanied by general physical examination to determine whether other conditions coexist or complications have developed.

In its own right, hypertension is a major risk factor for the development of cardiac, cerebrovascular and renovascular sequelae, and it is important to determine whether other risk factors coexist. Computer program such as Risk disk and Heartscore deliver risk scores when they prompt for, and are supplied with, all relevant patient details. The Framingham risk score is an accurate predictor of coronary events and takes into account data on age, sex, total cholesterol, HDL cholesterol, BP, smoking, diabetes, and left ventricular

hypertrophy as determined by ECG. All these data should therefore be entered on the patient's computer record.

Default monitoring

Although it is possible to identify most defaulters to hypertensive surveillance by searching for gaps in the repeat medication file, prescriptions are sometimes renewed at home visits or during temporary residence elsewhere. A similar consideration applies to failed appointments. Provided that the surveillance record itself is invariably updated after home visits or on receipt of a temporary resident notification from another practice, then monitoring of surveillance records will provide the most accurate indication of default.

9.15 EPILEPSY SURVEILLANCE

Introduction

In the UK the average GP cares for 10–20 ongoing cases of epilepsy, and sees two or three new cases each year. The risk of epileptics dying prematurely is three times greater than normal. The National General Practice Study of Epilepsy, in which 2000 practices participated, showed that 80% of cases went into remission for the remainder of the 10-year survey. Of the epileptics whose condition is resistant to drug treatment, a further 80% can expect remission with stereotactic surgery. One in 20 uncontrolled epileptics may have congenital benign tumours for the detection of which an MRI scan is required. Efficient consistent shared management between practice and hospital is therefore vital to outcome. Shared care arrangements have also been shown to be more acceptable to patients.

Management guidelines

Standards for the management of epilepsy are set by the British Epilepsy Association, the National Society for Epilepsy, the Joint Epilepsy Council, and authoritative international bodies. Guidelines entitled *Adults with Poorly Controlled Epilepsy* are obtainable from the Royal College of Physicians and published by them in association with the Institute of Neurology and the National Society for Epilepsy.

Computerized surveillance records and the process of care

The epilepsy surveillance record must prompt for, and validate, the entry of all data required by the process of care protocol.

Although accurate diagnosis requires an initial consultation with a neurologist, most subsequent surveillance is undertaken in general practice. The framework for this is:

- the organization of surveillance clinics with their attendant educative and administrative procedures
- a seizure diary to be kept by the patient, which also contains the name and contact number of the designated carer
- a specialist nurse, preferably trained to ENB standards, who monitors seizure frequency, checks drug compliance, arranges blood levels and counsels the patient. The counselling check list can be stored on computer and must include advice on:
  - repeat medication and free prescriptions
  - precipitating factors – alcohol, lack of sleep, television, lack of food, stress and fever
  - first aid
  - water, heights, driving and machinery
  - fears for the future
  - contraception and pregnancy
  - self-help groups and Epilepsy Association membership
- a practice register of epileptic patients which identifies carers and distinguishes women of childbearing age.

- The computer record will titrate seizures against therapy dosage and blood levels over time and display the results graphically. The condition orientated record should also contain the following details:
  - date of first fit, and whether pyrexial
  - date diagnosis confirmed by neurologist
  - date of last review by practice
  - ability to fulfil requirements at work or school
  - lifestyle risk factors including alcohol intake.

The computer record is updated at each review. A printout may be given to the patient if a neurologist's review is pending.

- Referral is best considered in all new cases, but especially those of late onset, those in childhood and those accompanied by focal manifestations. Re-referral will be necessary if signs of raised intracranial pressure, or focal symptoms or signs develop, if there is retarded motor or mental development, or if control proves difficult. The presence or absence of these factors should be noted on the record.

Audit by computer

Audit should check the process of care records and show whether blood monitoring, referral to confirm diagnosis, and all annual checks have been carried out. It should also determine the proportion of patients on monotherapy and those driving vehicles. Outcome audit should investigate seizure frequency, drug reactions, and epilepsy related injury or death.

9.16 MENTAL HEALTH

Community mental health records on computer

The wholesale closure of long-stay mental hospital beds that occurred during the 1990s precipitated some startlingly inappropriate patient discharges into community care. To make matters worse, facts that were known at the time to individual hospital-based care professionals were seldom shared with other members of the mental health team. To overcome this problem, Central Manchester Health Care Trust implemented a multidisciplinary electronic patient record system with PCs and portable computers connected over a wide-bandwidth wireless network. Called the AMIGOS system (Advanced Medical Information Guidance and Organisational System), the radio network allows all clinical staff to record case notes electronically, to share those records with all other responsible colleagues, and to produce reports which are forwarded to GPs, medical staff and Community Psychiatric Nurses. Members of the 'Deliberate Self-harm and Homeless' team carry a full complement of records on their portable machines and upload amendments to the main network system. The consequent improvements in the coordination of care have been dramatic – no patient now slips through the net. Audit by computer checks process (positive care plan goal achievement) and outcome (mental state improvement estimated by a scoring system using validated tests).

NHS IT strategy now stipulates that linkages will be built up between the Electronic Patient Record (a minimum data set for health care maintained by general practitioners) and community mental health records. Provided that this fusion is achieved, then the community health record will become a further condition-orientated record within the practice patient record.

Schizophrenia

While the most efficient method of managing schizophrenia in the community still remains to be defined, it is estimated that a quarter of all patients are managed solely by their GPs. Many more are cared for jointly by GPs, who renew their repeat medication, and consultants, who review their progress and treatment once or twice yearly. Some GPs are members of community mental health teams and are thus involved in the decision-making process. All GPs should receive care programme approach (CPA) record documents (a form of individual care plan) from consultants to whom patients have been referred, so that continuity of management can be maintained. The contents of CPA documents could, with advantage, be transmitted and accessed electronically.

15% of schizophrenics commit suicide. The condition itself may be confused with the effects of the 'recreational' drugs angel dust and amphetamine. Side effects of pharmacotherapy for schizophrenia include a reversible parkinsonian state and an irreversible tardive dyskinesis resulting in tics, spasms and tremors. For all these reasons, close supervision at GP surveillance clinics is imperative and default must be closely monitored by computer.

Dementia

Needs assessment must embrace social needs, housing, employment and state benefits as well as physical and psychological health care requirements. The standard care needs assessment pack Carenap D (Dementia Services Development Centre, University of Stirling) is suitable for use on computer display or as printout.

Use of the 'Mini Mental State Examination' (MMSE) protocol in the diagnosis of dementia was advocated by the Audit Commission Report entitled 'Forget me not', dated January 2000.

Depression

National and local guidelines are available for the treatment of depression, and self-help materials such as booklets and audio-tapes are obtainable from the Royal College of Psychiatrists with further support from the 'Defeat Depression' Campaign. A CD-ROM-based, interactive, self-help computer program was launched in 1998 by the Institute of Psychiatry entitled 'Beating the Blues'. Based on cognitive behaviour therapy, which research suggests is as effective as medication, the computer takes each patient through a series of questions. Responses are used to produce a recovery plan with instructions on how patients can change their thinking and actions to overcome their illness.

Obsessive compulsive disorder (OCD)

An innovative self-help service for registered patients with OCD, organized by the Institute of Psychiatry in London, enables them to use a touch-tone telephone to activate a variety of recorded voice messages stored on a central computer. The patient selects choices with the touch tone keys in response to questions posed by the system. Practical exercises with which to confront the obsession are provided, together with goals to be achieved. The patient is also enabled to weight the severity of the disorder, the level of attendant depression, and the degree of social and financial disruption experienced.

By the end of the self-assessment procedure, the patient will have been trained to understand how the relapse has been triggered and to appreciate the principles of 'ritual prevention'. If needed, further therapy can be provided either by computer or by a clinician.

Anxiety

An interactive CD-ROM-based self-help programme that can be run on a practice's or patient's computer has been developed for patients suffering from anxiety by the Glasgow Community and Mental Health Services NHS Trust. Patients use the programme over three sessions each lasting 40 minutes, answer questions, and learn about the causes of anxiety and the problems associated with it (such as panic attacks, phobias, and insomnia). All participants in a pilot trial showed improved psychiatric rating scale scores, and half showed significant improvement.

9.17 CONTRACEPTION

Contraception is a form of surveillance that is usually conducted at routine consultation rather than at dedicated clinics. As with other forms of surveillance, responsibility is often shared with the practice nurse and repeat medication is usually required. Blood pressure readings and details such as smoking habits and body weight should be entered on the surveillance record.

Contraception, like antenatal care, requires the completion of a claim form, and the contraception claim must be renewed each year. Because of this, some practice systems provide an opportunistic reminder when the claim form should be signed afresh. Default does not usually endanger the patient's health, as it would do in many forms of surveillance.

9.18 ANTENATAL CARE

Antenatal records housed on the doctor's desk display have the ability to prompt for the inclusion of all necessary data, and also to prompt for the completion of time-sensitive procedures. Reminders for items such as patient information, welfare benefits, blood tests, pelvic examination, checks due at 28 or 36 weeks, and claim completion, assist in making antenatal care punctilious (Figs 9.9, 9.10) The system can also highlight procedures that are overdue or have been omitted.

Patient histories taken by midwives who employ a computer-based protocol have proved to be more comprehensive than those taken by conventional means. Important items are not omitted and details elicited can be refined by the ramification programmed into the computer questionnaire.

Automated referral letters that include all required details, and automated claims, can be completed, provided always that the system incorporates the necessary data and prompts for any that are outstanding.

Remote monitoring of maternal blood pressure and fetal heart rate from the patient's home through

Fig. 9.9 Data entry screen: Antenatal Assistant System (Dr P Wilson, Watchet, Somerset, http://www.ds.dial.pipex.com/brenhillsurg/index.htm)

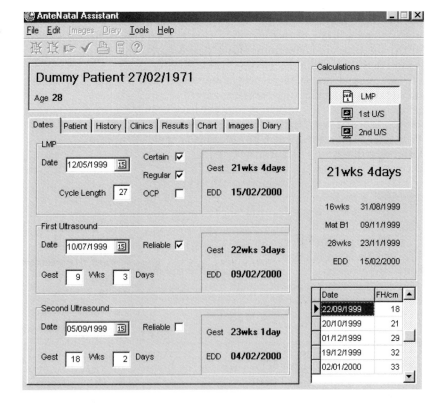

Fig. 9.10 'Shuttle' electronic record used jointly by GP and hospital: Torex's Orfeus system's obstetric history screen

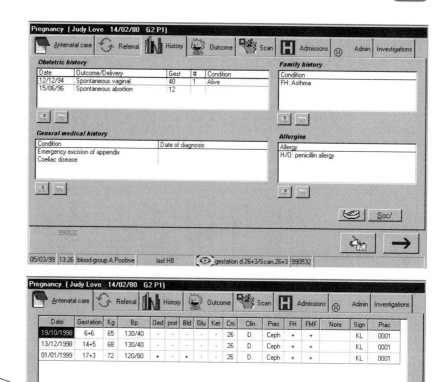

Press this to see a summary of clinical observations

telephone channels to a hospital computer has enabled some cases of pre-eclamptic toxaemia to be supervised without hospital admission. Reflectance meter results can be added to obtain the exceptional control needed for diabetic expectant mothers.

9.19 INFLUENZA IMMUNIZATION

Patients attending a cohort clinic for hypertension, diabetes or asthma may be offered influenza immunization each autumn.

The cohort clinic brings together patients who are at special risk, thus sparing the need for recall letters. Batch purchase of influenza vaccine by the practice is profitable, although no item of service is paid by the PPSA for this procedure.

SUMMARY

- Improved health care in developed countries increases longevity, which in turn increases the prevalence of chronic morbidity and the need for ongoing medical control, both by supervision and medication. Surveillance of chronic disease is a task the size of which demands that the practice nurse should take over some of the doctor's workload. This can be done safely and effectively under the doctor's supervision if s/he specifies requirements in terms of control criteria to be met, issues repeat medication and arranges for patient default monitoring.

- Item of service funding for surveillance is restricted to contraception and antenatal care. Diabetes and asthma care attract their own specific management fee. The greater part of the nurse's chronic disease management pay can be reimbursed under the NHS. Health care performance-related payments are being introduced.

- Basic surveillance clinics may be conducted with manual procedures, when it is best to maintain a ledger or card index register for patients under review. Both the manual record and the register must be updated separately. Manual procedures cannot cater for the requirements of protocol and audit implementation.
- Surveillance encounter forms can be produced by a practice computer situated in the secretary's office, upon which both surveillance records and repeat medication systems are stored and linked. This is probably the most worthwhile example of an encounter form system. It removes the need for a manual surveillance register, but is prone to the problems of transcription delay and error, and fragmentation of medical data between the computer and the remainder of the patient record if the latter is maintained manually.
- The fully computerized patient record system, to which both doctor and nurse have access through visual display units, overcomes the problems of both manual and encounter form systems.
- Surveillance records may need to be shared with the hospital, and this can be done if a patient-held paper record, a smart card, a patient-held electronic monitoring device with memory, or an electronic 'shuttle' record is used as an intermediary.
- Protocols assist in the assembly of surveillance clinics and records, and expert protocols assist in the referral decision-making process as well as other forms of case management. Practice surveillance strategies and process protocols must be agreed with PCG+T/HAs and providers. Payment for authorized surveillance clinic management is dependent upon HA approval of these practice policies.
- Representation in graphic form and in colour can enhance data presentation in surveillance records.
- Asthma, diabetes, cardiovascular disease, epilepsy, mental health, contraception and maternity surveillance records now have exacting computer system requirements but are an essential part of the practice database portfolio.
- Influenza immunization can usefully be incorporated into some surveillance clinics each autumn.
- The surveillance process, like prevention, will increasingly be controlled by protocols that originate from the National Institute for Clinical Excellence and are mediated through PRODIGY.
- Audit of process and outcome using MIQUEST or equivalent extraction software will be required for

reports to the PCG+T/HA and the CHI. Audit of a practice's performance as measured by government indicators of health care will be compared with peer results, will be exhibited in 'league tables' and will help to determine performance related pay. Overall scores of practice performance will depend heavily upon the effectiveness of practice surveillance procedures.

FURTHER READING

Bowling A 1981 Delegation in general practice. Tavistock Publications, London

British Hypertension Society 2000 Guidlines for the management of hypertension – brief summary 2000. 127 High Street, Teddington, Middlesex TW11 8HH

British Thoracic Society, Research Unit of the Royal College of Physicians of London, King's Fund Centre, National Asthma Campaign 1990 Guidelines for management of asthma in adults: 1 – Chronic persistent asthma. British Medical Journal 301: 651–653

British Thoracic Society, Research Unit of the Royal College of Physicians of London, King's Fund Centre, National Asthma Campaign 1990 Guidelines for management of asthma in adults: 2 – Acute severe asthma. British Medical Journal 301: 797–800

Consensus Group 1992 Asthma: a follow up statement from an international paediatric asthma consensus group. Archives of Disease in Childhood 67: 240–248

Hull F M 1982 Watching nurse practitioners. Update 15 July: 242

British Thoracic Society 1993 Management of chronic asthma in adults and children. British Medical Journal 306: 777–778

Medeconomics 1981 Capitalise on nurses. Medeconomics, July: 18

Asthma Working Party of the RCGP 1986 Protocol for the care of patients suffering from asthma: proceedings of the asthma working party of the RCGP. Royal College of General Practitioners, London

Reedy B L, Metcalfe A V, de Roumanie M et al 1980 A comparison of the activities and opinions of attached and employed nurses in general practice. Journal of the Royal College of General Practitioners 30: 483

Reedy B L, Philips P R, Newall D J 1976 Nurses and nursing in primary medical care in England. British Medical Journal 2: 1304

Silverberg D S, Batluch L, Hermoni Y, Eyal P 1982 Control of hypertension in family practice by the doctor-nurse team. Journal of the Royal College of General Practitioners 32: 184

Wallace H, Shorvon S D, Hopkins A, O'Donohue M 1997 Adults with poorly controlled epilepsy. Royal College of Physicians of London, London

10 Repeat prescriptions

10.1 INTRODUCTION

The prescribing instruction 'the mixture as before', much revered by our medical predecessors, struck the public at large as being so autocratic a piece of buck-passing that it remains to this day a cliché of the English language. The effect of the instruction was that the pharmacist had to keep repeat medication records in order to stay in business, while the doctor noted the medication once only, at the time of the first consultation. Times have changed. The onus is now on the doctor to write all prescriptions in full and to keep both initial and repeat medication records.

10.2 THE SIZE OF THE PROBLEM

With wide variation between individual practices, repeat prescriptions range from 9% to 60% of all prescriptions issued. Repeat prescribing is on the increase and is predominant among the elderly. No less than 55% of those over 75 years of age use repeat medication, and the difficulties that older people experience in remembering to take consistent dosage are compounded by the multiple preparations that are often necessary for them. Yet, without consistent dosage, control of what may well be a life-threatening condition will be sacrificed. The issue of repeat prescriptions is usually associated with the need for periodic reassessment of the case and, unless the number of repeats between reviews is monitored, the doctor will be condoning any default attributable to the reluctance which many patients have for consulting in the absence of symptoms.

The doctor in single-handed practice, acquainted with his own patients and his own handwriting, has fewer problems in determining the appropriateness of continuing medication between consultations, and in respecifying it. If he insists on seeing every patient before renewing treatment, he increases his workload to a significant degree. If he issues a prescription without seeing the patient, then he gambles with the possibility that the details of the drug requested as a repeat by the patient may be inaccurate, that the drug may no longer be appropriate or that it is being misused.

In the past, psychotropic drugs have been extensively prescribed as repeat medication, but an increasing awareness of the dangers of addiction has led most practices to confine the use of these drugs to issue under direct supervision. Controlled drugs, requiring handwritten specification by the doctor, are also unsuitable for inclusion in repeat prescribing systems.

Without adequate repeat medication records and control, various types of error may occur (Fig. 10.1).

10.3 MANUAL METHOD OF REPEAT MEDICATION CONTROL

The first step towards control is to introduce repeat medication cards. Although the drug's identity and regimen will be the same as those entered in the patient consultation record, the card allows recording of successive repeats and often shows the date after which no further repeats should be allowed without review of the patient. The repeat medication card is kept in one of three places:

- in the patient's record
- in a card index on the receptionist's desk
- by the patient.

When the patient requests a repeat prescription, the receptionist refers to the repeat medication card (24–48 hours notice is usually expected). Details are then faithfully copied by the receptionist on to a blank prescription form, together with the patient's

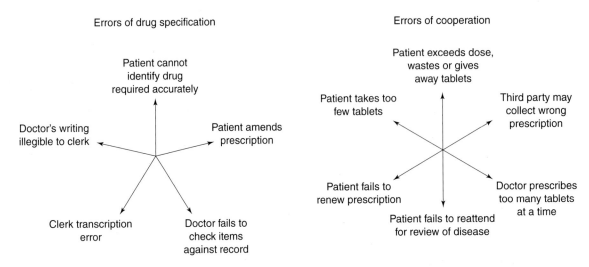

Errors of drug specification

Errors of cooperation

Fig. 10.1 Errors likely to occur in uncontrolled repeat medication procedures

name and address for later signature by the doctor. The repeat card is updated with the renewed medication. The prescription is then collected by the patient or is returned to him in a stamped addressed envelope, together with the repeat card if this is held by the patient. If the repeat card shows that authorization of repeats has expired, the receptionist reappoints the patient to see the doctor.

Manual methods overcome some of the difficulties in control of repeat medication, but they fail to resolve the following problems:

- There may be transcription errors.
- The prescription may be adulterated by the patient.
- They require duplication of medication records, one for consultation and one for repeat control.
- Although the receptionist saves the doctor time and effort by entering the patient and drug identity on the prescription and by updating the record, her own task takes correspondingly longer. There is, of course, no economy in the pulling and refiling of manual records, a task that takes approximately one minute per record.
- Patient-held medication cards are a useful source of information to other doctors or hospitals treating the patient; the patient may lose them or fail to bring them to the surgery.
- If the patient does not hold the repeat medication card, s/he may forget when reauthorization or case review is due. Some designs of patient-held card fail to incorporate these data.

10.4 PRINCIPLES OF COMPUTERIZATION – MAIN OBJECTIVES

Computerization seeks to underpin the economy in professional time achieved by issuing repeats between consultations, and to remove the disadvantages listed for manual systems.

The main objectives are:

- to provide accurate, authorized reduplication of drug details in printed type, with 'blocked out' spaces between items to preclude false additions by the patient
- to place a time limit on authorization for repeats, or else to limit the total number of repeats authorized
- to update the computer repeat medication record automatically
- to provide a patient-held record of repeat medication
- to monitor the rate of consumption of drugs issued as repeats
- to prompt the receptionist to re-appoint the patient as authority for repeats expires, or as case reassessment becomes due
- to save time by generating all output from a single entry transaction, by avoiding the need to pull and refile manual records, and by the speed of system operation as compared with manual methods

10.5 THREE LEVELS OF SOPHISTICATION

Repeat prescribing was the first computer application to become generally accepted in UK general practice, and it remains one of the most appropriate ways to begin stepwise implementation of a practice system. Amateur system developers were invariably attracted towards the construction of what is, in essence, a simple piece of program writing, yet the full potential of a repeat medication module cannot be realized unless it is integrated with a total prescribing package, a computerized clinical record and the shared surveillance of chronic disease.

The earliest repeat prescribing systems were little more than faithful reprinters of prestored prescriptions, but the fact of printing gave them the obvious advantage of legibility over the use of handwriting with carbon copies.

With systems of intermediate complexity, the doctor wishing to initiate repeat medication uses the manual record to note the treatment s/he is about to prescribe, and also to note the fact that in future s/he authorizes its re-prescription without consultation. S/he then handwrites the first prescription and gives it to the patient with the instructions as to how to obtain repeats and when, after using the repeats, the patient should reattend for assessment.

The manual notes are then handed to the secretary, who enters the prescription details and authorization details on the patient's computer record. When subsequently a repeat is requested, the computer record is summoned, the drug and its repeat authorization are checked for the patient in question, the computer prints both the prescription and the accompanying patient-held medication record (usually in the form of printed details on the right-hand side of form FP 10 comp), and the patient's computer record is automatically updated. If patient compliance in taking regular medication is suspect, this fact may be highlighted by a comparison of daily dosage, drug supply and repeat intervals. This comparison may be emphasized by methods of computer display that bring it to the receptionist's notice. If authorization will expire after the prescription being issued, then the system will warn and the warning will be passed to the patient.

10.6 THE PRESCRIBING MONITOR

It is possible, by using drug data stored on computer and with reference to details already stored in the patient's clinical and medication record, for the system to monitor the doctor's selection and specification of a drug for a given patient. As the doctor enters the drug details on the patient's computer medication record for the purpose of constructing a first prescription which the computer will print, the system supervises the correct spelling of the drug name and offers alternative varied options for formulation, strength, dosage and supply in relation to that name – details that are derived from the drug dictionary. The system then checks the patient's computer record to ensure that the drug selected is not inappropriate in terms of: known patient allergy; reduplication of action of, or interaction with, repeat drugs or other drugs recently prescribed; and conditions for which the drug is contraindicated. Dosage checks for age, and the addition of any special administrative instructions are undertaken. Checks for indication are also possible.

These automated checks form the basis for total prescribing validation by computer. The requirements for the facility are an adequate clinical and medication computer record for the patient, an up-to-date drug database, and a practice policy of writing all prescription through the computer. A later chapter describes the manner of operation of the prescribing monitor in greater detail, its links with protocols to assist the doctor in selecting a drug for the condition to be treated, and its link with prescribing audit.

10.7 SOPHISTICATED REPEAT PRESCRIBING SYSTEMS

The most sophisticated repeat medication systems operate as part of a total prescribing module, integrated with the computerized clinical record and with shared care surveillance. Because the doctor writes all prescriptions and enters all records through the system, a single medication entry simultaneously suffices to update the computer medication record, to generate the first prescription and to print the accompanying patient-held medication record. All the checks of the prescribing monitor will have been used, because all necessary data are available to the system. The doctor adds to his medication entry the authority to allow the prescription to be repeated, and specifies the duration of that authority – information that is also transmitted to the patient-held medication record. In sophisticated systems there is no intermediary data entry on the part of the secretary, although the secretary's tasks in generating repeats on demand remain similar to those performed with systems of intermediate complexity.

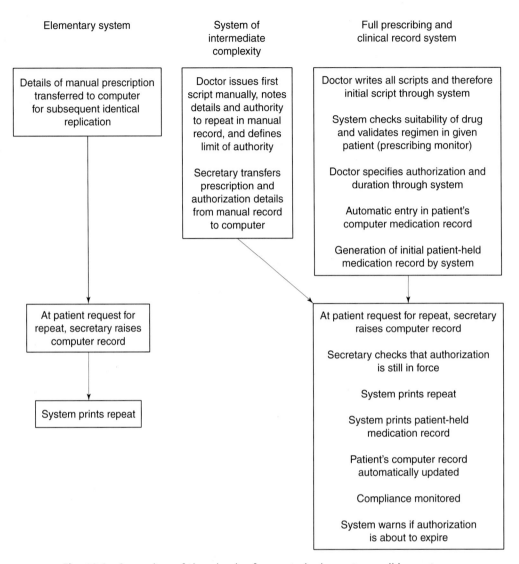

Elementary system

Details of manual prescription transferred to computer for subsequent identical replication

↓

At patient request for repeat, secretary raises computer record

↓

System prints repeat

System of intermediate complexity

Doctor issues first script manually, notes details and authority to repeat in manual record, and defines limit of authority

Secretary transfers prescription and authorization details from manual record to computer

Full prescribing and clinical record system

Doctor writes all scripts and therefore initial script through system

System checks suitability of drug and validates regimen in given patient (prescribing monitor)

Doctor specifies authorization and duration through system

Automatic entry in patient's computer medication record

Generation of initial patient-held medication record by system

↓

At patient request for repeat, secretary raises computer record

Secretary checks that authorization is still in force

System prints repeat

System prints patient-held medication record

Patient's computer record automatically updated

Compliance monitored

System warns if authorization is about to expire

Fig. 10.2 Comparison of three levels of computerized repeat prescribing system

Checks by the prescribing monitor on the suitability of drug choice and the validation of regimen in a given patient are virtually useless unless practised on the first prescription. It is dangerously misleading to run an interactions check on repeat prescriptions if one ignores the first and all acute prescriptions. Similarly, prescribing audit, and the ability to list and recall all patients on a specified drug in the event of its withdrawal by authority, suffer from severe limitations unless applied to all prescribing. Only the most sophisticated systems have the power to perform these functions satisfactorily. Figure 10.2 compares systems of differing complexity.

10.8 DATA REQUIRED IN PRINTING PRESCRIPTIONS

All prescriptions whether new, repeated, manual or computerized require:

1. patient's name, address, age if under 12 years
2. drug identity (name, formulation, strength)
3. drug schedule (dosage, frequency, and any other instructions for drug administration)
4. drug total supply (total quantity, or number of days of treatment)
5. date
6. doctor's signature.

On computer systems, 1 and 5 are selected automatically from prestored data; 2, 3 and 4 are prompted for at entry and dictionary-validated by computer.

The DHSS authorized the free supply of continuous 'fan-fold' stationery (FP 10 comp) to general practice through its Family Practitioner Committees (subsequently FHSAs, now Health Authorities), for printing computerized prescriptions (FPN 279 March 1981). Computerized systems must comply with specific requirements in order to obtain and use this stationery, and these constraints include the printing of the health authority name, and the doctor's name, address and prescribing number in an agreed standard format at the bottom of the prescription.

Since the last doctor to authorize a repeatable drug for the patient is held in law to be liable for the repeats that follow, a computerized repeat medication system must always store that doctor's name and print it at the foot of a repeat prescription.

10.9   RECORDING REPEATS AND MONITORING THE RATE OF CONSUMPTION

Computerized repeat medication systems must record the issue of repeats on the medication record, and the recording process may be designed so as to assist appraisal by eye of the general level of drug consumption. Alternate methods demonstrate the dates of all repeats, the dates of the first and last repeat compared with the total authorized and the authorization expiry date, or a count up to or down from the total number of repeats authorized (expressed as a fraction), together with the date of authorization. Rough and ready rate monitoring of this sort can be applied to regular or intermittent treatment regimens alike.

When dealing with continuous and regular administration of drugs, a more rigid monitoring process may be applied, because the number of units of drug consumed can be predicted accurately per unit time. Working from the date of authorization, the control factors here are date of expiry of authorization, number of repeats authorized, and days' duration of treatment per prescription – any two of which factors are sufficient to calculate the third factor. When the calculated rate of consumption is compared with the date on which a repeat prescription is requested, discrepancies can be monitored automatically. This process has no meaning in the case of topical, or systemic 'as required' (PRN) drugs.

10.10   THE PATIENT-HELD MEDICATION SLIP

The FP 10 continuous stationery provided for printing prescriptions by computer is almost twice as wide as a conventional prescription. The reason for this is that printers originally used in general practice could not accommodate narrow continuous stationery. The extra width was provided by a blank area to the right-hand side of the prescription form, almost as large as the form itself and separated from it by a perforated line. Even though alternative printers are now available, provision of the blank page has proved to be so useful for printing a patient-held medication record that the design of the FP 10 (comp) has not been changed, other than to add a serial number and to use a different background colour to deter fraud. Future changes may express the serial number as a bar code.

The FP 10 blank page may be printed with the details of all authorized repeat medication for the patient and given out with the repeat prescription. The patient may carry this as a means of medication identification in case of emergency, dental treatment, or temporary resident care elsewhere. Other details, such as patient drug idiosyncrasy or special instructions connected with medication, may be included and the form should show the patient's and the doctor's identity. The form can be used to identify drugs when the patient requests repeat medication, and should warn when authorization is about to expire and reassessment is necessary (Fig. 10.3).

In systems where the initial prescription of a series is handwritten, the blank page may be turned back to lie behind the prescription, carbon paper inserted, and the duplicated prescription details used to request the first repeat.

Although its role as a patient-held medication record is the most common one played by the FP 10 blank page, many other uses have been found for it during the extensive experience that repeat medication systems have provided.

- It may supply detailed instructions for the patient on the administration of drugs whose schedules are too complex to be accompanied on the label of the dispensing bottle. These instructions may be elaborated so as to constitute a condensed form of individual self-management plan.
- It can be used to carry computer-generated information back from a reception area installation to the doctor before he signs the repeat prescription (e.g. compliance monitoring data).
- It can be used in a doctor's desktop system to carry computer-generated information from the doctor to medical centre ancillary staff – e.g. re-

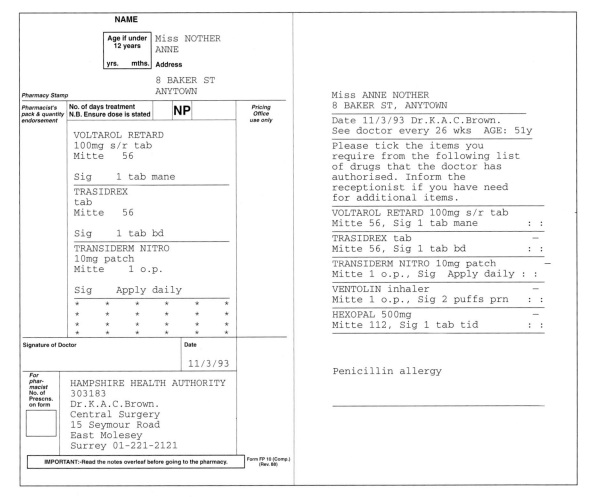

Fig. 10.3 An example of a repeat prescription in which the blank right-hand page has been used to print a patient-held list of all medication authorized for repeat (Courtesy of David Gunter, Ciba-Geigy)

appointment instructions, the need for screening or immunization by the practice nurse, or the need for claim completion.

- It may be used as an encounter form. In systems that do not print acute prescriptions but do print encounter form summaries, the patient summary history has been printed out on the right-hand blank page and the prescription left empty for completion by hand. The doctor sees the patient, writes the prescription and gives it to the patient, then amends the encounter summary and gives it to the secretary, who updates the system.

A more pertinent use of the blank page as an encounter form is in shared surveillance of chronic disease. In the supervision of maintenance treatment in chronic disease it is possible to share review of stabilized cases with the practice nurse.

The doctor presets strict criteria to which the nurse must adhere before allowing continuation of medication. It is convenient to print these criteria on the right-hand FP 10 blank page, and to print on the left side, at the same time, the repeat medication to be used at the clinic. As well as showing the control criteria, the right-hand side will contain other details necessary to surveillance. If the control criteria are met, the prescription is issued to the patient and the right-hand page, duly amended by the nurse, is passed to the secretary who updates the patient's computer record.

- The blank page may be used for the printing of private prescriptions.
- When authorization of repeats has expired, the blank page may be used to print out a summary of

a patient's repeated medication for inclusion in the manual record.

10.11 'CASH-POINT'-TYPE TERMINALS FOR REQUESTING REPEAT PRESCRIPTIONS

The GP system supplier Aremis Soft (formerly L. K. Global) has designed a computer terminal that provides 24-hour access for patients who wish to request repeat medication. The patient inserts a 'smart card' into the terminal to enable the system to identify the patient and his/her authorized repeatable drugs. These details are checked, and displayed on the terminal's screen in a format that allows the drugs required to be selected. Instructions as to how the prescription may be obtained are also appended.

10.12 ADVANTAGES AND DISADVANTAGES OF COMPUTERIZATION

The success of computerized repeat prescribing, despite the fact that it does not generate extra practice income, underlines its importance as an administrative tool. There are considerable savings in professional time – doctor, nurse and secretary can all benefit, especially if the level of confidence is such that pulling and refiling of manual records for cross-checks are deemed unnecessary. The verification of authorization for repeats is much faster if a VDU is used. The end

product is a fully legible prescription that is unalterable by the patient. An unwavering accuracy of patient and drug detail taken from stored data is matched by a high level of efficiency in monitoring compliance with regular medication, and in encouraging patient reattendance for assessment when this is due.

In more sophisticated systems, a single entry procedure suffices to generate an entry in the patient's computer record, a repeat prescription and a patient-held medication slip. If all prescriptions, both acute and repeat, are issued via the computer, then extensive checks on the appropriateness of prescribing become possible, patients taking drugs that are withdrawn by authority at short notice can be identified and recalled, and audit of prescribing may be undertaken.

It is possible to run search programs on computerized repeat medication records to detect those who have defaulted from reassessment, but this information is obtained more effectively from search of the surveillance files if these have been conscientiously maintained. Monitoring of default from renewal of repeats per se is vitiated by those who obtain prescriptions at home or whilst away from the district.

Developmental projects are now at an advanced stage that explore the possibility of using GP–pharmacy links in which electronic transmission of a prescription will be directed to the pharmacy of the patient's choice, will enable the pharmacist to increase customer loyalty and build prescribing records on computer, and will offer the patient the prospect of

Fig. 10.4 Repeat prescribing screen: Global Clinical System (Aremis Soft Healthcare)

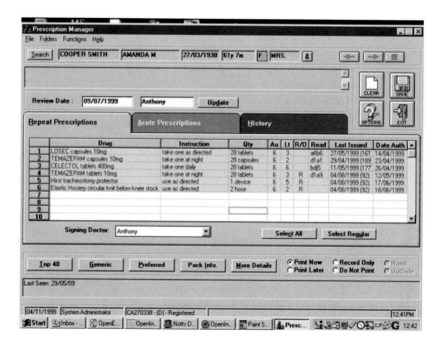

Fig. 10.5 Repeat prescribing screen: new GPASS system

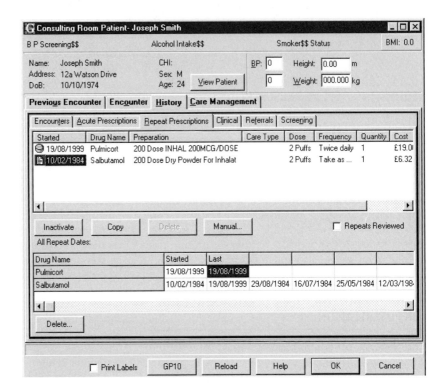

being able to request repeat medication from the pharmacy.

SUMMARY

- Repeat prescribing systems bring control by the practice to a process in which patients otherwise take the initiative for better or worse.
- Computerization has the distinct advantage of producing a fully legible, faithfully reproduced prescription which cannot be adulterated.
- The more sophisticated the computer system, the more saving there is in time for the doctor, nurse and secretary, and the more accurately compliance can be monitored.
- Sophisticated systems constitute part of a total prescribing package in which all prescribing is subject to automated checks by the prescribing monitor, and in which a single medication entry produces the first prescription and authorizes a specified number of repeats.
- Prescription printing is coupled with the production of a patient-held medication slip and updating of the medication record.
- There are close links between repeat prescribing, the shared care surveillance record and prescribing audit.
- Repeat prescribing constitutes the best introductory application for stepwise computer implementation in practice.

FURTHER READING

Balint M I, Hunt J, Joyce D et al 1970 Treatment or diagnosis – a study of repeat prescriptions in general practice. Tavistock Publications, London

Bligh J G 1981 A survey of repeat prescribing. Update 15 November: 1453

Bradshaw Smith J H 1980 Proceedings of symposium on automated records in primary care, Oxford, 1 July. Oxford Community Health Project H3

Difford F 1985 A question of communication. Practice Computing 4(1): 8

Drury V W M 1982 Repeat prescribing – a review. Journal of the Royal College of General Practitioners 32: 42

Garber J R, Fitter M 1984 Is it worth it? Practice Computing 3(3): 19

Madely J 1974 Repeat prescribing via the receptionist in a group practice. Journal of the Royal College of General Practitioners 24: 425

National Health Service 1981 FPN 279 On computer compatible prescription forms FP 10 (Comp).

Stoddard N 1983 The case for repeats. Practice Computing 2(3): 26

11 Writing all prescriptions by computer

11.1 INTRODUCTION

Nowadays we are repelled by accounts of the leeching, blood letting, purge and clyster of old medical regimens, which did more to harm patients than to help them. The ghost of those days still haunts our ministrations in the form of iatrogenic disease, disease caused by treatment that does more harm than good.

As general practitioners, we value very highly the double checking of our prescriptions by the pharmacist before the drugs we have specified are dispensed. Apart from verifying the identities of the patient, drug and doctor (as best he may), the pharmacist checks against inappropriate dosage for age, and potential interactions of drugs on the same prescription. Ratification of the doctor's choice of drug with regard to indications, contraindications, previous idiosyncrasy and previous medication (save where customer loyalty is dependable) is beyond the pharmacist's reach, since this would require knowledge of the full medical record.

Despite the care taken in prescribing and dispensing, and for a variety of reasons, standards of accuracy in drug use by the patient fall far below an acceptable level. The awesome toll in morbidity and mortality among the elderly that is attributed to iatrogenesis is a constant indictment upon the medical profession, with whom responsibility for this problem primarily rests. The problem is not limited to old age.

Because the distinction between medication and poisoning may become blurred, despite efforts to the contrary made by the doctor and pharmacist, we must design and employ new methods to assist us in the selection and use of drugs. The complementary processes of selecting a drug that will cure, and avoiding one that will poison, can benefit from the exploitation of new technology, just as surely as orthopaedic surgery can harness robot procedures or ophthalmic colleagues can use lasers.

11.2 THE COMPONENTS OF THE PRESCRIBING PROCESS

The act of prescribing, which may appear to the patient to be a one-stage process, in reality requires a sequence of steps to be taken. Each step may be assisted by the computer.

Steps taken when issuing a prescription

- The drug must be appropriate for the treatment of the disease.
- The drug must not be inappropriate for use by virtue of the patient's age, physical condition, other pathological conditions present, previous drug idiosyncrasies or concomitant treatment.
- The cost/benefit/risk ratios of alternative products should be considered.
- The drug name, formulation, strength, dosage and supply must be accurately specified.
- Details of the patient's, doctor's and health authority's identity, and the date, must be accurately reproduced.
- Administrative instructions for the drug must be conveyed to the patient.
- The patient should be warned of potential side effects of the drug.
- Patient compliance must be encouraged, and checked where possible.

Steps taken after the preparation has been issued

- The patient's cure must be assessed.
- Adverse drug reactions must be assessed and treated.
- Adverse drug reactions must be reported.
- If a drug is generally withdrawn from use, no further prescriptions must be issued, and those taking the drug must be warned to discontinue it.

113

The principal tools that we must employ in order to provide automated assistance in each of the above steps in the prescribing process are:

- a comprehensive, structured patient medication record on display which distinguishes between acute and repeat prescribing, and which provides links between medication and diagnosis
- a comprehensive, structured patient morbidity record using terms identifiable by a computer search
- an authoritative electronic database of drug information, structured so that targeted data may be pinpointed instantly for either textual display or automated electronic interrogation
- a software package that guides the doctor during prescription writing, making all necessary checks on data in the database and in the patient's clinical and medication records, so as to eliminate all known sources of error and print a legible document
- a software package for recording responses to treatment in a form which can be used in future management of the patient, and which can be communicated to agencies responsible for collecting drug intelligence in the field.

11.3 THE MEDICATION RECORD DISPLAY

The medication display – one of the six primary screens of the patient's clinical record – has three main components:

1. Stacked statements of prescribed items. Each statement must show the date, authorizing doctor's initials, drug name in full, terms such as 'enteric coated' or 'effervescent' used to qualify the drug name, formulation, strength, dosage, supply, administrative instructions, and repeat factors. An acceptable degree of condensation of terms other than the drug name allows the statement to be accommodated within one 80-character line of a visual display.

A clear way to distinguish between acute and repeat medication is to display the latter as double-intensity or colour-coded text, provided that authorization is still in date. It is preferable to show each repeated item as a fresh line entry stacked in chronological sequence below previous issues of the same drug. Other than for repeat medication, opinion is divided as to whether new statements should be stacked in chronological or reverse chronological order – the latter conforms with the design of the consultation log, and allows the most recent statements to be viewed most readily. Repeat medication entries will be replicated by themselves in the repeat medication record.

It is important to retain the linkage between prescribed drug and diagnosis when viewing medication entries. This can be programmed in such a way that, if the user first places the cursor on the prescribed item statement and then presses a function key, the relevant diagnosis will be displayed immediately below the drug statement. Within the consultation log, the linkage between diagnosis and condensed medication statement is preserved by the horizontal correspondence each shares with the date of entry.

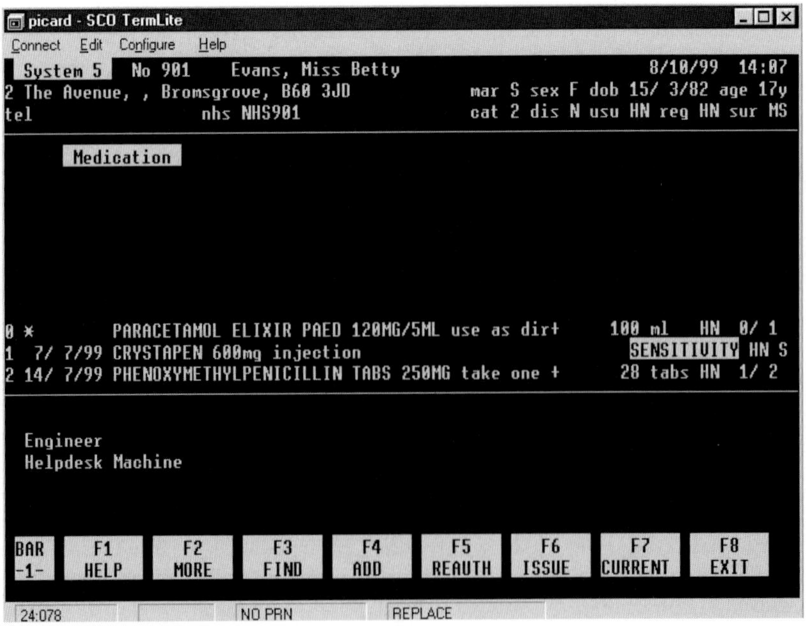

Fig. 11.1 Medication record screen: Torex Meditel System 5

2. *Circumstantial details needed when writing a prescription* are accommodated at the top and bottom of the medication display. These will include the patient's identity data, previous drug idiosyncrasies, and status with regard to prescription fees, dispensing, or private treatment.

3. *Display of text generated while a new prescription is being constructed* is best accommodated in an inset window or 'dialogue box' – a small, rectangular 'notepad' area of the screen temporarily cleared while the background of the full medication display remains in place. Option lists, prompts and warning messages are all displayed within the window and, when the newly prescribed item statement has been completed, the latter is added to the stack and the window disappears.

11.4 DRUG DATABASES

There are four essential components in a fully functioning electronic drug database:

- textual reference data describing drug attributes in a structured format for browsing on display
- drug lists with pack sizes and prices ('drug line' data) such as are used in pharmacy stock control, and by the Prescription Pricing Authority for reimbursement of pharmacies and the provision of PACT reports
- electronically coded and structured details of the attributes of each drug (indications, contraindications, dosage, etc) for use with prescribing software
- an electronic drug interactions matrix.

Textual reference data

Given that there are over 2500 brand-named products on offer and at least 30 000 other preparations that doctors are at liberty to prescribe, it is not surprising that most practitioners confine themselves to a small repertoire of tried and trusted drugs. The price of such a defensive policy, however, is the loss of therapeutic potential. A doctor who limits him/herself to 50 preparations would be using a mere 2% of the branded market. In order to enlarge their therapeutic armoury, prescribers need fast access to appropriate, authoritative and carefully structured drug data.

Manual sources of drug information are many and diverse. They include the *Monthly Index of Medical Specialities* (MIMS), the *Data Sheet Compendium*, the *British National Formulary* (BNF), drug house representatives and promotional mailings, medical meet-

ings, medical journals and textbooks, official directives, hospital contacts and drug information centres. The volume, content and style of presentation of drug information in manual reference is not suited to general practice. Many sources are at variance with each other and show bias.

The manual source with the most succinct presentation is MIMS and this is, consequently, by far the most frequently used in general practice, but its information on contraindications, precautions and drug interactions is so brief that it cannot be held to be legally binding on prescriber or manufacturer. By contrast, the wealth of detail given to the description of these and other attributes in the Data Sheet Compendium impedes its use during a busy surgery.

A further impediment to access from manual data sources is, of course, that a labour-intensive search of bookshelf, index, page and paragraph is required before target data are located.

MIMS, the BNF and the Data Sheet Compendium are all now available on CD-ROM and provide textual reference data but, of course, no interactive electronic support for prescribing software. The BNF is also available on CD-ROM in combination with the *Drug and Therapeutics Bulletin* (which provides drug line data) and the *MeReC Bulletin*. Martindale has been available on-line for over two decades.

E-MIMS was launched in 1999 and is supplied to NHS practices free each month in a CD-ROM format that self-negates after 5 weeks so as to prevent the use of outdated information. In addition to its structured text describing drug attributes, it has been embellished by the addition of a news section, drug monographs, data sheets with easily accessed subsections, images of tablets and capsules, lists of foreign preparations with ingredients, lists of self-help groups, clinical guidelines, access to manufacturers' websites and e-mail, and a number of useful reference tables, calculations and educational facilities. Patient instruction leaflets on drugs and fact sheets on diseases can be displayed or printed, and provision is made after downloading the data on to the GP system hard disk for the user to flag products in order to select a practice or group formulary. Minimum system requirements are a 486 150 MHz processor with 60 Mb free hard disk space, a sound card, a CD-ROM drive, a 600 × 800 screen setting and Windows 95.

The text that is accommodated by most computer visual displays consists of 20 lines, each of 80 characters. This format proves to possess suitable visual appeal, and the optimal text volume for assimilation before the interruption caused by page turning. Experience has shown that in almost every case it is possible to condense the contents of drug data sheets to fit this format without detriment, as judged by both the prescriber and manufacturer, and integral purpose-built electronic databases adopt this concept. Carefully structured product attributes should be arranged in standard order, under headings where necessary, to produce a parcel of information that is at once more useful and more convenient than existing manual sources.

11.5 FULLY FEATURED ELECTRONIC DRUG DATABASES

Multilex and the Doctor's Independent Network Coding (DINC) are electronic databases that provide textual reference, drug line data, interaction matrices and electronic support for prescribing software modules as combined features for UK general practice systems. Multilex has been the longer established of the two, covers over 32 000 products, and has been incorporated into the systems marketed by nearly all UK systems suppliers. DINC's Safescript claims coverage of 25 000 preparations, was launched in 1996 and has been adopted by several of the smaller GP system suppliers. In addition to the two fully featured drug databases for prescribing support, two other important projects offering comprehensive patient management protocols have been developed that take the patient's diagnosis as a starting point, and include decision support for prescribing as one of their func-

tions. These are PRODIGY and MediDesk, both of which incorporate electronic drug databases and are described more fully in Chapter 23.

The PRODIGY project was planned and funded by the Department of Health for the purpose of retaining control over drug selection by computer. The other three concepts were the direct result of innovation by individual British GPs, and have been supported by the pharmaceutical industry in terms of both finance and data validation.

The approach to prescribing support adopted by all four of these modules is broadly similar, though Multilex, by virtue of its superior refinement, market penetration and comprehensiveness, continues to set the standard in its field.

11.6 MULTILEX

Preece, EDB's first chairman, was responsible for the concept and original specification of the prototype GP drug database and prescribing module that was originally entitled the ABPI-Whipton project, later renamed Philex, and ultimately Multilex (Preece 1984). From the outset, pharmaceutical industry participation was considered essential, because of its ownership and validation of the branded data that the system used. The project has, however, always enjoyed political independence.

The Multilex module provides textual reference data, drug line data, an interaction matrix, electroni-

Fig. 11.2 The Drug Dictionary: Multilex drug data in use on the Practice Made Perfect GP system

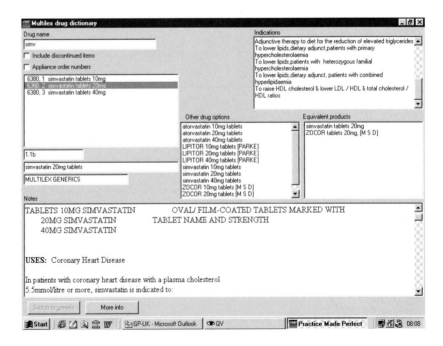

Table 11.1 Product attributes accessible through Multilex

'Drug line' data	Textual pharmacological data
Drug name	Uses – licensed indications
Qualifier (e.g. 'effervescent')	Contraindications
Formulation	Precautions
Strength	Prescriber warnings
Company	Side effects
Order number (appliances)	Active and inactive ingredients
Flavour (where appropriate)	Mode of action
Links to Read 2, Read 3, PIP, EAN codes	Drug–drug interactions
NHS reimbursement price	Drug–food interactions
England & Wales part VIII price (Scotland part 7) in drug tariff	Dosage
	Equivalent products – by product, use or action group
Tray size	Patient counselling advice
Packs	Label warnings
Prices	Action groups
Legal classification for prescribing category (e.g. CSM, controlled drug)	
Storage conditions	

Automated cross checks available for indications, contraindications, interactions, idiosyncrasies, reduplication of action, and dose for age. Relevant precautions, prescriber warnings and drug–food interactions are triggered and displayed textually when a regimen is proposed.

---

cally structured drug attribute data and driver software for prescribing support in the production of 200 million prescriptions yearly. The attributes stored are listed in Table 11.1. Interactions may be interrogated as one to one or all to one.

Validation software used during prescribing compares the proposed prescription with data in the patient record and drug dictionary to expose contraindications, precautions, prescriber warnings, side effects, patient sensitivities, interactions, doubling of ingredient action, and inappropriate dosage. All checks dovetail with the Read coding system.

Price comparisons may be made by pack, by unit within the pack, or by a comparative price index. Alternative equivalent products may be accessed by product, use, or action group. The system can suggest a suitable dose for age at two alternative levels of therapeutic intensity, and can compute the optimal dose related to age, gender, rate, height, organ function, pre-existing morbidity and concurrent medication.

Multilex provides a tool kit for integration with all commonly used operating systems and can link with MS-DOS, Windows or Internet-type browsers. 'FastTrack' is a special facility for embedding new product launch data in a suppressed format on GP systems, to be triggered on the due launch date.

The pharmacy version of Multilex software provides for label printing and stock control, and incorporates all prompts needed to maximize the chemist's income.

Multilex data are updated monthly and issued to GP system suppliers, who integrate them with their own regular system upgrades.

11.7 SAFESCRIPT (DOCTORS' INDEPENDENT NETWORK CODING)

Roger Weeks, an East Sheen GP, spent 8 years developing his World Standard Drug Database in cooperation with Dr Ivan Stockley, an eminent authority on drug interactions, together with pharmacy and computing colleagues. As a module incorporating prescription monitoring software, the database was first marketed under the name SafeScript in 1996, targeting GP system suppliers, hospitals and pharmacies. It can be integrated with all commonly used operating systems, has a Windows user interface, and links with all UK and US coded pharmaceutical ingredients. SafeScript checks and warns for indications, contraindications, side effects, toxicology and interactions, using Read code linkages. It also provides messages relating to pregnancy, lactation, and renal or liver disease.

Searches can be initiated by keyword on all drug, clinical and procedural terms, and drug attributes are accessible both textually and by electronic interaction.

11.8 PRESCRIBING SOFTWARE – THE PRESCRIBING MONITOR

Repeat prescribing was one of the earliest successful uses of the computer in practice: the function of monitoring all prescribing is proving to be one the most important uses in mature systems.

The computer that is used for all prescribing can monitor for all prescribing errors, but it must be able to access authoritative drug information, and it must access relevant data in the patient's computer record. All prescriptions must pass through the computer if the monitoring of each is to be effective. Partial information in this context is dangerously misleading, and systems that only cross-check repeat medication, because they do not automate other prescriptions, live in a fool's paradise.

In a fully developed computerized prescribing system the steps taken to construct a prescription are as follows:

1. The doctor starts to key-in the name of the drug to be prescribed. When a sufficient number of letters has been entered to render the word unique, the system completes the name. Alternatively, the doctor can enter the first two or three letters, depress a key to call a list of all those names beginning with the same few letters and select the one required.

2. The system automatically checks the name of the drug against previous patient–drug idiosyncrasies held in the patient record, against potential interactions with other current medication, against conditions shown in the patient record for which the new drug is contraindicated, and against the concurrent use of two drugs with the same action. The system can check that the condition for which the drug is to be used matches one of the drug's approved indications. Appropriate warnings are displayed if they apply. If the patient has a history of self-administered overdose, this fact is also displayed.

At this stage, the system will also warn as to the drug's legal category and take any necessary action that is consequent. A controlled drug name entered will allow details to be completed for the record but calls for the prescription to be handwritten. 'Blacklisted' drugs are not permitted, 'generic only' drugs invoke generic substitution of brand name entries, and 'ACBS' entries warn the doctor that additional justifying data will need to be supplied on the prescription. Private patients will have their prescription printed on blank paper such as the counterfoil of the FP 10 (comp) form. If the item to be prescribed would be cheaper to buy

without a prescription, given the patient's prescribing fee status and standard dosage schedules, then the system can indicate this.

3. If the drug name does not provoke warnings, the system accepts it and automatically displays a list of all formulations and strengths available under the product name. From these the doctor makes a final choice by the use of one key depression.

4. The system then suggests a treatment schedule for the product, both as regards the dosage with frequency, and the supply. If appropriate, dosage may be suggested at two alternative therapeutic levels, both of which must lie within the recommended range for the age of the patient. (The dosage schedule quoted by Multilex relates to a drug used for its commonest indication.) The supply suggested takes into account the average duration of a course of treatment, if this applies, and the quantity provided in an original pack size. The doctor has the option to accept one or other suggested schedule by a single key depression, or of overwriting and thereby changing the dosage and supply details with his/her own requirements by typing them in. If the doctor over-rides the suggested schedule, then the system checks the new dosage (quantity per 24 hours) to ensure that it lies within the recommended range for age.

5. The system adds, automatically, those further administrative instructions that are mandatory to the use of the drug. The doctor has the option to augment these if s/he so wishes.

6. The system provides the patient's surname, one forename and other initials, address, title, and age if under 12 years (details taken from the patient record). It also provides the doctor's name, address, telephone number and prescribing reference number (linked to the password he used when signing on with the system), the health authority name and address required at the foot of the prescription, and the date.

7. The doctor checks the prescription on display and, if s/he approves it, presses the print key. The details are added automatically to the medication record.

Apart from keying in the first three to five letters of the drug name, the doctor need only make two further key depressions in order to compose the prescription, and one more to print it. Computer prescriptions are constructed more rapidly and with much less effort than their conventional manual counterparts. They eliminate all known potential errors of prescribing, and produce a printed, and therefore legible, prescription that cannot be adulterated by the patient. The computer medication record for the patient is updated

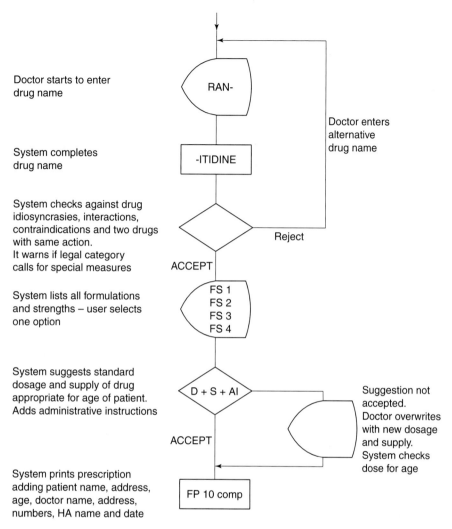

Fig. 11.3 Computerized assistance in prescribing – the prescribing monitor; the system may also check indications and suggest a suitable alternative drug

automatically. The doctor has the option of authorizing repeat issues of the prescription s/he has just entered.

Figure 11.3 shows the stages in computer-assisted prescribing.

Some practical points

If all reported drug interactions are included in the reference matrix of the database, then an overload of unsubstantiated anecdotal material will be included that cannot be considered significant from the practical standpoint. A further problem encountered in setting up the interactions matrix is that, where a possible interaction exists between the products of two

pharmaceutical companies, each company may take a differing view as to the interaction's existence and importance. These problems can only be overcome by the mediation of a nationally respected authority on drug affairs. Multilex prioritizes interaction warnings into one of four categories according to severity and significance, and the prescriber may elect not to view those that are not considered clinically significant.

When total prescribing first begins on a computer, a lead-in time of 3 months must elapse to ensure that renewal of all practice repeat medication has been recorded on the computer medication file before interactions and reduplication of action can be checked automatically. Thereafter, a decision has to be made as to how long following prescription a drug

Fig. 11.4 Acute prescribing data entry screen: In-Practice Systems' Vision system

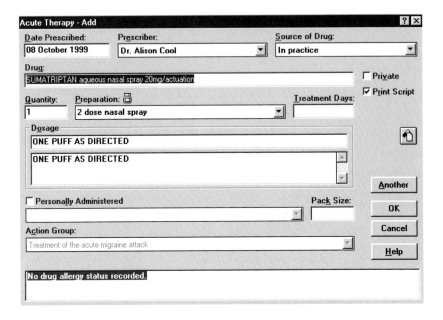

Fig. 11.5 Prescribing data entry screen: Torex Meditel's System 6000

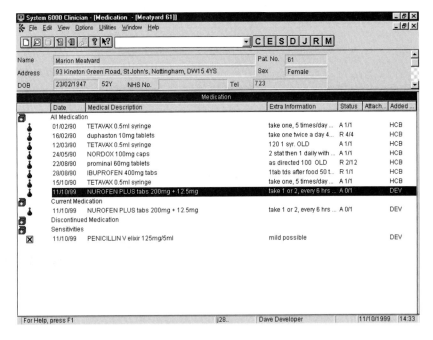

will be checked against subsequent prescriptions. Some computer systems allow this trigger period to be defined by the user. Obviously, 'current' therapy against which a new prescription must be checked will include all acute medication within its span of administration, and all repeat medication within its authorization dates. Uncertainty remains in the case of acute or repeat medication that is to be taken 'as required', the expiry date of which may be as much as 2 years from the date of issue. Another difficulty arises over drugs obtained from the pharmacy without a prescription. It would be safest to legislate that all drugs where interaction with other concomitant therapy is possible should require a prescription, but too many such products have now been deregulated. As an alternative, package inserts should be provided with all 'as required' and 'over-the-counter' products warning patients that those products should not be taken with concomitant treatment except under medical or pharmacist's advice.

Both the interactions check and the check against the use of two products with the same action occur at active ingredient level, although the prescriber will be dealing solely with product names. Dosage for age checks are usually calculated in terms of drug quantity administered in a 24-hour period. Indications and contraindications checks require standardized clinical terms, and the adoption of Read codes has been instrumental in making these checks possible. Older GP systems that had not adopted Read morbidity entry were obliged to list all contraindications, whether relevant or not, on display – a time-consuming distraction for the prescriber.

Patient instructions for drug administration

Instructions for the administration of a drug will be conveyed to the patient verbally, but there is increasing appreciation of the need to reinforce verbal advice with printed instructions. Official standards for the provision of these instructions now apply in many countries.

Printed administration instructions may be conveyed:

- on the prescription itself
- on the dispensing label (an adhesive label attached by the pharmacist to the outside of the drug container)
- on the blank right-hand side of the FP 10 (comp) prescription (the PRODIGY project expands this use of the blank by including information on the nature of the disease for which the drug is being used)

- as a package insert provided by the manufacturer (now a European legal requirement).

The Consumer Protection Act 1988

Any patient who establishes that drug treatment caused them damage can sue without having to prove negligence. If the manufacturer cannot be identified the supplier is liable, and if the supplier cannot be identified the doctor is liable. It is therefore necessary for personally administered drugs to have maker, batch number, pack size and wholesaler logged in relation to supply. Dispensing practices must log these details on all drugs supplied, and this should be done through their computer system. These details should be retained for at least 10 years.

11.9 DRUG RESPONSE REPORTING

Because each practice in the UK consists of registered patients who have contracted with their doctor for the provision of health services, defined populations are created. Only a defined population can be used as a backdrop against which occurrence of disease can be measured to give rates. Hospital populations, and patient distributions in health-care systems without registration, do not share this advantage. Assessment of the outcome of drug treatments, and of the need for other health-care resources, also depends heavily upon the consistency offered by defined practice populations. So important are these data to the surveillance of drug products by the pharmaceutical industry that the acquisition of them has, in the past, prompted the setting up of a number of expensive

---

Box 11.1   Requirements for computer-issued prescriptions (Source: BNF)

1. Date, patient's surname, one forename, other initials, address, title
2. Age if under 12 years
3. Name of doctor responsible for prescription; address, prescribing reference number, telephone number, HA
4. Drug name in full taken from drug dictionary, formulation, strength, dosage in numbers, frequency in words, supply quantity in figures between brackets. Alternatively, supply can be specified as length of treatment in days
5. All instructions for administration given in full in English. If 'when required' is instructed, maximum daily dose must be specified. Supplementary warnings to be in line with those given in BNF
6. Unused space in the prescription should be cancelled by overprinting with non-specific characters
7. The total number of items on the prescription should be specified as a numeral shown elsewhere than in the box provided for the pharmacist for this purpose
8. Handwritten amendments should not be made. It is preferable to print out a new prescription
9. Controlled drug prescriptions should not be printed
10. The prescription must be signed. Deputizing doctors must also write their name in block capitals beside their signature

computerized electronic networks with terminals in general practices.

Manual methods of drug response reporting

The principal paper-based schemes for monitoring drug responses in the UK have been:

- reports of recognized or suspected drug reactions to the Committee on Safety of Medicines ('yellow card')
- event monitoring ('green card')
- postmarketing surveillance undertaken by, or on behalf of, the pharmaceutical industry.

Each scheme has its shortcomings.

Yellow cards

The yellow card system that is used to report recognized or suspected adverse reactions to the CSM has been estimated to record a mere one-tenth of all reactions that occur. Moreover, posted reports submitted in handwriting have to be checked and transcribed on to computer prior to analysis – a manual procedure that causes delay. At the time when one offending product was withdrawn from the market, there proved to be a backlog of 4000 yellow card reports that had been received by the committee but were still awaiting analysis.

Although Prestel sets and other terminals that complete facsimiles of paper forms – the 'electronic yellow cards' – provide central agencies with computer-readable data, they do not overcome the main problems associated with yellow cards.

These are:

- the completion of a yellow card or Prestel frame requires the doctor to interrupt a busy consultation session for 5–10 minutes (the same time as it takes to see another patient). If doctors operate an appointment system they usually defer, and may then forget, the need to complete the yellow card.
- the doctor feels some diffidence in exposing to general scrutiny any possible prescribing errors s/he may have made, especially if adverse reactions have occurred, because there may then be the complication of legal liability.
- the doctor may not recognize an association between the use of a drug and an unusual adverse effect.

Event monitoring

Event monitoring was introduced in 1982 by Dr Bill Inman of the Drug Safety Research Unit in an attempt to overcome the last of the above problems. In effect, event monitoring searches prescriptions identified by

the PPA for the first-time use of a limited number of specified drugs under scrutiny and, having located them, asks the prescriber to reduplicate from the patient's medical record any event that followed the use of each drug under investigation.

In describing the term 'event' the net is cast wide, but comes to mean a subsequent record entry or series of entries to that at which the drug was first prescribed. Event monitoring claims to obtain a 50% response from general practitioners; manual processing of handwritten reports is still required, and the number of drugs scrutinized by the method is disappointingly small because of the labour involved. The drugs selected tend to be those upon which suspicion has already alighted – a policy that is both the method's strength and its weakness.

11.10 THE DATA COLLECTION SCHEMES

Paper-based recording schemes for post-marketing surveillance (PMS) of drugs in general practice began in the 1950s and were employed over four decades with varying degrees of success. Some of these schemes were thinly disguised exercises in the promotion of new products, a practice that prompted the medical profession and drug industry to join in introducing stringent guidelines for the conduct of further studies. Notable early electronic network reporting took place under a scheme launched by the University of Surrey, and also on the BARIC computer using the PRESTEL network.

In 1987 the GP system suppliers VAMP and AAH Meditel launched their 'no-cost' option schemes whereby general practitioners were offered virtually free computing services if, in return, they allowed the extraction of day-to-day anonymized prescribing and clinical data from their systems. Problems with logistics and a dearth of early data customers caused both schemes to founder in 1991, after which VAMP offered its participating practices the option to continue providing data on a profit-sharing basis – an offer for the most part accepted. Subsequently the VAMP Data Collection Agency was renamed the General Practice Research Database and it was adopted by the Department of Health. In 1999 control of the Database passed to the Medicines Control Agency, for whom it provided postlicensing drug information.

AAH Meditel participants had to buy or return their equipment, and the company ceased data collection. Some AAH Meditel participants subsequently formed the 'Doctors Independent Network' whose data were collated by Compufile on a profit-sharing basis. Other former AAH Meditel participants linked with Intercontinental Medical Statistics, a company that transferred its long-standing paper-based operations to electronic data collection and offered equipment or cash in return for data. Whereas VAMP, DIN and IMS extracted anonymized data from the electronic practice record and therefore did not make demands upon the doctor's time, a fourth agency, INCA (International Network for Clinical Assessment), requested the completion of facsimile PMS forms on the practice computer. INCA's enquiries were confined to patients on specified drugs under investigation, and replies were recorded on diskettes that were returned to the company each month, attracting cash payments. INCA was set up by the system supplier AMC (Advanced Medical Communications) in 1991.

The quality and specificity of data provided to the data collection agencies still needs further refinement, but has very considerable potential. It will be of the greatest importance for pharmaceutical companies, epidemiologists and health service management alike to have access to first-hand evidence obtained from within defined populations. For the purpose of drug assessment, data provision will need to be extended beyond the simple extraction of clinical and medication records – a method that relies on the demonstration of increased or reduced morbidity following a prescription, to indicate whether the drug has acted harmfully or beneficially.

A drug may cure a patient and at the same time cause an adverse reaction. It is important for further patient management that both types of response should be recorded in the patient notes, and both types of response are important to PMS. If an adverse reaction has occurred, it may preclude further use of the drug, and the occurrence must be noted. Cure responses are useful in guiding the doctor towards successful future treatment in recurrent conditions, and away from repeated failures.

Adverse and cure responses must of necessity be recorded at a patient attendance subsequent to the one at which the drug was prescribed, and should be prompted for by the doctor's computer system. In addition to their benefits in assisting future patient management, these recordings provide the process of centralized automatic response reporting with the data that are essential to its operation. By interrogating a combination of non-confidential demographic details, medication, morbidity, adverse and cure responses, all the requirements of the yellow card and the green card systems can be satisfied, and the principal needs of PMS can be met. Even the US Food and Drug Administration's searching Drug Experience

Report Form can be completed in all important respects by these data.

By using fully automated methods of response reporting, not only are data provided in computer-readable form but, as no separate reporting exercise is required on the part of the prescriber, information is obtained on all use of all drugs prescribed. Moreover, the doctor who has specified drugs through the use of the prescribing monitor, and may also have checked automatically their indications for use when prescribing through the computer, need fear no qualms in releasing information about his prescribing policies. He will know that mistakes in prescribing have not contributed to his patient's adverse reaction.

Automated computer response reporting highlights both those adverse reactions that the doctor attributes to drug use, and those in which s/he does not recognize an association – a combination of *ad hoc* adverse reaction reporting and event monitoring, but it does more. It is not limited to one point in time, as are manual systems, and it adds information about the success of a drug as well as its failure.

Data may be conveyed from general practice to the collating computer either on diskette or through modems and telecommunication lines. The size of the total patient population base needed to give mathematical significance to the results of analysis has been the subject of controversy between the agencies and their critics, but is of the order of at least 1 million. It will in any case vary with the incidence of disease and size of discrepancy under investigation.

11.11 CHDGP AND MIQUEST

The Collection of Health Data from General Practice (CHDGP) national project set up pilot local data collection schemes in 1997, developing MIQUEST software to provide a standard method for expressing queries and extracting anonymized data from records housed on disparate GP computer systems.

It established training methods and standards for data collection and analysis, and explores ways in which data can be used by practices, health authorities and researchers. The method will be used to support improved control of needs assessment, commissioning and purchasing, and clinical audit. Clearly, it could also be extended to include drug monitoring.

CHDGP is one of the national facilitating projects within the NHS Executive's IM&T strategy designed to enquire into the demand for, and use of, acute, community and primary health care services, and the morbidity and other relevant characteristics of local populations.

Software with a design broadly similar to that of MIQUEST is also required by Primary Health Care Groups and Trusts for the extraction of individual practice data in order to enable the audit of performance. Once again, MIQUEST software could be adapted for this purpose, but results would necessarily have to be identifiable rather than anonymous. Reports suitable for submission to HAs and the CHI need to be housed in a standard format.

MIQUEST (an acronym for 'morbidity information query and export syntax') is an NHS copyright suite of software that is able to extract data from disparate GP practice systems and export those data to off-the-shelf analysis packages such as Excel or Access. Potentially, any data lodged on the practice database can be scrutinized, though the process is facilitated if those data have already been Read-coded. However, in order to preserve confidentiality, the identification of a patient's name, address and NHS number has been disabled, the software can only extract age rather than date of birth, and only the first part of a postcode can be read. The data's practice of origin cannot be identified.

Diagnoses, previous history and all prescriptions are retrievable. The software comprises four modules – Health Query Language Editor, Query Manager and Response Manager, which are provided by the Clinical Information Consultancy (http://www.clinical-info.co.uk), and the MIQUEST Interpreter, which is provided by the individual GP system supplier (through whom the use of MIQUEST must be commissioned).

Three types of query can be initiated:

- the identification of cases given one criterion
- a count of cases given multiple criteria
- extraction of several types of information from previously selected records (Johnson et al 1999).

PCG+Ts can use MIQUEST to monitor practice adherence to policies and guidelines. Provision to incorporate MIQUEST and PRODIGY within GP systems is now a mandatory requirement for accreditation (RFA99).

11.12 WITHDRAWAL OF A MARKETED DRUG

When a marketed drug is found to have important adverse effects and is thereby banned from further use, it may suffice for the practice to bar the prescribing of further supplies, and an amendment to the drug database will ensure this. If the adverse effect is of serious immediate importance, or if the drug is one that is only taken intermittently, then it will be necessary to institute a computer search for all patients who have received the offending preparation. As this situation usually arises in relation to recently marketed preparations, and because of considerations of expiry date, record search need not extend further back than 1–2 years in most cases. Patients listed in the search must be contacted by phone or by computerized standard letter.

11.13 PRACTICE FORMULARIES AND GENERIC SUBSTITUTION

In order to minimize costs, and in dispensing practices to simplify stockholding, many practices have introduced practice formularies – shortlists of drugs to be used preferentially as a matter of practice policy. These lists may be compiled by the practice, by the system supplier, or by the local hospital or health authority. Audit has shown that reductions in prescribing costs of up to 10% are obtainable by the introduction of practice formularies, a result influenced by the predominance of generic products in the selection process.

Computer systems can be programmed to substitute the name of a preferred drug on display for any equivalent product that may be entered by the user. Similarly, a generic name may be substituted automatically when any brand product name is entered.

SOJA, a computer program model for supporting the selection of appropriate drugs to be included in a formulary, was designed by Janknegt and Steenhoek in 1997. The selection criteria used include clinical efficiency, the incidence and severity of adverse effects, and costs (Janknegt R, Steenhoek A 1997 Drugs 53: 550–562).

The electronic MIMS drug database can be downloaded to the hard disk of the practice system, and allows users to flag those drugs required for a practice or group formulary.

Four well established practice drug formularies are now in general use:

- The Grampian Formulary 1995 (a joint formulary for hospital and GP use): Drug Monitoring Unit, General Office Administration Block, Aberdeen Royal Infirmary, Forester Hill, Aberdeen AB9 2ZB. Update reference: Ferrow L, Hickey FM, Jappy B et al 1996 The Grampian Joint General Practice and Hospital Formulary – an update. Pharmaceutical Journal 257: 124–125
- Grant G B, Gregory D A, Edwards C 1994 A basic formulary for general practice. Oxford Medical

Publications, Practical Guides for General Practice. Oxford University Press, Oxford

- The Practice Formulary 1997 (4th edn) Royal College of General Practitioners, Northern Ireland Faculty, Dunluce Health Centre, 1 Dunluce Ave., Belfast BT9 7HR
- The Lothian Formulary 1992 (3rd edn) Lothian Liaison Committee, Ladywell Medical Centre, Ladywell Road, Edinburgh EH12 7TB

11.14 PRESCRIBING AUDIT

During the past 30 years, successive schemes have been devised and introduced by government to exert downward pressure on prescribing costs. Indicative prescribing budgets were renamed indicative prescribing amounts with the introduction of the 1990 contract, since when fundholding has come and gone in a costly surfeit of political new-broomery.

The advent of locality commissioning requires multiple practices to form Primary Care Groups and Trusts in a concerted attempt to implement budget restrictions. Cost control policies decreed by authority will be mediated not only by the PPA and Health Authority Pharmaceutical Advisers, but also by the National Prescribing Centre (NPC) which was set up in 1996 to encourage rational and economic prescribing.

The implications for practices are that primary care locality group protocols for prescribing have to be agreed and adhered to by individual members, and that the use of group formularies will assist in this process. Personal responsibility for cost containment requires that each prescriber has a notional amount to spend per unit of time.

The practice system can be used to audit actual expenditure in relation to a notional ceiling. Given that drug prices are already stored in the electronic drug database, it is relatively easy for ratios to be expressed as percentages where 100 represents parity.

When comparing the cost of prescriptions issued through the computer with the prescriber's notional ceiling rate, it must be remembered that, except in fully dispensing practices, up to 15% of those prescriptions issued will be unredeemed – the patient will either fail to take the prescription to the pharmacy or fail to collect the dispensed items. A corresponding adjustment must be made in practice auditing software.

In the days of indicative prescribing amounts, ceilings could be renegotiated if the practice considered that all relevant factors had not been taken into account, and similar considerations apply to group budgets. In support of this reappraisal, the practice computer could be used to identify:

- especially expensive patients and their drugs
- the impact of changes in practice policy for treatment of conditions such as asthma, migraine, shingles or hypertension
- expansion of practice activity into new forms of screening, new clinics or nursing homes
- a disproportionately large number of patients aged 45–65. Because the PPA age dynamizing factor for drug cost comparisons is not applied until old age, it discriminates unfairly against the middle-aged, in whom costs are already beginning to rise.

PACT data constitute a detailed audit of practice prescribing, and relate individual doctor and practice costs by therapeutic category to local health authority and national averages. A similar exercise can be undertaken by the practice computer, but with the additional advantage that drug use can be linked with specific diseases and patients. This means that concepts such as audit of outcome, and comparison of the cost effectiveness of alternative treatments can be investigated.

Most prescribing is related to the long-term control of chronic disease in the following subgroups:

- cardiovascular category: hypertension, angina, heart failure
- respiratory category: asthma
- alimentary category: peptic and reflux disease, bowel dysfunction
- central nervous category: psychotropics and analgesics
- musculoskeletal category: non-steroidal anti-inflammatory drugs.

There is therefore a strong economic case to be made out for prescribing the cheapest equivalent product in chronic disease. Provided that this is done, then comparisons between practice, local and national prescribing costs allow some interesting generalizations to be made. Higher than average prescribing costs in the cardiovascular and respiratory categories suggest a better quality of care in these areas, and lower prescribing costs suggest underdiagnosis of hypertension and asthma. Higher than average costs in the infections and musculoskeletal categories suggest inappropriate use of antibiotics and non-steroidal anti-inflammatory drugs respectively.

Stringent economy in prescribing tends to inhibit the use and development of new drugs, which are necessarily more expensive. Therapeutic advances involving increased drug costs therefore need to be agreed with the health authority before they are implemented in practice.

11.15 PACT AND GP ELECTRONIC PACT (GPEP)

The Prescription Pricing Authority has been costing English prescriptions since the inception of the health service. In 1988 it began to issue computer printouts to practices detailing their drug costs. These analyses avoid the discrepancy between drugs prescribed and drugs dispensed, and as such are a more accurate assessment of primary care drug expenditure than any data that can be generated at practice level (dispensing practices excepted).

However, paper-based reports that are issued quarterly suffer the obvious disadvantage that they are retrospective and cannot be used for concurrent audit in relation to restrictive practice drug budgets. In 1994, in order to overcome this disadvantage, the PPA developed software (general practice electronic PACT – GPEP) derived from PACTline, an analysis package that had originally been used by professional prescribing advisers.

The central PPA database, which accumulates details on more than 500 million prescriptions each year, is now available for enquiry by remote users through modem and NHSnet. While health authorities can examine data on all practices for whom they are responsible by using HEAPACT, general practices are restricted to their own data.

General practice access is provided by GPEP software obtainable from the PPA, which requires a minimum 486DX 66 MHz processor and 8 Mb RAM using DOS, or DOS running under Windows. The system allows analysis of PACT data by total, BNF chapter, or BNF section, and is applicable to individual prescriber or practice for comparison with local health authority and national norms (with adjustment for PU equivalence), and with previous years' figures. The number of items in each category, net ingredient cost, actual cost, total generic cost, percentage of generics prescribed, and especially expensive drugs are shown. There are five options for graphical analysis of level 3 data.

GPEP's financial analysis section shows detailed figures on performance, which include comparisons against the same month in the preceding year, expected performance against an average partner, and forecast out-turn.

In contrast to the retrospective analysis provided by paper-based PACT reports, GPEP can produce concurrent audit of costs, which can be compared with a notional ceiling limit. Although charges are made for the purchase and upkeep of GPEP software, these are in part reimbursable.

The Prescribing Information System for Scotland (PRISMS) is broadly comparable with GPEP.

11.16 OTHER COMPUTER APPLICATIONS RELEVANT TO GP PRESCRIBING

Three other computer applications associated with the use of pharmaceuticals are worthy of mention.

- The Toxicology Unit of St George's Hospital, Tooting has produced a database on CD-ROM that describes and illustrates the physical characteristics of loose tablets and capsules for the purposes of identification by health professionals. Although the CD-ROM, entitled TICTAC, is not generally available, GPs can obtain indirect access to it through regional drug information centres. A similar identification facility is also provided by e-MIMS.
- The Addicts Central Enquiry System (ACES) enables registered health professionals through ISDN to access a central server containing a database of the physical characteristics of drug addicts. In this way it is possible for networked addiction clinics to prevent addicts from obtaining prescriptions concurrently from more than one clinic.

  The database stores name, date of birth, gender, postcode, height, weight, eye colour, hair colour and records of distinguishing marks such as scars or tattoos. Where an addict shares similar characteristics with others on the database, colour photographs of all are shown on the screen (Garfoot 1998).
- Plans are being drawn up for the transmission of electronic prescriptions between GP and pharmacy, and between pharmacy and the PPA, which will in future avoid the need for the pharmacist and PPA staff to repeat those keyboard data entries that have already been performed by the prescriber. These developments will both save time and effort, and increase the accuracy of prescription processing.

The PharMed project (PharMed, Orchard House, Newton Road, Bromsgrove, Worcs B60 3EA) is already piloting trials of an encrypted, Internet-based e-mail system linking prescribers and dispensers. PharMed software integrates with existing GP clinical systems, and can also access NHSnet. The connection will be used to allow patients to request and collect repeat medication on a single visit to the pharmacy.

OTC data may be included, and with patient consent compliance could be monitored. Prescription fraud will be abolished by this system.

PharMed was established in 1997, is a non-profit-making organization and has a target date of 2002 for the implementation of its designs.

Practice Resource Systems, with their product Health Plus, are also engaged in providing GP–pharmacy networks (Pharmaceutical Journal, 1996 24 May: 718).

In the USA there is widespread use of computer systems linking dispensers with prescription pricing agencies.

SUMMARY

- Avoidable iatrogenesis is an indictment upon the medical profession and can be banished by computer. The computer makes checks on all steps involved in the prescribing process, and needs to be able to access a drug database and the patient record.
- The electronic drug database can be used to obtain visual information on all or separate attributes of a drug, and on interactions against all other drugs or another specified drug. The database provides rapid access to more appropriate and better structured information than can be obtained by manual methods.
- The database is also accessible electronically by a software prescribing package (the prescribing monitor) the function of which is to assist the entry of prescribing details that will be used to print the prescription. The prescribing monitor ensures the correct specification of the drug name, formulation, strength, dosage and supply. It checks that the choice of drug is not unsuitable for the patient in terms of known drug allergy, interaction with other medication, indications or contraindications. It also checks dosage for age and warns if two drugs with the same action are proposed. Administrative instructions, the patient's name, address, and age (if under 12 years), the doctor's name and address, telephone and prescribing numbers, the date and the Health Authority name are all added to the prescription automatically.
- Automated response recording requires doctors to enter adverse and cure responses for the drugs they have prescribed. It overcomes all defects from which manual methods suffer. Response data abstracted electronically from the patient record may be collated centrally from multiple sources.

- Prescribing audit is required to monitor practice prescribing costs in relation to a notional budget, and to assist economy in prescribing. The practice computer can offer more varied forms of prescribing audit than those provided by the Prescription Pricing Authority, but practice audit suffers from the disadvantage that it measures prescribing rather than dispensing, and so does not allow for prescriptions that are unredeemed. GPEP is a software package marketed by the PPA that allows GPs to interrogate the PPA central database for concurrent information on their own practice drug expenditure and to compare this with locality practices, national norms and previous years' figures.
- General practice computer-based data describe events in a defined population, and are therefore very valuable to epidemiologists and pharmaceutical companies. Extraction software such as MIQUEST has been developed and is being used to tap data from disparate GP systems. For broad epidemiological purposes these data will be anonymized, but for use at PCG and PCT level doctors' identities and patient NHS numbers must be verifiable.
- Practice and group formularies can be purchased 'off-the-shelf' or constructed at practice level with the assistance of purpose built software or the e-MIMS CD-ROM-based drug database. Formularies assist in reducing prescribing costs and in regularizing prescribing across a group.
- In future, electronic prescriptions will be transmitted to pharmacies and processed automatically by the PPA. Pharmacies will also benefit from software that helps them to optimize their income.

FURTHER READING

Beeley L 1976 Safer prescribing, 2nd edn. Blackwell Scientific Publications, Oxford

Caranasis G J, Stewart R B, Cluff I E 1974 Drug induced illness leading to hospitalization. Journal of the American Medical Association 228: 713

Crooks J 1981 The Committee on Safety of Medicines and the prescribing doctor. British Medical Journal 282: 385

D'Arcy P F, Griffin J P 1979 Iatrogenic diseases, 2nd edn. Oxford University Press, Oxford

Davies D M (ed) 1977 Textbook of adverse drug reactions. Oxford University Press, Oxford

Garfoot A 1998 Doctor 30 April

Head S 1992 Audit of prescribing. The art of Kaizan. Medical Monitor 13 March: 93

Johnson K, Roberts R, Wright L 1999 Prescriber 5 October: 35–44

Martys C R 1979 Adverse reactions to drugs in general practice. British Medical Journal 2: 1194

Mowat D 1992 A decade of development – a formulary and an audit. Prescriber, Feb: 5

Oxmis problem codes for primary medical care 1978 Oxford Community Health Project, Oxford

Preece J 1984 A new interaction. Practice Computing 3(2): 14

Richards D J, Rundel R K (ed) 1972 Adverse drug reactions. Churchill Livingstone, Edinburgh

Rogers J 1992 Data collection: good for GPs and their patients. Practice Computing, September: 17

Stockley I 1974 Drug interactions. Pharmaceutical Press, London

Wade O L 1970 Adverse reactions to drugs. Heinemann, London

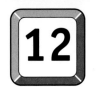 # Pathology and radiology requests, reports and records

12.1 INTRODUCTION

During the Second World War it was common practice for attacking aircraft to drop a shower of metal foil tags to thwart detection by radar. The multiplicity of signals received on the radar screen caused confusion, an effect similar to the 'white-out' experienced by mountaineers in heavy snowstorms. The principle has since been used in anti-missile defence.

Since the inception of the UK National Health Service, the throughput of pathology departments has increased to an extent several fold greater than that experienced by other service areas. A demand for tests that used to be met by a handful of staff working in one room now calls for manpower, premises and funding 20 times as great. Each test on each patient is reported on a separate document, and the plethora of reports of varying shape and size that has to be accommodated in the disorderly manual record wallet confounds retrieval. There are too many reports and, at consultation, too little time to unfold, sort and search through them when all we may be seeking is a single test result. We have been foiled.

12.2 MANUAL PROCEDURES AND THEIR PROBLEMS

- Using manual procedures, GPs do not make the most effective use of pathology investigations. In January 1991 the Audit Commission reviewed the £330 million spent during the previous year on NHS pathology services, and reported to government. It concluded that there was a very large disparity in the use made of those services by individual GPs, and that no correlation between laboratory usage and primary care disease detection could be demonstrated. The commission strongly recommended that protocols should be developed and used to refine the selection of tests requisitioned.

- The conventional procedure for requesting and reporting on a pathology test usually employs a combined request-report document (a 'turn-around' form) with one or more copies. Both the specimen label and the request section of the form are handwritten, and their contents may prove incomplete, misleading or illegible. Patient details have to be copied out from the clinical notes.

- All specimens and request forms have to be checked for correlation on leaving the practice and on arriving at the pathology laboratory.

- When processed at the laboratory, all specimens are given a new identity code and have to be decanted from the conveying container to a test container. If more than one test is required, then the specimen may have to be split into multiple containers. Specimen handling incurs contamination risks for laboratory staff.

- Reports have to be married with the request form, which now becomes a combined request and report. The day's reports for each practice must be collated and posted. It is not unusual for individual reports, and even the whole day's reports, to be sent to the wrong practice. Turn-around and postage will incur between 1 and 3 days' delay.

- Incoming reports received each day by the practice must be viewed by the doctor who requisitioned the tests. Reports must be compared with normal values, which the doctor may remember or may have to look up. Report forms are often endorsed at the practice with the action that the GP requires to be taken, but confirmation of whether this action has been taken is often lacking. Especially significant reports are often retained on the doctor's desk to ensure that they are not overlooked, should the patient fail to enquire for them. However, until reports are filed in the manual record wallets, the receptionist is frustrated in searching for them when attempting to respond to patients' enquiries as to whether they have been received. If the doctor must answer the patient's queries in person, then s/he often needs to refer to clinical notes as well as the test result.

Doctors who are temporarily absent from the practice must either arrest the filing procedure, and thereby disrupt the use of records, or else lose track of pathology reports received during their absence.

Many practices keep aside from the normal filing process those test results that are used solely as a guide to drug dosage. Prothrombin times, blood counts used to monitor penicillamine or chlorambucil treatment, and lithium levels are often discarded after a suitable interval.

- When the reports are filed in the patient record wallets, problems of identification arise with common surnames and this may cause misplacement.
- No facility for the graphical display of serial test results is available, and there is no provision for enhancing the significance of test results by incorporating other variables in their interpretation.
- Form printing, mail handling and postage all incur expenses that can be considerably reduced by electronification.

12.3 REFORM OF THE SELECTION/REQUEST/TEST/REPORT/AUTOFILE CYCLE

Data exchange between general practice and pathology laboratory is currently undergoing extensive reform, in which electronification plays a key part. However, accurate planning for data processing cannot be achieved without fundamental redesign of all the components of the selection, request, test, report and autofile cycle. The principal requirements for redesign and modernization are:

- electronic requesting, with autoassisted entry of data
- electronic reporting, with autofiling of data
- the introduction of a unique identifier, which follows both the specimen and the request/report throughout the whole cycle
- increased automation in the laboratory, with reduction or elimination of the risk of contamination of personnel
- decision support in the selection of tests requisitioned, and in their interpretation
- audit of process, outcome and costs.

The emergence of new cost-effective near-patient testing procedures will also have an impact upon the GP's interchange with the laboratory.

We must now examine these features in greater detail, and it is appropriate to consider them in the order that they occupy in the cycle.

Protocols for test selection

Protocols codify expertise, and can be applied to the selection of appropriate pathology tests in a given situation just as well as they can to other forms of patient management. Unlike paper-based protocols, computerized protocols can be consulted rapidly, discreetly, and in either broad or fine detail in the presence of the patient. Only the hierarchical node of immediate relevance to the decision in hand need be exhibited. Computerized protocols can be readily updated and expanded from diskette or e-mail upgrades, and can be inverted for teaching purposes. Protocols can be trimmed to suit the user's level of expertise.

Test selection protocols proceed from the input of Read-coded clinical presentations, recommend useful tests and the way specimens should be taken, stored and transported, and support results with interpretative data and any recommendations for secondary tests. Protocols were initially constructed for hyperlipidaemia, diabetes, thyroid function and prostate-specific antigen tests (Batstone 1991) but have since been expanded to cover the majority of biochemical, immunological and haematological procedures. Many laboratories provide handbooks in diskette format with details of test selection (Ryan 1992).

Protocols reduce the number of unnecessary tests requested, thus saving laboratory costs, staff time and resources. They refine the process of investigation so that faster and more accurate diagnoses may be made.

Test selection protocols will constitute a section of the protocol library which all GP systems will house, and which will be regularly updated.

Printing the specimen label and request form

Various approaches to the printing of the specimen label and request form by computer have been attempted. These include printing the label and request separately, or adding the request details to the specimen label. The advantages of computer printing are that details are not omitted, that they are legible, and that most can be taken directly from data already stored on the practice computer.

Currently, on reaching the laboratory, both label and form are invariably given a fresh identity, which is usually a serial number determined by the order of receipt of the specimen during a particular 24-hour period. It would be much simpler for the practice to print a unique identifier for the specimen label, and thus avoid the need for the laboratory to re-identify the sample. The extent to which decanting the specimen from a transportable to a separate test container can be avoided is of course dictated by the design of equipment, and the frequency with which multiple tests must be performed on the same sample. However, increasing automation within the laboratory will lead to less direct handling by laboratory personnel and increase the importance of the unique identifier.

The unique identifier could with advantage be a bar code, printed on a self-adhesive label by the practice computer, that incorporates the practice identity, the patient's new NHS number and a serial number signifying the ranking of the specimen taken from the particular patient on a particular day. If the laboratory divides the sample for multiple tests, then further digits could be added, otherwise the identifier would suffice for the complete request/test/ report/autofile cycle.

The electronic request form would also carry the unique identifier, but in addition bear the following uncoded data:

- doctor's name, practice name
- patient's names, address, whether high risk of cross-infection
- patient date of birth, gender
- specimen type, test required
- Read-coded presentation, current pharmaco-therapy
- time, date.

All data can be provided automatically from information already available on the system, with the exception of the nature of the specimen and test required, which can be selected from a picking list (and in future from a default option embedded in the test selection protocol). It is no longer necessary for the requesting doctor to sign requests, as his password has already controlled access to the system. Although requests will usually be transmitted electronically, the option exists to print them and enclose them with the specimen.

The above data categories must be regarded as a minimum data set for test requisitions, which can be expanded to include other data available on the practice system, if the laboratory so wishes.

Testing, and the availability of results

The specimen is conveyed to the laboratory by courier as one of a batch, and tested. Read-coded results are married up with the request data, which have already been stored on the laboratory computer, and which are located through the unique identifier. The results of all tests undertaken on the practice's behalf during the 24 hours are stored in the laboratory server as a batch and transmitted to the practice mailbox in time for the nightly download.

Urgent requests can be interrogated on the laboratory server from the practice system using the unique identifier. All tests undertaken for the practice on the same patient on the same day can be interrogated on the laboratory server by using the date and the first two components of the unique identifier (practice identity and patient new NHS number). Given appropriate safeguards, it should also be possible for other authorized health professionals such as hospital staff to access all previous tests undertaken on an individual patient, using the patient's new NHS number.

Processing results at the practice

Each night, automatic dial-up to the practice's mailbox results in downloaded reports being stored on the practice server to await viewing. On the practice system, results for the previous 24-hour period can now be accessed, either as those requested by an individual doctor or those for the whole practice. Within either of these modes of access, results are classified by test. Under each test heading normal reference values are shown, then lists of patients divided by their results into normal and abnormal. Results can also be interrogated as all tests pertaining to a particular patient on the day in question. As any number of practice staff can access report data simultaneously through individual VDUs, results once received by the practice are permanently available and never misplaced.

Each doctor checks the results of the tests s/he requisitioned and appends an action indicator which determines whether, as a result of the report, the patient should be instructed that no further action is needed, a prescription should be collected from the medical centre, an appointment should be made to see the doctor or nurse, or direct advice should be provided over the phone by the doctor. When the patient phones and receives the recommended instruction, the fact of receipt is also recorded beside the result. After the passage of several days, a computer search will reveal those patients who have not contacted the medical centre for their results, and a decision can then be made as to whether further action should be taken. When the processing of results by practice staff has been completed, tests need no longer be viewed in the mode of the day's batch.

Storing results in the practice files

Using the unique identifier, results are also autofiled by the computer within individual patient clinical records, and here it is useful to consider the economies that can be made in the volume of data presented to the doctor who wishes to review historical pathology records.

- Compaction in the manner of presentation of results is required – synoptic recording. When certain types of test are reported, particularly the more complex type of report, compaction can be obtained by the use of a simple convention. Results of urine tests, full blood counts or 12-channel biochemistry, for instance, can be quoted as all normal, if this is the case, or as those results that are abnormal. When this convention is used, it is to be understood that those results not specified as abnormal have nevertheless been tested and are normal (e.g. differential white count: monocytes 20%, Turk cells 3%). Synoptic recording is not required in tests whose results are quoted as simple numerals, and the method does not bar the storage of the full pathology report in another area of the patient record if elaboration is required.
- Practices may also have an agreed policy of archiving certain categories of pathology report so that they are not routinely presented on historical review. The last normal test should be retained, but previous normals may be relegated. All abnormals need to be retained.

- Within the patient record the pathology section is subdivided by test, and under each test heading normal values are quoted for reference. Reports are then listed by date and result, and are stacked in reverse chronological order so that the latest result, which is most frequently required, is most easily accessed. Because the computer rearranges pre-existing text in context around a new entry, there is no problem of space allocation in anticipation of further record entries such as obtains on paper. The pathology record on computer remains compact. Extensions to the screen are accommodated by scrolling upwards.
Some subdivisions of the pathology record are held in common with the preventive medicine record – cervical cytology and triglycerides, for example.
- Results can be enhanced by computer. The compaction achieved by synoptic reporting and computer insertion have already been mentioned. Abnormal results can be highlighted by the use of double-intensity characters, underlinings, colour coding, or the use of black characters on a white background when most of the display shows white on black ('reverse video').
- Result significance can be enhanced by referring to previous results in the same patient. Thus a result that is only just outside the normal range may represent a marked swing from a former result in the individual concerned – a fact that changes its interpretation. Similarly some tests, such as thyroxine and TSH, enhance each other's results.

Fig. 12.1 Incoming pathology test results listed for processing on receipt by practice, prior to autofiling in patient records: In-Practice pathology screen

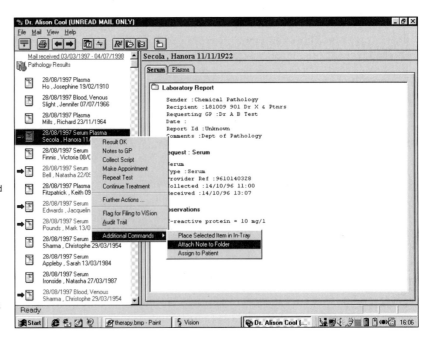

- Pathology messages will be posted to the requesting GP by the system and are automatically matched to the patient record
- Messages can be selected by date, view status and message type
- Individual messages can be selected from a summary list and the full contents displayed
- Comments may be added to each result
- During a consultation the patient's pathology results can be directly accessed from the transaction prompt
- Abnormal result lines are highlighted
- Mail forwarding and copying assists in mail management

Fig. 12.2 Multifactorial analysis. The mutual support given by the results of a series of different tests enhances probability in diagnosis (Courtesy of Dr P D Welsby, City Hospital, Edinburgh)

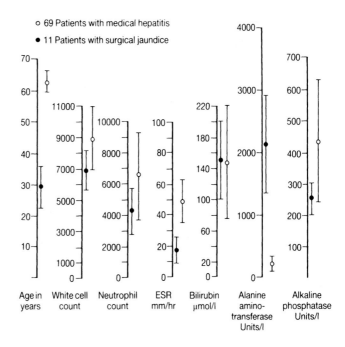

○ 69 Patients with medical hepatitis

● 11 Patients with surgical jaundice

The calculations involved in these comparisons can be both effected and demonstrated by computer (Fig. 12.2). Another calculation that can be made is to convert a numerical result into units of standard deviation – an expression of the degree of swing of abnormality away from the norm.

- Serial numerical results may be displayed by graph or histogram, a method of particular value where two variables other than time are involved – e.g. phenytoin levels, dosage and the incidence of convulsions; or prothrombin times and anticoagulant dosage. Such displays are really surveillance screens and carry implications for repeat medication.

12.4   DOES ELECTRONIFICATION REALLY HELP?

It is fair to conclude that manual routines for requesting pathology tests, transmitting specimens, and receiving results are poorly targeted, error prone, dilatory, labour intensive, and carry risks of contamination. It is therefore disappointing to note Dr Jonathan Kay's conclusions, reached in 1995 after 5 years' experience with computerized pathology reporting in Oxford, that no savings in administrative time had been achieved and that, in any case, speedier reporting was of doubtful advantage because GPs seldom read test reports immediately (Pulse, 4 November 1995).

A Netherlands study reported in 1992 was somewhat more encouraging, in that, although it concurred that few (33%) doctors read their e-mail pathology reports within 8 hours (and some took more than 48 hours to do so), report delivery time was reduced from upwards of 4 days to 1 day, and the error rate for entering tests into GP notes was reduced from 0.5% to zero (Branger et al 1992).

Further studies of benefit and cost are required before final conclusions can be drawn, but such studies cannot be undertaken until all the reforms listed in Section 12.3 have been introduced.

12.5   AUDIT

In as much as it constitutes one form of patient management, the techniques and objectives of process audit are applicable to the use of pathology tests. Practices may wish to check how many of their diabetic patients had glycated haemoglobin estimates within the previous 12 months, or the proportion of patients on ACE inhibitors who had urea and electrolyte estimations within a given period.

Outcome audit can also be employed in order to determine the effectiveness of policies such as anticoagulant INR estimations in preventing embolic sequelae, or thyroid function tests in assaying the control of thyrotoxicosis.

The appropriateness of use of pathology services made by individual doctors can be assessed in relation to the number of newly diagnosed cases for which they are responsible, and the results can be compared with peer performance. In the past, this exercise has enabled improvements in requisitioning to be made.

As test procedures can be accurately costed, audit of the practice's laboratory costs became a feature of fundholding, and is of comparable importance in locality commissioning.

12.6 OTHER COMPUTER FACILITIES LINKED TO THE PATHOLOGY RECORD

What further facilities may we find linked to the pathology record in future?

- Indicators may be used in the clinical record in relation to episodes of disease to show that pathology investigations have been carried out, and these will be summoned for viewing by hypertext linkage.
- Schedules may be prepared automatically for certain treatments, such as intramuscular iron injections based on haemoglobin or serum iron levels, with the computer prompting for the entry of the body weight value.
- Some screening schedules may be based on the pathology record – biochemical screening for the middle-aged or elderly, and urinary glucose in diabetic families. Cervical smear clinics are operational at an early stage in computer use.
- Surveillance of established disease such as blood dyscrasias, pernicious anaemia, post-gastrectomy anaemia, menorrhagia, and past thyroid surgery or irradiation, may all be linked to the pathology record and will be monitored by using a surveillance format.
- Research requiring epidemiological or workload statistics in general practice will often access pathology results. The numerical units in which many tests are recorded make search and evaluation of data a more straightforward task than is the case with language. The computer's in-built arithmetic functions are a further advantage in this field.
- Billing in relation to pathology procedures is required for private practice and in some health services in other countries.

12.7 GP–PATHOLOGY LINKS

Professor F V Flynn of University College Hospital, London pioneered the provision of electronic pathology reports to general practice in 1982, and Dr Jonathan Kay's seminal work at Oxford in supplying 50 practices with e-reports in the early 1990s provided the pattern for the technology adopted by 100 laboratories during that decade. Other pioneering projects were undertaken at Kettering and at Sandwell.

Ryan (1992) and Peters of the Wolfson computer laboratory designed early protocols for the selection of tests by GPs.

GP–Pathology Links began at Oxford in 1991, used Avon as a trailblazer site in 1996, and is now being rolled out to all computerized practices in the UK. Messages are sent using EDIFACT and X400 (88) communication standards. GP suppliers, in conjunction with Racal HealthLink, are responsible for establishing the necessary software for, and connections between, practices and laboratories. Services, for which there are itemized charges, include:

- registration with Racal
- the provision and rental of a mailbox
- carrier usage (charges for which are related to time spent on the network, the volume of traffic, and storage for any information not downloaded from the mailbox within 24 hours)
- Pathology Links modular software
- communications software
- installation
- training
- support line provision
- a modem
- a bar code printer (where the laboratory accepts bar code input).

BT Syntegra has also contracted to provide Pathology Links and other network services, and uses a more sophisticated technology, access to which requires an upgrade in GP system software.

Comprehensive pathology computer systems, such as Bayer LMX, are now operational. These coordinate all the laboratory's input, assay and output data, report direct to hospital wards, and report to GP practices through HealthLink and the GP's system.

12.8 RADIOLOGY

Computerized management of the selection/request/test/report/autofile cycle for open access radiology is closely similar to that used for pathology, except that no specimen and no courier service are involved. Instead, the patient must be given an appointment to attend the Radiology Department, and this appointment can be allocated at the time that the request is received electronically by the department. It is, of course, adroit to transmit the request while the patient is still in the GP's consulting room, so that the patient can confirm that the time and date of the appointment will prove convenient.

The factors upon which effective computerization depends are as follows:

- A central fileserver is set up in the radiology department to accommodate patient radiology records. The unique identifier used to access these records is the new NHS number augmented by extra digits which identify the client practice, and the ranking of all radiological investigations requested for the individual patient on an individual day.
- Protocols that assist the GP in selecting investigations may be used, such as those pioneered by Wirral Hospital NHS Trust (1996).
- The electronic request form includes: the doctor's name and practice name; patient names, address, date of birth and gender; Read-coded presentation, investigation requested, and time and date of request.
- The patient is issued with an appointment.
- The investigation is carried out and the Read-coded report transmitted via the practice mailbox. *Ad hoc* interrogation of the Radiology Department server may be made with authorized access; and by use of the patient's new NHS number.
- The day's incoming reports are viewed on the GP computer, with the responsible doctor appending 'action required' instructions, and the secretary flagging the report as and when the patient has enquired and has been appropriately instructed. Each day's reports are retained as a batch for 2 weeks, after which the reports of patients who have failed to enquire are considered for further action.
- All reports are autofiled in the appropriate patient records. It is common practice for newly received reports to be kept in a prominent position within the computer record for a limited period.
- Audit of process, outcome and costs may be undertaken.

SUMMARY

- The multiplicity and disorderly storage of pathology test results in the general practice manual record wallet bedevil the search for an individual report.
- Conventional postage is slow, and manual procedures for the transmission of samples, collation of reports in the laboratory, and assimilation and filing of results in practice are labour-intensive, expensive, error prone and subject to delay.
- The implementation of computers by pathology laboratories and general practices, together with communication technology, has the potential to correct all the defects of the manual procedures and also to offer enhancement of data presentation.
- Test requesting on computer merely requires the selection of a test from an option list or the depression of a confirmation key when viewing a selection protocol. All other details will be entered automatically by the computer.
- Practices seldom condense manual pathology results on to summary cards, nor, as a rule, do they take-on old results when computerizing records, and the transition to electronic mail will find general practitioners unprepared for the design changes required. Careful system planning, and liaison with laboratories are needed.
- Simultaneous viewing by different users, presentation of data in alternative formats, result enhancement, automatic filing of results within the patient record, and control of patient default are all bonuses to be added to the greater efficiency obtained when pathology results are reported by computer.
- Protocols refine the process of investigation and eliminate wasted tests.
- The key to successful use of electronic services in the cycle of selection, requesting, testing, reporting and autofiling is the adoption of a unique identifier, which will be allocated automatically by the practice computer, will avoid re-labelling by the laboratory, and will enable GPs and other authorized health professionals to interrogate the central pathology department server with precision.
- The same container should be used for collection and testing of samples wherever possible and, when decanting is required, mechanical methods should be used in order to reduce the possibility of contamination of laboratory staff.
- Radiological investigations also involve a cycle of selection, requesting, testing, reporting and autofiling, but do not require courier services nor the use of bar codes. Appointments for radiology should be made electronically by the GP in the presence of the patient.

FURTHER READING

Batstone C 1991 Pulse 20 April: 12

Branger P J et al 1992 Electronic communication between providers of primary and secondary care. British Medical Journal 305: 1068–1070

Brumfitt W, Hamilton-Miller J M T 1986 The appropriate use of diagnostic services. Investigation of urinary infections in general practices: are we wasting facilities? Health Trends 18: 57

Flynn F V, Ball S G 1982 Comprehensive computerised data management in a chemical pathology laboratory with *SOCRATES*. Medical Informatics 7(4): 275

Goldman L 1979 The unreliability of 'reliable' laboratory tests. Doctor, February 22: 23

Healthcare I/T Effectiveness Awards 1996 Wirral Hospital NHS Trust. Incorporating radiology guidelines into doctor ordering pathways. Computer Software and Services Association Press Release London WC1V 6LE March 96 RW + NB

Houghton M 1998 Prescriber, May: 47

Meson I 1981 Haematology in the 1980s. Pulse, June 6: 45

Ryan M 1992 Breaking down the barriers between the path lab and GP. Practice Computing, September: 24

Whitehead P 1983 Which test to request? Medical Digest, March: 28

13 Appointments

13.1 OVERVIEW

The word 'patient' derives from the Latin for 'to suffer' (*pati*), and implies an element of endurance, a necessary virtue for those waiting to see a general practitioner prior to the 1950s, when surgeries universally operated on a 'first come first served' basis.

Appointment systems are now used by the great majority of UK practices and bring the following demonstrable advantages:

- a reduction in patient waiting times
- fewer home visits
- freedom for the doctor to buffer surges in demand
- less risk of cross-infection between waiting patients
- a reduction in the area needed to accommodate waiting patients.

There are also disadvantages. These are:

- longer delays between the patient's decision to seek advice and his opportunity to do so; this disadvantage can be largely offset by 'block' booking arrangements whereby long-term forward appointments are interspersed with vacancies for last minute acute demand
- the practice must accept a large number of extra incoming telephone calls which require extra staff time and, often, a dedicated line
- patients without access to telephones are placed at a disadvantage.

13.2 ADVANTAGES OF COMPUTERIZATION OF APPOINTMENT SYSTEMS

British GPs were slow to adopt, and adapt to, computerized appointment systems, largely because early software-driven appointment-making in US practices had been shown to take twice as long as its manual counterpart, and because system failure, a not infrequent occurrence in those days, caused havoc.

However, during the last 15 years, pioneering work by AMC, Informatica (Front Desk Pro) and Phenix system developers has set the standard, and the appointment module is now a cornerstone of all major GP systems. Improvements in software flexibility and refinement now deliver an electronic appointment-making process that is not only more expedite and accurate than its paper-based alternative, but to which can be added bonus features. Principally these are as follows:

- Appointments can be made from any site that has a terminal.
- The appointing patient's identity can be verified with reference to registration details held on the practice system. This ensures that the patient is registered with the practice, that the correct name is entered on the appointment list, and that the correct record will subsequently be accessed. The starting point for an interrogation of the registration files may be patient surname, previous name, forenames, date of birth, NHS number or post code.
- If electronic patient records are used in conjunction with an electronic appointment system, the doctor need employ only one key depression to toggle between the patient's name on the consultation list and the individual patient record.
- The throughput of attending patients can be assisted. The colour coding of the background of the appointment slot on the consultation list can be changed as the patient checks in with reception, and as the doctor toggles between consultation list and patient record. This will enable system users to determine whether the patient has arrived at the medical centre, has entered the consultation room, or has left the consultation room.

Fig. 13.4 Appointments – 'receptionist's view': Global Clinical System (Aremis Soft Healthcare)

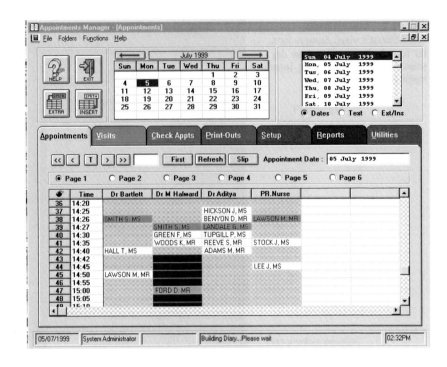

provided to allow a 1-, 2-, 3-, 4-, 8- or 12-week shift in date in either direction.

Slots show list-holder times and patient names, to which a variable number of other data categories can be linked. These will include address, post code, date of birth, date of making appointment, reason for making appointment, the name of the person making the appointment and the method of request used. These additional details are held in the background, and are only entered or displayed by use of a superimposed 'added detail window' which is summoned to appear on the screen as required.

Slot list screens are configured either to show one session for one list-holder (for use by the health professional), several consecutive sessions for one list-holder, or parallel sessions held on the same day by several list-holders (for use by the receptionist). Each view is summoned by its own dedicated command and can be browsed by any or all users simultaneously, although lists can only be written to by one user at a time.

D. Appointments can be made while browsing session lists, or can be selected by a program that summons the next available slot selected so as to accord with one or more of the following criteria:

- a specified list-holder
- any list-holder

- a morning or an evening consultation
- a specified date
- a specified day of the week or time of day.

Individual appointments already made can be checked by date, time or name, and changed or cancelled. All appointments in a session can be changed, and notification can be sent by automated mailmerged letters.

A macro-driven facility exists to allow a doctor to re-appoint a patient at the end of a consultation merely by specifying the required latent interval. When a patient needs to see two health professionals synchronously, the appointments can be automatically juxtaposed.

E. Opportunistic reminders, which are made available to reception staff when the patient checks in, prompt for the completion of temporary resident or maternity claims, or for any outstanding personal details required on the record. They also bring to attention any health promotion or immunization procedures that are due or overdue.

F. Appointment slips or cards can be printed automatically for re-appointed patients or those requesting an appointment in person.

G. Lists of defaulters can be compiled, and if the reasons for the appointments have been added to slot details, these can be quoted in order to enable staff to determine whether further action should be taken.

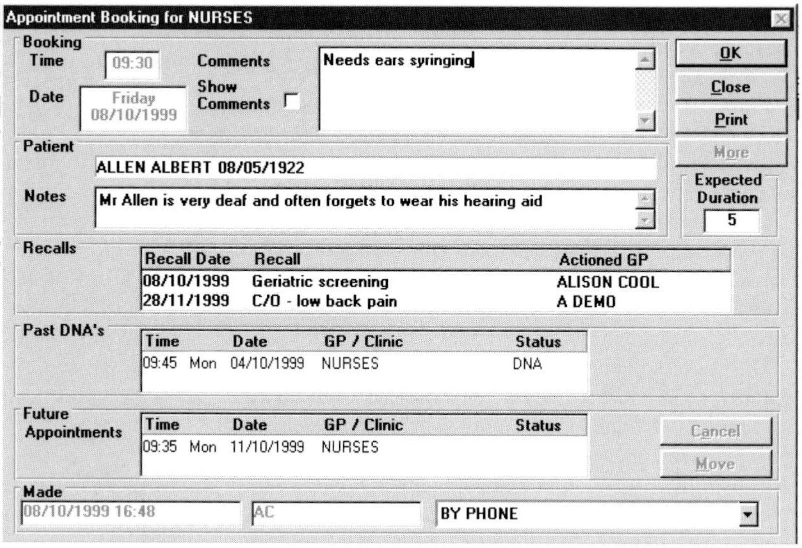

Fig. 13.5 Booking form for individual appointment: In-Practice Systems

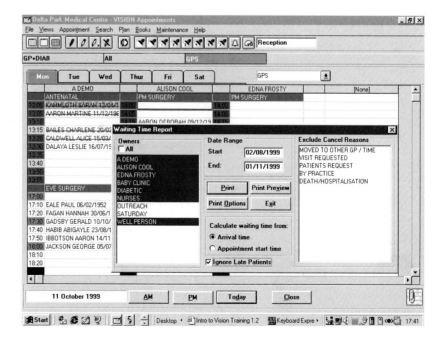

13.4 FURTHER CONSIDERATIONS

A. Some practices have found it useful to install a large-screen colour monitor at the desk of the receptionist who is primarily concerned with telephone appointment-making. Because computerization allows relocation of this staff member from the front desk to an independent office, the work will be free from background noise and other distractions. Correspondingly, pressure on the front desk will be relieved.

B. The patient-summoning LED display located in the waiting area shows the summoned patient's name,

and the consulting doctor's name and room number. The summoning message is triggered by the toggle action by which the doctor selects the next patient from the current consultation list. When not used for calling the next patient, displays can carry health promotional or other practice initiated messages, which have been recorded by the software provided with the display and housed on the practice server.

Messages provided on the LED display marketed by Jayex Technology Ltd (21 Wadsworth Business Centre, Wadsworth Road, Perivale, Middlesex UB6 7LQ) are shown in characters of either 30 mm height,

Fig. 13.6 Setting up an appointment waiting time audit: In-Practice Systems

visible up to 8 m, or 50 mm height, visible up to 25 m. Two lines of up to 30 characters per line are exhibited. The display is usually mounted above head height and is visible from widely oblique angles. An audio signal alerts patients to a change of message. Messages persist for 120 seconds, and the software queues messages that overlap.

C. In a similar manner to consultation lists, visiting lists can be prepared and printed out on the system. Theoretically these could be defined by doctor or by geographical area. Printout can be ordered alphabetically for support in pulling manual records.

D. Help screens are available, and training in system use is usually provided. Whereas list-holders can familiarize themselves rapidly with their own use of the system, each member of reception staff whose responsibility includes setting up templates requires up to 24 hours of training. When a practice inaugurates computerized appointments, it is wise to confine data to those of a single list-holder until all staff have become fully conversant with the use of the system.

E. Daily backup is essential, both to diskette and as printout that downloads data for the following 3 days.

The contents of diskette-based backup should be checked weekly for integrity.

F. Audit can be undertaken on:

- *bookings*: when appointments are made; whether appointments are made by phone, in person or by re-appointment; the number and pattern of appointments; default rate
- *consultations*: the numbers, time, distribution and duration of consultations, showing values for the longest, shortest and average, by list-holder and by practice
- *waiting times*: lapses between booking and attendance, and between attendance and consultation.

Campbell and his co-workers (1996) compared their appointments procedures before and after computerization. They found that the times required to make appointments either by telephone or in person were reduced. The time taken for the check-in process itself was unchanged, but the times spent by the patient queuing for check-in and appointment making were both reduced.

Fig. 13.7 Appointments – 'receptionist's view': new GPASS system

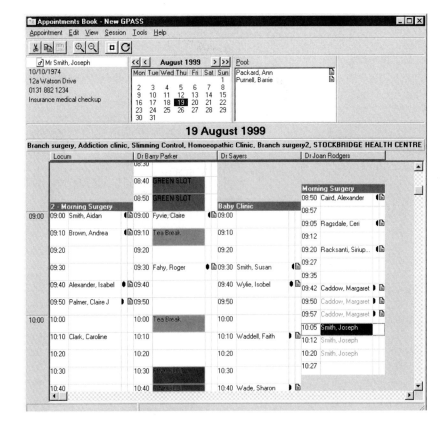

G. A graphical representation is available on some systems to display the pattern of the uptake of appointments and the workload of each list-holder.

SUMMARY

- GP appointments reduce waiting times, reduce home visits, reduce the area required for patients awaiting consultation, reduce the risk of cross-infection, and enable the doctor to buffer surges in demand. They may, however, extend the time that elapses between the application for, and provision of access to, the doctor. They increase the number of telephone calls to a practice and disadvantage patients who do not have a telephone.

- Templates must be set up that will mould computerized appointment schedules to the pattern of work in a practice, and due allowance must be made for holidays. In an operational system, there are two principal forms of presentation – the 'health professional's view', which shows all appointments for one list-holder for one or more sessions, and the 'receptionist's view', which shows appointments for several list-holders simultaneously on the same screen.

- Appointments can be allocated when browsing successive lists, or by a program that searches for the next available slot in accordance with criteria specified by the user

- Patients' identities can be checked accurately against the practice's database when they apply for an appointment. Appointments can be made from any terminal on the system. Appointment slips or cards can be printed out, and visiting lists compiled using slots in a similar manner to that used for appointments.

- Appointment slots are colour-coded to signify whether the patient has arrived at the medical centre, has arrived in the consulting room, or has left the consulting room. On the doctor's screen, clicking on a patient's appointment slot serves to call up the patient record and light up an LED display to summon the patient from the waiting area, whereas refiling the electronic patient record causes the appointment list to be re-presented in its newly amended form.

- The changes in patient location logged on the system can be time-and-date-stamped to allow comprehensive auditing of the appointment process. Lists of defaulters to appointments can be compiled, and additional data that may be contained on the system in relation to an appointment will allow judgement to be made as to whether further action should be taken.

- Opportunistic reminders in relation to appointment slots give the system the power to prompt receptionists to enquire after missing patient data, or to suggest action for procedures due or overdue.

FURTHER READING

Becan J M, Draper G T 1967 Appointment systems in general practice. Oxford University Press, London

Bickler C B 1985 Defaulted appointments in general practice. Journal of the Royal College of General Practitioners, January: 19

Campbell S M, Rowland M O, Gormanly B 1996 Evaluation of a computerized appointment system in general practice. British Journal of General Practice 46: 477–478

Grabinar J 1981 Appointment systems – are they worthwhile? Update 1 October: 941

Maclean D W 1972 An appointments system in trouble. Update, April: 1021

Marshall E 1986 Appointment systems cut back surgery delays. Medeconomics, September: 69

Oberst B B, Long J M 1987 Computers in private practice management. Springer Verlag, New York: 84

Preece J F 1972 Applications for the computer file in general practice. Update, July: 155

Ridsdill-Smith R 1982 Medeconomics, February: 42

14 GP–provider linkages 1: transactions initiated from general practice

14.1 INTRODUCTION

The interchanges of data between general practice and hospital outpatient or inpatient departments are considerably more complex than those required by the GP–HA, GP–Pathology and GP–Radiology linkages that have been considered in previous chapters. This is because a greater number of intermediary steps is usually involved in the request–test–report cycle, and because of the overburden of free text in hospital-generated data which has to be condensed, usually in two separate stages, before it can be Read-code-assimilated into GP computer records. Hospital outpatient and hospital inpatient notes are both voluminous when initially recorded, and have to be summarized in order that a more concise report to general practice can be formulated. This more concise report itself must then be further abstracted so that relevant keywords and key phrases can be matched exactly with terms in the Read classification for inclusion in the GP record as summary history statements.

Data interchange is, of course, a two-way process and, as with the linkages we have previously considered, requires the use of compliant systems at each end of the transaction, data entry templates, communications software, modems, mailbox, the use of the standard messaging conventions UN/EDIFACT and X400/88, encryption, and the services of a carrier such as Racal HealthLink or BT NHSnet.

The transactions we must consider in relation to GP–provider communications are listed in Box 14.1. Seamless shared care is vitally dependent upon their quality and timeliness. Those initiated from general practice will be dealt with in this chapter and those initiated from hospital will be detailed in Chapter 15.

The following facilities are in the process of development and implementation.

14.2 GP INTERROGATION OF ADMINISTRATIVE HOSPITAL DATA

Waiting list volumes and deferral periods for all hospital inpatient and outpatient department appointments can be inspected through on-line access to a database stored on the provider's server. An electronic 'notice-board' is also accessible, which details those hospital services that are available, together with their costs, clinic times and any further trust activities. One trust has made clinical guidelines available on line (Fountain Project 1996). The so-called 'Pink Book' is an electronic handbook which combines data on local services with the facility for

---

Box 14.1 GP–provider transactions

Initiated from general practice
- View waiting list volumes and delays, view costings; view the 'Pink Book'
- Outpatient bookings
- Day-case surgery bookings
- Patient transport requests
- Referral letters
- E-mail
- Pathology tests
- Radiology investigations

Initiated from hospital
- Notification of discharge
- Full inpatient reports on discharge
- A&E reports
- Outpatients attendance reports
- Subsequent referrals
- Notification of admissions to, and deaths in, hospital
- Interim inpatient report
- Contract invoices
- E-mail

printing out patient information leaflets, so that GPs may provide patients with explanatory details of specific diseases and their treatments.

In 1996, the Wirral Hospitals NHS Trust 'Pathfinder Project' provided 22 GPs with notebook computers which enabled them to use hypertext electronic books and browsers in order to access locally constructed patient management and referral guidelines. In 44% of cases this information led to modifications in clinical practice, and in 26% referral practice was changed (Pathfinder Project 1996).

14.3 ON-LINE BOOKING FOR DAY-CASE AND OUTPATIENT APPOINTMENTS

On-line booking for day case surgery was pioneered by Dr Ian Greaves of Stafford in 1995 (GP Magazine 1998b, Doctor Magazine 1998). Subsequently the method he had established was widely adopted as the National Booked Admissions Programme, and extended to outpatient appointment booking. While it is logical to check the convenience of a prospective hospital appointment with the patient during a GP consultation, and fewer missed or amended appointments will ensue, the applicant GP cannot be aware of the relative priorities that should be accorded to his own and other waiting cases. Appropriate ranking must therefore remain the prerogative of hospital clinical staff.

14.4 REQUESTS FOR PATIENT TRANSPORT

Requests for patient transportation will be available on line.

14.5 REFERRAL LETTERS AND ELECTRONIC APPOINTMENT REQUEST PROFORMAS

In the USA a well-known brand of cake-mix powder failed commercially because it left the American housewife nothing to do except to add water before baking. Cooking had become depersonalized to the extent that it had no appeal for the cook. The situation was rectified by redrafting the recipe so that the mix needed an egg as well as water; the housewife felt that she had made a contribution, and honour was satisfied.

At the risk of sacrificing individuality, the baker of the cake mix is provided with accurately predetermined ingredients and a rapid labour-saving method for using them. The author of computer-written referral letters finds himself in a similar situation.

Assuming that general practitioners refer one in 12 of their consultations and see all patients on average three times a year, then they will make 250 referrals per 1000 patients per year – one quarter of their practice. A handwritten, or audiotyped and visually checked letter may take 5–10 minutes of the doctor's time. This means that between one half and one whole working week per thousand patients is spent on referral letter construction alone each year – a cottage industry in itself.

Word processing is a form of computing that assists repetitive letter writing by supplying, in the correct context, those statements that the repetitive letters have in common, leaving the secretary the task of typing in those statements that vary. 'Standard' letters in which the text does not vary at all do not require this facility, other than that authors must specify their own and the recipient's identity. The computer prints standard letters *en bloc*.

It often comes as a surprise to general practitioners when they realize that, of the 15 components most often required by consultants in referral letters from general practice, 13 can be assembled by automatic processes, given an up-to-date patient record on computer. Moreover, although all 15 components are commonly regarded by GPs as relevant and important to the referral letter, the chance of the doctor forgetting to include two or three of these components is high, unless a check list is used, which it seldom is.

Although surveys of consultants' views on referral letters are not unanimous in their recommendations as to what should be included, there is general agreement that the following items should appear:

- Registered and referring general practitioners' names and addresses
- Date
- Consultant's name, department and address
- Patient's name and address, title and sex
- Patient's date of birth
- Patient's new NHS number
- Patient's hospital number (until this has been displaced by the new NHS number)
- Introductory statement (e.g. Dear ..., I would be very grateful if you would kindly see this patient, who has presented with the following problem)
- Present complaint, history of present condition and physical findings on examination
- All past medical history, suitably condensed and arranged
- Medication, including long-term medication
- Drug and other allergies
- Remarks on family or social background when relevant

- If the GP requests the consultant to play a particular role (such as inviting support of the GP's views that tonsils should not be removed, or that a surgical belt should be renewed, or that the patient's overanxiety should be allayed), then this request should be clearly stated in the letter
- Coda to letter (e.g. I would be glad to receive your views on further management. Many thanks, Yours sincerely).

Commissioning practices must also provide the patient's treatment code and contractual details – see Chapter 17. Fundholding additionally required ethnic origin to be included.

Automated letter assembly

If a full patient record is held on computer, then 13 of the above constituents, plus commissioning contract details, can be assembled automatically by programs that search out blocks of data from within the record and print them in letter format. The sequence is as follows:

1. During consultation the doctor has the patient's computer record on display. S/he elicits from the patient the presenting symptoms, history of the present condition and physical findings, and enters them on the consultation area of the record.
2. The doctor decides to refer the patient for consultant opinion, and holds the patient record in reserve while s/he refers to waiting lists and costs

data, and calls up a list of consultants' names and addresses from which to choose. The doctor need only press one key to select a choice, initiate the referral letter process, and display the consultant's details on the letter in the appropriate position. The letter that is about to be created will first be shown on the visual display screen, and will subsequently be printed if the doctor approves it.

3. The general practitioner's name and address are known to the computer from the coded password s/he keyed in when the workstation was switched on at the beginning of the consultation session. The current date is known to the system. The patient's name and address, date of birth, NHS and hospital numbers are known from the patient record. The introductory statement and the ultimate statement will have been composed by the practitioner when the referral letter facility was first set up – these are registered on data entry templates and stored by the computer in readiness for use. The system may also have recorded instructions to address the consultant by first name.
4. Details of the present consultation are now obtained from the consultation record. They are followed by the summary history record (which functions as the past history in this context). Repeat medication and patient drug allergies are printed from their unique area in the computer record.
5. At this juncture, the computer invites the doctor to add any relevant remarks on the patient's family or

Fig. 14.1 Semiautomated construction of a referral letter using overlapping data boxes: Torex Medical's Premiere system

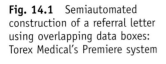

Referral letters are linked to the patient record for easy retrieval and viewing

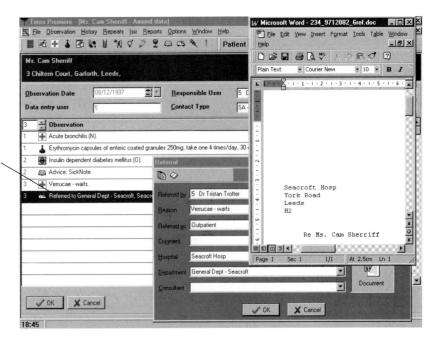

Fig. 14.2 'Patient Information Folder' used as an electronic referral letter (Courtesy of Professor R Kitney, Imperial College, London and *GP* magazine)

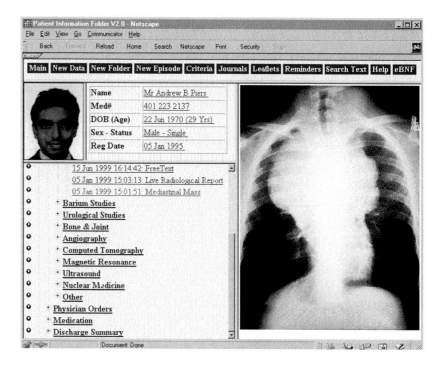

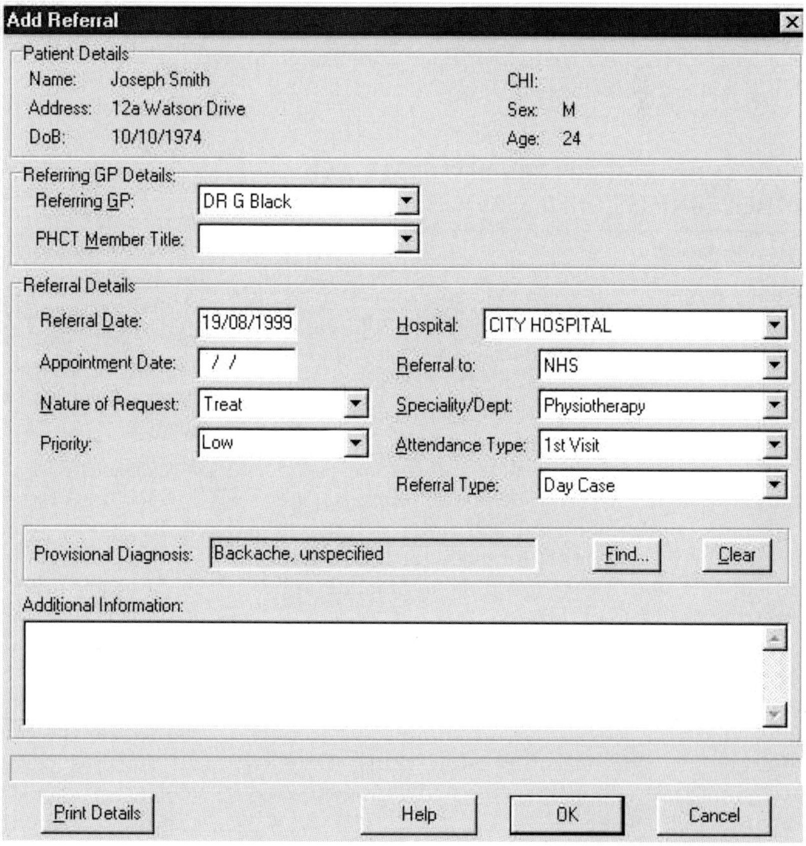

Fig. 14.3 Electronic referral letter: new GPASS system

social background, or on the particular role requested of the consultant. All that remains is for the coda to be reproduced from the referral letter protocol stored on template in memory. Contract details are appended, and the letter is then ready for signing by the doctor.

As the electronic referral letter already contains all the information usually required for the completion of an outpatient appointment request form, or its equivalent electronic proforma, this subset of data too can be provided automatically if the Trust requires it to be printed as a separate exercise.

In addition to their request for the essential ingredients of a referral letter, the consultants' main plea is for legibility. This is never a problem with computer printout or electronic mail.

For those who are concerned that the flavour of originality in their letters to consultants will be sacrificed by the computer, there is the consolation of knowing that the opening and closing statements will have been written in their own individual style. Moreover, the practitioner will be adding constituents 13 and 14 (patient background and the role the GP requests of the consultant) freestyle through the keyboard, prior to printing or transmission. Finally, the practitioner has the power to amend any statements in the letter on display by overwriting. With the computer you can both have your cake and eat it.

14.6 AUDIT RECORDS FOR REFERRALS AND OTHER COMMISSIONED SERVICES

With the introduction first of fundholding and now of commissioning, it is clear that government scrutiny and downward financial pressure will continue to be exerted on the point of referral, and that the GP will continue to be held responsible for providing the data on which that scrutiny is based. To this end, the practice system must be used to keep audit records.

A categorized log of all commissioned services should be kept. This must include all referrals, pathology tests, and radiological and other investigations instigated by the practice. Annually these results must be collated and incorporated in a practice annual report to the PCG+T/HA.

Commissioning practices are able to use their own dedicated referral software, which initiates ledger entries, and dovetails with referral appointment making and referral letter construction, in order to track referral data and establish audit trails. Detailed accounting procedures are associated with each referral made (see Chapter 17).

The referral log

The 1990 contract required all practices to log and tally all referrals, categorizing them according to their inpatient or outpatient hospital department. Self-referrals to the Accident and Emergency department, and pathology and other investigations commissioned by the practices were included in the trawl. Regulations for practice annual report compilation specified that these data might either be related to the individual referring GP, or jointly to all doctors within a practice, and the ability to do either is important for commissioning audit. The purpose of the exercise is to identify those GPs requesting an above-average number of referrals, who may be making unnecessary use of hospital facilities, and those GPs making below average referrals, who may be underdiagnosing or failing to treat some diseases. The Government White Paper *Working for Patients* purported to show a 20-fold variation in GP referral habits, but most later research reports instead suggest a fourfold range of discrepancy.

Anomalies in referral rate analysis have arisen in respect of the fact that some workers, like health authorities, investigate referrals per capita of practice population, whereas others quote rates as referrals per 100 GP consultations. Distortions occur in rates calculated per GP in practices where partners refer each others' registered patients. Some GPs specialize in obstetrics and gynaecology, or practise in areas where a high proportion of patients are referred privately. One study (Coulter) showed that two-thirds of surgical outpatient referrals resulted in admission, whether sent from high- or low-referring practices. Clearly, we should be looking for criteria that indicate the effectiveness of referral rather than its rate.

As pressures will be applied to over-referring practices, 'defensive' data should be included with the data logged at referral. Fry (1991) has suggested the following data set, which includes referral justification details:

- Patient's name, sex, age
- Diagnosis or clinical category
- Reason for referral – diagnostic, therapeutic, investigative, reassurative
- Urgency – immediate, urgent or non-urgent
- Hospital, department and consultant
- Retrospective data – waiting time and outcome.

Commissioning practice software collects all data needed for the practice annual report and basic referral audit as part of its referral routine, but some 'defensive' data such as diagnosis, reason for referral, urgency and outcome are not included. This is a defect that should be corrected by system suppliers. Commissioning referral data entries capture the date, the referring GP, patient identity (including sex and date of birth), hospital, department and consultant, treatment category code, and expected treatment date.

Diagnosis, reason for referral, urgency and outcome are also parameters important to the practice's audit of referral policy for its own internal use and for PCG+T purposes. These data can also be used as a measure of performance in secondary care provision. Reason for referral and urgency should be obtainable from GP records, but diagnosis and outcome derive from hospital data, are already coded by Data Extraction (formerly HAA) clerks, and thus are obtainable electronically after hospital discharge.

14.7 PERSONAL MEDICAL ATTENDANT REPORTS FOR INSURANCE

Although PMA reports are not a communication between GP and provider, and although they are not yet transmitted on line, it is appropriate to consider them here, as their method of automated construction resembles that employed in compiling referral letters.

A multitude of insurance companies ask for PMA reports, but they all speak with one voice if their reports are not completed and returned with alacrity. PMA reports are tedious to complete, have to be attended to outside consultation time and, if delayed, may prejudice the patient's house purchase arrangements. The close similarity of all PMA questionnaires received from the various insurance companies suggests that the risk factors that they all take into account are the same, even though the weighting given to those factors may vary between companies. The following details would appear to be *requested by all companies*, although the precise wording of the questions often differs.

1. Date registered (How long have you known applicant?)
2. Date last seen
3. Record of previous illnesses, operations, and accidents (with dates)
4. Record of X-rays or other special investigations (with dates).

The majority of companies require:

5. Reason last seen
6. Date of first record entry/date records initiated
7. Present drugs taken
8. Latest blood pressure readings

9. Latest urine tests for albumen and sugar
10. Misuse of drugs, alcohol or tobacco
11. Lifestyle risk of contracting AIDS (or possession of positive test).

A few companies require:

12. State of health when last seen
13. General state of health
14. Predisposition to nervous illness
15. Knowledge of consultations with other doctors
16. Weight, actual or assessed in general terms
17. Female functions – periods, pregnancies, gynaecological problems
18. Family history prejudicial to health.

Once again, we are faced with writing a document in which most of the sections deal with data already held in the computerized patient record in a structured form. Only the details 10–13 and 16 are not explicitly contained on the computer record; 12 and 13 can be inferred from a full knowledge of the last entry in the consultation record, and the summary history, respectively. This leaves three outstanding details to be completed from general knowledge of the patient rather than recorded detail.

The use of manual summary records for PMA reports

Manual summary records provide a useful source of data from which past illnesses, operations and investigations can be obtained when completing PMA reports. For this reason alone, as well as for patient management, it is prudent to include blood pressure measurements, and urine sugar and albumen tests in summaries (the latest normal, and selected abnormal readings). Summary records considerably reduce the time taken to complete PMA reports, as they avoid the need for a total record search. It is also possible for suitably trained ancillary staff to complete most of the PMA report from summary records.

Record driven systems and PMA reports

After the patient record has been fully transferred to the computer, the system is capable of reproducing all details except 10–13 and 16 as a printout in sequence when a PMA report is required.

From this printout, the practice secretary may complete the PMA report by hand, highlighting those questions in the original questionnaire for which the printout does not provide answers. The doctor must then complete these remaining questions and sign the report. Ultimately, as a result of negotiations in progress with insurance companies, it is probable that the computer printout taken from the GP record will be accepted as the basis of the report, albeit with a few extra questions which the individual company poses, and which are particular to that company. The burden of writing PMA reports in his off-duty hours will then be lifted from the shoulders of the general practitioner.

14.8   OTHER REPORTS WHOSE ASSEMBLY CAN BE ASSISTED BY COMPUTER

Other types of report may be written with partial help from the computer. Thus, the notification of infectious disease may be prompted for by the system when the relevant diagnosis is entered on to the patient record. The ensuing facsimile form for notification, shown on the display in readiness for completion, will have nine or 10 possible questions answered by the system and will prompt for one or two questions for which the record does not provide an answer.

Reports to the Committee on Safety of Medicines and to drug companies were dealt with more fully in Chapter 11, and the preparation of claims was described in Chapter 8.

SUMMARY

- Although the automated writing of referral letters by computer requires the presence of structured patient records on computer, the increase in efficiency and convenience, and the saving of general practitioners' time that are achieved by computerization are considerable. Consultants would also receive, consistently and legibly, virtually all the details they require from referral letters.
- A log of all referrals should be kept by all practices, and a yearly tally of these must be provided for the practice annual report and locality commissioning, categorized according to their hospital inpatient and outpatient department. Self-referrals to the

Accident and Emergency department, and pathology and other investigations commissioned by the practice, must be included. Although many of the data required for this audit can be derived automatically from the commissioning process itself, it is wise to supplement them with elaborative categories, which will help to justify the individual doctor's and the practice's referral policies.
- Some help in completing PMA insurance reports can be obtained manually from the use of summary records that avoid the need to search the full manual record, and the form can be completed, in part, by ancillary staff. Once insurance companies have reached agreement on the principle and contents of automated reports from general practice, then these reports may be created with minimal human intervention and with greatly improved promptness, efficiency and legibility.
- Other reports can be considered for completion on the computer using the general plan of producing, automatically, those details that are stored in memory and prompting for those that are not. Notification of infectious disease provides one example of this procedure.

REFERENCES AND FURTHER READING

Doctor Magazine 1998 Pilot plan enables GP referral on-line. Doctor 8 Oct: 20

Fountain Project 1996 The Fountain Project. Practice Computing, September: 5

Fry J 1991 How to monitor hospital referrals. Update, March: 472

GP Magazine 1998a GP electronic information network wins award. GP 10 July: 20

GP Magazine 1998b GPs to book operations via computer. GP 31 July: 2

Office of Health Economics 1990 Variations between general practitioners. OHE Briefing 26, July

Pathfinder Project 1996 The Pathfinder Project. Practice Computing, Summer: 7

Wilkin D, Smith A G 1987 Variations in general practitioners' referral rates to consultants. Journal of the Royal College of General Practitioners, August: 350

15 GP–provider linkages 2: transactions initiated by hospitals

Clinical reports from hospitals to general practice divide into five main categories:

- Notification of discharge (NOD)
- The full inpatient report on discharge (FIRD)
- Outpatient reports
- Accident and Emergency Department (A&E) reports
- Subsequent referrals.

15.1 NOTIFICATION OF DISCHARGE, AND A&E REPORTS

At the outset of this chapter it is essential to discard terms such as discharge summary, discharge report and discharge letter, which may refer to either NODs or FIRDs and thus cause misunderstanding. An NOD is a note given to the patient at discharge for transmission to the GP which contains, in addition to the date and patient identification details, two other essential subsets of discharge data. These are the diagnoses and clinical procedures ('the clinical subset'), and the details of prescribed drugs, if any, to be taken home (DTTO – 'the medication subset'). The classes of data contained in A&E reports, which may also be given to the patient, are essentially the same. As both NODs and A&E reports are given to the patient, the prescription details recorded on them can also be used to requisition drugs from the hospital pharmacy.

It is both feasible and desirable that hospital computer systems should code diagnoses using the ICD-10 classification, and code procedures using the OPCS classification. ICD-10 and OPCS are both used by hospital clerical staff to log throughput for hospital activity analysis, and both classifications map to Read codes. Drugs require coding using the Read classification, and the Multilex drug database, which is rapidly expanding within secondary care, provides for adequate linkages with Read. Both subsets are

therefore potentially capable of being transmitted electronically to general practice in a format that can be autofiled, and it is precisely these subsets that need to be incorporated within the summary history and medication sections, respectively, of the computerized GP patient summary record.

While both NODs and A&E reports allow for additional freestyle comment, this need not as a rule be transferred to the GP record, so the only annotation that the GP need make to either type of report prior to autofiling is to 'flag' it with an electronic marker to trigger 'reminders', and so prevent the omission of any follow-up procedure s/he deems necessary.

15.2 FULL LENGTH HOSPITAL NOTES AND THEIR TWO-STAGE CONDENSATION

When a detective investigation is under way, a very considerable amount of information may be collected that later proves to be irrelevant to the course of events. In summing up at the end of the trial, the judge will concentrate only upon those details that are salient to proof – giving these details, which may be positive or negative, preferential treatment.

Cases of patients admitted to hospital for investigation are submitted to an in-depth study that pursues a similar process of resolution. A great deal of fine detail, much of which has no further relevance, is generated in the ward notes, which must undergo two stages of reduction and condensation before pertinent data can be incorporated into a summary history section of the GP record.

- The first reduction occurs at patient discharge, when junior hospital staff construct a precis of the ward notes to produce the FIRD.
- The second reduction starts with the FIRD and is a further abstraction that produces the clinical and

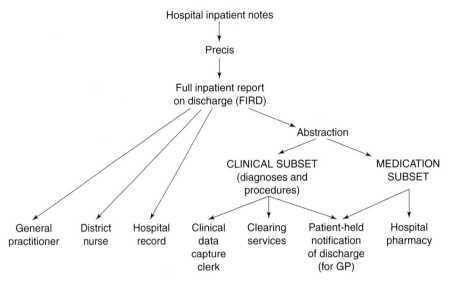

Fig. 15.1 Dissemination of the full inpatient report on discharge and its subsets

medication subsets, undertaken by the same junior doctor when writing the NOD.

- An identical abstraction to produce the clinical and medication subsets is performed by the GP on receipt of the FIRD, for the purpose of updating summary history and medication records.
- Abstraction to produce the clinical subset is undertaken independently by the hospital Clinical Data Capture clerk for required statistical returns, and also by the Clearing Services clerk, who matches them with contract details for invoice returns.

Since the NOD, the GP summary history and medication record, the hospital pharmacy, the Clinical Data Capture clerk and the Invoices clerk all share either the clinical subset, the medication subset or both, it is a gross misuse of NHS manpower to perpetuate a system in which each party to the subsets is obliged to make his or her own individual abstraction from discharge data. If the junior doctors who construct the FIRD had access to software that coded the subsets as they were entered, they could not only provide for all other users of the subsets, but also save themselves the trouble of writing a separate NOD, since this could be provided automatically by computer program as hard copy.

Why does this not happen? There are five cogent reasons:

- Most hospital staff still write freestyle letters and have not addressed the need, nor assessed the advantages to themselves, of converting to closely structured, protocol-driven FIRDs.

- The task of writing FIRDs is delegated to junior hospital staff who receive no training in this skill.
- By 1999 only 25% of UK hospitals had achieved any significant level of computerization, so the necessary data entry terminals have yet to be installed in wards. If data obtained on admission, and data relating to investigations and operations were to be entered as and when they were generated, on to the nascent FIRD, FIRD construction would be greatly facilitated, as would all other IT-dependent procedures.
- Although ICD-10 and OPCS can be mapped to Read, none of these three coding systems is readily available on hospital computer dictionaries, except in a very few locations.
- The various parties whose tasks involve use of the subsets work in isolation and do not appreciate the need to confer in order to coordinate their data transactions.

Pilot trials of subset abstraction by hospital staff

Experience in the field has already shown that it would be a very simple task for hospital doctors to structure their reports in such a way that the clinical and medication subsets were readily identifiable. In 1974, a pilot study on hospital output produced self-adhesive labels on which the necessary summary statements and patient identity were reduplicated and enclosed with the full hospital report. These labels were later inserted into the GP manual record to assist in building a summary document. The opinion of the 32 general practitioners who received summary data on labels during the study was that this form of data presentation was very useful (Exeter and District Health Services 1974).

15.3 THE FULL INPATIENT REPORT ON DISCHARGE (FIRD)

As with the NOD, the principal components of the FIRD are the clinical subset (diagnoses and clinical procedures) plus the medication subset. However, instead of presenting its data as the 'headline'-style codable terms used for NODs, FIRDs elaborate data to the extent required by fully informed continuation of care.

Consistent, precise and adequate FIRDs can only be constructed if a protocol is used. Standard terms and a succinct style must be used, data categories must be defined, and data fields must be ordered.

In general, there are two basic models of FIRD – surgical and medical. Although the two possess many features in common, they differ in the following ways:

- Surgical FIRDs deal primarily with one physiological system of the body. Medical FIRDs often deal with several systems.

- The focal point of the surgical FIRD is the operation, which is the principal, and may be the only, procedure. Its date and title are the most important entries in the FIRD, with the diagnosis usually ranking as the indication for operation.

- Problem-orientated records are particularly appropriate in medical cases, in which multiple problems, each of which requires its own approach, are common. Case resolution is usually a gradual process, which spans the inpatient period.

Procedures in any type of case must include imaging, endoscopies, transfusions, and such measures as epidural anaesthesia and electroconvulsive therapy. Histology is also usually included under this heading.

Hospital Clinical Data Capture clerks must record all these items in their returns, and the data are equally relevant to GP history summaries.

The data categories usually included in each of the two main types of FIRD are listed in Table 15.1.

Subsequent referrals contain the same clinical data categories as FIRDs, but add the details of the tertiary consultant and department, and transfer dates, if any. Outpatient reports may not need summary extraction, or else may require similar data categories to the medical FIRD. As all these types of hospital report

---

Table 15.1 Data classes for full inpatient reports on discharge

Surgical	Medical
Patient ID	Patient ID
Date of admission	Date of admission
Date of operation	Date of discharge
Date of discharge	Consultant + dept
Consultant + dept	GP
Operative surgeon	Problem summary (diagnoses)
GP	Active 1
Name of operation	2
Indications	3
Patient drug or other	Inactive 4
idiosyncrasies	5
Current details of:	6
1. Primary system	
2. Other systems	
Past history	
Other procedures	
Subsequent progress in hospital	
Recommendations	
Drugs TTO	
Points for review	
Waiting list or emergency admission	
Discharged to:	
Hospital follow-up	
Told/not told of diagnosis	

Problem no.	Clinical notes	Procedures	Medication	Duration to continue drugs after discharge
1				
2				
3				
4				
5				
6				Duration TTO

have similar implications for subsequent patient management in general practice, it is convenient to refer to them all collectively as 'full reports'.

15.4 CHANGING PATTERNS OF USE OF THE FULL REPORT IN PRACTICE

Just as there is an important and fundamental difference between the reference made by the general practitioner to his own current consultation notes while the current episode of illness lasts, and that made to notes recorded during episodes closed months or years previously, so the use made of hospital reports in general practice changes with time.

Here the distinction is between the general practitioner's use of hospital data for immediate aftercare following hospital discharge, and the call for the salient facts of the hospital episode, rather than the fine detail, in the long term.

Summarization of hospital reports

The need for a summary of past morbidity applies equally strongly to hospital-originated and general-practice-generated data within the GP record.

A further similarity exists. During construction of either the hospital report or the GP's own record, it is possible to distinguish and earmark those data required to summarize the case at the time when the record is actually written. Of course, in the GP's own notes the conclusive summarizing entry may have to wait until the last consultation in a sequence, just as the final details in the summarization of the hospital case must wait until discharge.

In both manual and computer records, summary data that have originated from radiological and hospital reports must be clearly distinguishable from those originating in general practice. This usually involves labelling secondary care data with markers or 'flags'.

Summarization of hospital reports, whether undertaken by hospital or general practice staff, is a form of streamlining that no reformer of the general practice record can ignore. Summary records are meaningless without it. Manual record systems seldom employ summarization of hospital reports but, when they do, the summary form of the report is used to the virtual exclusion of the full report once initial aftercare has been completed.

Three phases

It is possible, therefore, to define three distinct phases in the use of hospital reports received into general practice (Fig. 15.2).

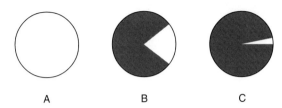

Fig. 15.2 Eclipse in the use of the whole hospital report if a summary report is available   (a) All whole reports read on receipt by practice   (b) 2 months after receipt of report, most immediate aftercare recommendations will have been implemented; a few whole reports will still be read again by the GP at this stage as initial aftercare phase draws to a close   (c) After 3 months from time of receipt, the use of the whole report dwindles to one in 250 consultations

1. Initial receipt, when the whole report is read by the GP.
2. Immediate aftercare following hospital inpatient or outpatient attendance. For this purpose, the GP will usually re-read the hospital report in the presence of the patient to ensure that all specialist observations and recommendations have been given due consideration.
3. Long-term use, for which summary material is always necessary, but for which access to the whole report is rarely required.

Further considerations

There are two further considerations:

- Quite apart from summary morbidity recording for future record use, it is necessary to note hospital recommendations for further treatment, including drug treatment. This may require that repeat medication be transcribed into the appropriate area of the general practice record.
- If the patient fails to attend and cooperate in the general practice aftercare recommended by the hospital specialist, then some means of monitoring is required to check default.

Changes in priority given to the components of a report – a simple experiment

If we adopt the practice of highlighting clinical summary ('clinical subset data') and medication statements in the hospital inpatient or outpatient report at receipt, and apply 'action' flags where default monitoring is considered appropriate, we are in a position to run a simple experiment. This experiment will test the natural history of the use made in practice of the whole report and of its three subsidiary components: clinical subset statements, medication statements, and action indicators.

Each time a hospital report is referred to, a tally is kept of those components that have been accessed. If we take each category – total record, clinical subset component, medication component, and action flag – we find that not all reports require extraction of clinical subsets, and only a few have medication components relevant to further general practice record use. Some reports from outpatients, for instance, will merely say that the patient is progressing satisfactorily and that he need not reattend hospital. The number of reports requiring action flags proves to be very small. For the purposes of the graph we intend to draw (Fig. 15.3), it is convenient to show the number of times each component is accessed as a percentage of the total number of items in that particular category of component, and to plot this percentage against the time since receipt of the report.

This graph shows us that the use of the whole report starts at 100% at receipt, falls steeply to 2% by the third month and falls away progressively thereafter, provided that a clinical subset summary alternative is available. By contrast, the use of the clinical subset alternative, rather than the whole report, is nil at the time of receipt, rises to 9% in the second month and falls to a smaller but permanent level as it supplants the use of the whole report for long-term

record use. The medication component of the hospital report as a separate entity from the whole report is usually accessed in conjunction with the clinical subset component. It is accessed at a rate of nil at receipt, 25% during the first month, 37% during the second month, falling to 3% during the third month and thereafter tails off. The action flags are allocated at receipt of the report by the general practitioner. 100% of actions should have been carried out within a time limit determined by practice policy – say 2–3 months.

When the 3 months of immediate aftercare have expired, the rate of access to either the whole report or its clinical subset summary alternative is so small when expressed as a rate per document received, or in the manner shown in the graph, that we need a change of scale to compare further use. In terms of the rate of access per consultation, we now find that any clinical summary history in the record is accessed at consultation at a rate of one in every two consultations, whereas the rate of access to the whole report or reports in the record is reduced to 1 in 250 consultations or less.

The implications for the summary record are clear. Once the immediate aftercare situation has passed, and provided that the general practitioner has summary clinical records at his disposal, then access to the whole hospital report becomes a rarity. In terms of computer take-on from concurrent paper transmission, the user has the choice of taking on all hospital output, or else of holding hospital output in a manual bank until immediate aftercare is complete, and only taking on to the computer a clinical summary alternative to the full report.

15.5 PROBLEMS WITH MANUAL RECORD PROCEDURES

General practitioners are required to read incoming paper mail before it is filed in the manual records. If they do not, they miss consultant opinion in cases where no further immediate action is required, and in other cases are entirely dependent upon the patient's promptness and compliance in reattending the practice to become alerted to the recommendations of immediate aftercare. Patients often attend practice to implement consultant recommendations shortly after the receipt of the hospital report. The scramble to file hospital reports in the records within a short time of receipt, in order to facilitate their retrieval at patient reattendance, is in conflict with the need for all doctors to read incoming mail. If hospital reports are not stored together, centrally, the receptionist cannot check, when asked, whether they have arrived. When GPs are absent from practice for even short intervals, they must choose either to fail to

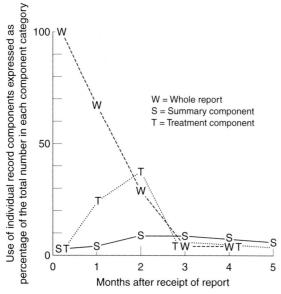

Fig. 15.3 Changes in the use made of the clinical summary and medication components of the FIRD by GPs, as contrasted with the use of the full text of the report

read the backlog of reports or to interrupt the flow of filing. The need to file reports promptly for ease of retrieval in immediate aftercare conflicts with the need to abstract clinical subset summary statements, plus medication or other treatment statements, and to implement action default monitoring. Unless the manual record has an ordered system for hospital report filing, the practitioner has to unfold and sort hospital reports within the manual record in order to retrieve the latest one.

The 'latest report' bank

An alternative approach to filing hospital paper reports promptly is to delay filing into the records by 3 months and to retain reports in a special temporary filing system. This has several advantages to users of either conventional manual records, manual summary systems or computer record systems. The advantages are:

- The latest report for immediate aftercare is quickly available. The practice receptionist can be instructed to provide the latest hospital reports selectively for GP consultation sessions, thus saving retrieval time for the doctor. The receptionist may also respond, without delay, when patients enquire as to whether their hospital reports have arrived yet.
- There is time for the take-on of clinical subset summary and medication statements to manual or computer systems that transcribe these features.
- The temporarily absent doctor can catch up with the incoming mail without disrupting filing procedures.
- Action flags can be applied to reports and if, subsequently, patients have failed to attend for immediate aftercare, their absence will be noted and further action can be taken.

15.6　SUMMARY RECORDS AND FULL COMPUTER RECORD SYSTEMS

A suitable sequence of operations for dealing with incoming paper reports would be as follows:

1. A practice records officer must be trained in those methods of summarizing that are implemented in the practice (see Chapter 5)
2. Daily hospital output is received into the practice. The practice records officer processes all reports by highlighting clinical subset summary and medication statements. The doctor reads all hospital output within a day or two of receipt and approves the summary annotation of the records officer. The doctor applies action flags as s/he considers necessary.

3. Each month's hospital output is filed under the month in a rack or series of files, and ordered alphabetically by patient's name. Reports are withdrawn from the bank as required when patients attend the practice for immediate aftercare, but are subsequently returned to the bank. If the latest hospital reports are to be selected before the practice consultation session, then the receptionist must enquire as to a patient's recent hospital attendance when practice appointments are made.
4. Early in the 3-month holding period, the clinical subset summary and medication statements already annotated and approved are keyed in as Read-compliant entries within the patient's computer record by the record clerk. Paper-based pathology test results are entered promptly on to the computer record as they do not need to be summarized, and often must be read in conjunction with GP record entries in response to patient enquiry.
5. At the end of the 3-month immediate aftercare period, the paper reports are taken from the manual bank and relegated to the manual card record wallet. Any reports showing unredeemed action flags are brought to the attention of the doctor.
6. On the very rare occasion that it is necessary to access the original full hospital report after the lapse of immediate aftercare, this is retrieved in the manual card record wallet. Experience shows that when this happens, several reports in the same wallet are usually sought at the same time.

Although the above plan involves the retention of, and rare access to, the card record wallet, the trade-off in terms of saving the keying-in of large volumes of obsolescent text is enormous. Retention of the card record wallet is, of course, a statutory obligation that is likely to remain until all hospital output becomes computerized at source.

15.7　SCANNING HOSPITAL REPORTS

Instead of using a manual 'latest report bank' with subsequent filing of full hospital reports within manual record wallets, many practices now opt to scan all relevant incoming reports as they are received. Unquestionably this is the best interim solution pending the adoption of e-mail across the board. There are, however, a number of critical technological factors to be taken into account (see also Chapter 16):

- The choice of scanner lies between a flatbed model, which can only accept one original document at a time but will cope with thick documents or books, or else a sheet-fed scanner, which accepts a stack of single pages.

- A monochrome scanner will suffice for documents.
- Originals will be scanned in as images unless optical character recognition (OCR) is used. Images demand considerably more storage space than text, even if file compression is used. If the clinical summary and medication subsets have already been abstracted, then the fact that (as with most image packages) the image format of the full report cannot be intelligently searched by computer program may not matter. If, however, the practice intends to carry out data searches on text stored in full reports, then originals will have to be processed by OCR software at the time of scanning, in order to convert them into editable text. Even if it incorporates a spell-checker, OCR fails to recognize a small proportion of characters and substitutes spaceholder symbols in their place, which have subsequently to be edited out using the keyboard.
- In addition to provision of the scanner itself, scanning and paper management software must be obtained and installed on the computer. Most practices that store images will require that these should be available through networks; care must be taken to ensure that the software purchased provides for this to be done, and that the extra user licence fees charged are not prohibitive. Some word processing packages enable OCR-processed text to be spell-checked and stored as documents. As an alternative, off-the-shelf database software for indexing and storing scanned images must be obtained. In either case, care should be taken to ensure that the access routines are compatible with those used by the practice system. Fully integrated solutions are available, and practices are strongly advised to consult their GP system supplier when defining their requirements. The company PCTI Solutions specialises in providing fully integrated scanner solutions for all the main system suppliers (PCTI Solutions Ltd, Churchill House, Mill Hill Road, Pontefract, West Yorks WF8 4HY, tel: 01977 690977).
- Minimum host system requirements for scan input are usually Windows 95/98 or NT, and a Pentium processor with 16 Mb RAM.

15.8 THE IMPACT OF ELECTRONIC MAIL

Experimental communication systems have been set up in the UK, the USA and Australia to pass Prestel-type frames containing electronic reports from hospital and pathology laboratory to general practice. These systems used the telephone line and visual display units but had little or no processing power. Although they had the advantage of speed in message transmission, they missed the opportunities of presenting data in a variety of different formats to suit the needs of the user, and of filing those data automatically within a structured computer-held record.

As we come to accept conversion of hospital and pathology reports to electronic mail, our daily hospital letters and reports will be downloaded automatically from the hospital server to the practice via the latter's mailbox. These electronic documents will be shown to us in general practice as and when we summon them on to visual display, but will be manipulated and stored for us by the practice computer. All reports will be available to all users at any time and, if need be, simultaneously on display. Reports may be viewed singly or in any required grouping so that the receptionist can check for the arrival of a single report, all doctors can view the daily batched intake, and the temporarily absent doctor can review all reports received during a given period. Latest reports for each patient will be labelled and accessed as such, and there will be no need for a manual bank. Clinical subset summary and medication statements may well be indicated as such on receipt of the report from the hospital and, if the GP approves them, they will be inserted automatically in their appropriate station within the patient's computer record. GPs will allocate their own action flags, and an automatic default monitor will indicate those patients who have failed to reattend for immediate aftercare. The need for intermediary processing of hospital reports will at last disappear with electronic mail, but the distinction between summary material for long-term use and obsolescent material for immediate aftercare will remain with us.

SUMMARY

- Hospital inpatient clinical notes are voluminous and contain an overburden of obsolescent data. At patient discharge a condensate is prepared by junior hospital staff as the basis for a full inpatient report on discharge (FIRD) to be posted to the patient's GP. From this condensate a further abstraction results in the isolation of a 'clinical subset', which includes diagnoses and clinical procedures, and a 'medication subset' of drugs to take home. Both subsets form the basis of the notification of discharge (NOD) slip, which is given to the patient to pass to the GP promptly on release from hospital. The GP requires the 'clinical subset' to be added to the patient's computerized summary history record, and may need to add the 'medication subset' to the patient's repeat medication file.

- One or other of the subsets is also needed by the hospital pharmacist, the hospital Clinical Data Capture clerk and the hospital Clearing Services clerk. It would be logistically efficient for the junior hospital doctor to use a computer program linked to coding dictionaries to prepare the FIRD, and to abstract both subsets formally at patient discharge, in order to prepare the NOD automatically and pass the subsets to all other authorized users.

- The two basic forms of FIRD are those used in medicine and surgery, and the components of diagnoses, procedures and medication are common to both, although the weight given to each component differs with department. Protocols, standard terms, a succinct style, and defined data categories and data fields should be employed in the preparation of all FIRDs. Subsequent referrals and outpatient reports have much in common with FIRDs, and all three are conveniently considered under the heading of 'full hospital reports'.

- The general practitioner uses the 'full report' to be able to provide fully informed immediate aftercare following a patient's hospital encounter, but he uses the clinical and medication subsets as the basis for patient management months or years later. The process of immediate aftercare requires the GP to monitor the implementation of the consultant's recommendations, and to annotate 'full reports' with markers to indicate actions required when the patient contacts the medical centre for instructions.

- With conventional manual record procedures, the practitioner faces a dilemma. Efficient retrieval of the latest hospital report for immediate aftercare requires that the report should be filed within the patient record without delay. Unless storage of latest reports is centralized, the receptionist cannot check whether they have arrived. By contrast, the need for all doctors in a group to read the incoming mail, for a doctor to catch up with mail that has arrived during his temporary absence, and the need to ensure that patients do not default from important hospital recommendations, all require that some latest reports should not be filed away promptly.

- A solution to this problem is for the practice to institute a 'latest report' bank in which hospital reports for the previous 3 months are stored. The bank also allows time for the transcription of clinical summary and medication subset statements to summary records or full computer record systems. Summarizing hospital reports carries a significant advantage in long-term patient management in general practice. If practice records officers are trained to do this, then their work can be checked by the doctor when s/he reads the incoming mail, and the results can be transcribed on to summary records.

- Scanning of incoming hospital paper-based reports can use the computer storage of images (though this is extravagant of storage space) or optical character recognition to convert images to text – a process that requires editing via the keyboard. Additional software is required in both instances, and must be compliant with the GP system.

- With the help of the practice computer, and the use of hospital coding dictionaries, electronic mail is capable of solving all the problems associated with incoming hospital reports.

REFERENCES AND FURTHER READING

Archbold RA, Kooridhottumkal L, Suliman A et al 1998 Evaluation of a computer-generated discharge summary for patients with acute coronary syndromes. British Journal of General Practice 48: 1163–1164

Doctor Magazine 1996 GPs save cash in computer linkup. Doctor, 6 June: 34

Exeter and District Health Services Computer Project 1974 Internal report on hospital discharge data. Exeter and District Health Services, Exeter

Houghton M 1998 Trailblazing GPs help burn off excess NHS paper weight. Rx, May: 47

Medeconomics Magazine 1996 GPs test out provider links. Medeconomics, September: 41–42

NHSE 1997 GP/Provider Links. Memorandum 14 July

NHSE 1998 Memorandum – clinical links in general practice. May

Nuffield Orthopaedic Centre NHS Trust 1995 Memorandum – automated discharge summaries. Nuffield Orthopaedic Centre NHS Trust, Oxford, p 1–5

Practice Computing Magazine 1996 Trial run for fountain project. Practice Computing, September: 3

Practice Computing Magazine 1996 Editorial. Practice Computing, Summer: 3

Pulse Magazine 1992 FHSA sponsors GP/hospital computer links trial. Pulse, April: 30

Pulse Magazine 1995 GPs keener on electronic links than consultants. Pulse, 4 November: 36

16 Paperless practice

16.1 INTRODUCTION

Although the first steps in medical computing were taken by hospitals in both America and Sweden in the 1960s, the development and implementation of secondary care systems has been surprisingly slow and patchy. By contrast, GP clinical systems, in which the UK has always held the lead, have now become a prerequisite for efficient primary care in most developed countries. With the uptake of NHS GP–Pathology and Radiology Links proceeding apace, and with more and more practices loading and using all GP-generated data on computers, one obstacle alone prevents progress towards totally paperless general practice – the deficit in hospital computing and the knock-on effect this has on provider–GP data communications.

It is a sobering thought that if UK hospitals had chosen to put their data output on line at any time during the past 20 years, the abolition of GP manual records would have been an inevitable and prompt sequel. As it is, practices that aspire to become paperless are faced with implementing a laborious transitional method for processing paper-based hospital data, knowing that this will become obsolete once provider electronification has been completed.

Transitional methods have an unpleasant habit of creating difficulties, both when they are introduced and when they are superseded, unless sufficient thought has been given to the details of their design. It is critically important, therefore, that the file structures and data standards used during the transitional phase should, as closely as possible, match those that are to be introduced with e-reports.

16.2 STEPWISE CONVERSION OF PRACTICE APPLICATIONS TO COMPUTER

In the long run, paperless practice will be adopted universally. Progress towards this goal is necessarily stepwise. Conversion of paper-based routines to their electronic counterparts now commonly takes place in the following order:

1. Appointments
2. Registration
3. IoS claims
4. Organizer functions: rota, diary, address book
5. Prescribing
6. Summary GP and summary hospital data for patient records
7. Patient instruction leaflets
8. Pathology
9. Radiology
10. Comprehensive GP data entry and use within the patient record
11. Guidelines and protocols
12. Referral letters
13. Incoming hospital reports.

Conversions pending:

- PMA reports
- CSM and REM reports
- PACT (EPEP)
- Intake of electronic 'dawn reports' from cooperatives
- Transmission of electronic prescriptions to pharmacies
- Patient record transfer between practices.

For the first few months after each step in the process of application conversion has been introduced, it is wise to maintain a double system until all problems have been ironed out, staff are confident that computer procedures are reliable and the necessary skills to implement those procedures have been acquired. Thus appointment conversion will begin with the appointments of a single listholder, claims registration and pathology will retain reduplicated paper backup for a time, and pulling and refiling of manual notes will be needed when computerized records are first used at consultation. As the reliability of record summarization becomes apparent, doctors may require only manual records of selected patients from the surgery list before even these can be disregarded.

It is essential that all members of the practice team should be allocated precise responsibilities, and be trained for the part they must play in the conversion process. A log book should document these responsibilities and, as with computer operations in general, log all problems which arise, together with the action taken, and by whom, to deal with them.

16.3   TOTAL ELECTRONIFICATION

All practices taking this stepwise approach to conversion are faced with making the critical decision as to when they finally dispense with all paper altogether as a factor for practice communication and data retrieval. Some UK practices have already taken the plunge and, if they retain hospital reports, do so solely for archive purposes, for medicolegal reasons or for the benefit of other GPs in the event of patient transfer away from the practice.

However, it is obvious that the greater the proportion of data that arrives electronically at a practice from external agencies, the less effort that practice will have to make to complete the conversion process. To go paperless before Pathology Links have been implemented, for example, will mean continuing to transcribe the majority of incoming test results in addition to hospital reports, a process that requires a considerable degree of commitment. If pathology results are delivered electronically, then only paper-based hospital reports will need processing when they arrive at the practice. When, ultimately, hospital reports do arrive in electronic format, transcription will be dispensed with altogether. On the face of it, prudence would seem to suggest that the longer we put off the evil day, the less evil it will be.

Of course, the issue is not that simple. If GPs continue to use hospital paper reports there will be little incentive for hospital doctors to provide electronic ones. Hospitals that do consider providing electronic reports realize that many practices must still face the problem of converting all their old patient records, and of converting the records of all new patients, until electronic patient record transfer between practices becomes the norm. We face a stalemate that can only be resolved by a resolute initiative, and this must necessarily stem from general practice.

Assuming that a stage has been reached in electronic conversion at which a practice handles all pre-

scribing, summarized previous GP and hospital data, comprehensive GP data entry and use, and pathology and radiology results on a practice system, then a transitional method for coping with new hospital reports is required until such time as these become electronic. This interim measure will enable the practice to become paperless as regards internal data handling for patient management.

For this purpose the following procedures must be put in place:

* Hospital reports must be processed as described in Chapter 15, with the extraction and entry to computer of clinical summary subsets, treatment subsets and action flags.
* Full hospital reports must be scanned into the practice computer system preferably using optical character recognition (OCR) techniques.
* Practice policies must be agreed as to the disposal of paper-based hospital reports. Thus the procedure for this will be either:
  - to file them in manual record wallets in readiness for possible patient transfer to another practice
  - to file them in date order in boxes stored in a low priority area at the medical centre
  - initially, to file them in date order and later, after a lapse of 6 or 12 months, to shred them.
* The pulling and refiling of practice manual records can now be discontinued.

16.4   THE ADVANTAGES OF PAPERLESS PRACTICE

Conversion to electronic records saves:

* labour (e.g. for pulling or refiling records, or chasing reports)
* time – data access is both accurate and rapid
* space (previously occupied by manual records)
* raw materials – principally wood pulp
* record deterioration – no further wear and tear, less dust generated
* costs – paper manufacture, printing, postage, labour (a conservative Department of Health estimate suggested that an annual economy of £100 million would be realized by full NHS electronic conversion).

Conversion to electronic records increases:

* data accuracy, efficiency, and comprehensiveness
* legibility
* record accessibility – records are never lost or temporarily unavailable, they can be interrogated by

several users simultaneously, they can be accessed remotely and interrogated on a 24-hour basis
- security – backup copies can be multiple and stored in a fireproof safe
- staff job satisfaction (shuffling paper is a tedious task).

16.5 LEGALITY OF COMPUTER RECORDS

Recognition of computer records as legally binding vectors has been long overdue. It has had to await European Union deliberations before the outcome of these could at last be reflected in UK statutes.

The legality of computer records now depends upon:

- the presence of a read-only audit trail that logs the date, time, content and originator of all entries and amendments to electronic data
- a unique password with which the author logs on and from which s/he logs off (with default routines to close down access if logging off is omitted)
- a formally binding obligation for all partners and other health professionals to use computer records and to enter all their working data upon them
- the invariable use of automated backup routines
- a requirement that computer records must contain the same amount of information as was previously recorded on paper
- a requirement that clinical notes shall be made at the time of treatment, or else as soon as possible afterwards.

Although the Data Protection Act requires that personal computer records should not be kept for longer than is necessary, it has formerly proved difficult to put a time limit on the need to retain medical records. Recent cases of litigation now indicate that records should be retained in perpetuity. If patients change to another practice, their electronic records should therefore be copied and not relinquished.

GP system suppliers were originally granted a year's grace within which to bring their clients' systems into line with the requirements of the new legislation.

16.6 LEVELS OF ACCURACY IN GENERAL PRACTICE RECORDS

All forms of record contain errors and omissions, and the process of conversion to computer has enabled some of the inadequacies of GP records to be quantified.

Roscoe (1997) reported that summarization of practice records prior to computerization had revealed a number of instances in which important details, though present, had become obscured and were therefore overlooked as long as reliance was confined to the patient manual record. Examples were abnormal or questionable smear results, and tests demonstrating thyroid dysfunction.

Johnson and his co-workers (1991) found that approximately three-quarters of cases of acute illness such as influenza were unreported on the GP computer record.

Ward and his co-workers (1994) found that lifestyle data were poorly recorded, and socio-economic data were virtually absent from GP computer records.

Pringle and his co-workers (1995) used sophisticated procedures to check levels of recording within GP computer records in four practices known to prioritize data entry. Although 100% of prescriptions and 82% of chronic morbidity data were logged, only 67% of referral data, 42% of smoking data and 38% of alcohol consumption data were recorded.

The Data Protection Act requires computer users to maintain high standards of accuracy within personal records. Record computerization therefore brings with it a markedly increased degree of accountability. Omission rates will only be reduced by the increasing use of data entry protocols and opportunistic reminders.

16.7 THE FUTURE OF THE ELECTRONIC RECORD

In the early days of the NHS, general practice handwritten records were regarded by their users as strictly personal jottings, penned on the complementary stationery that had been furnished by a beneficent higher authority as a way of showing its gratitude for services it hoped would be provided. There was a distinct feeling that other GPs had no right to read one's own notes even if this proved physically possible, and some doctors went as far as to destroy the evidence if the patient changed to another practice. The suggestion that patients might want to see their own records was as dangerous as the idea that the common seaman might want to learn to navigate his own ship. It could well provoke mutiny.

Now the boot is on the other foot. Not only is the computer record to be the data engine for general practice patient management, but anything we say in it will be taken down, audit trailed, and may be used in evidence against us. The list of third parties who lay claim to the right either to shape or to interrogate the GP record grows longer by the month, and it is prudent to be aware of the influence these external interests may have on future record design and deployment.

Claims to have an interested right of involvement with the GP record have been exhibited by:

- the Department of Health through its accreditation and reimbursement policies, its own electronic input mediated through HAs, and its control of Read code developments and minimum data set specifications
- the Department of Health through its plans for the NHS Electronic Health Record (EHR), which envisage that the GP computer record should be available to all authorized health professionals throughout the NHS on a 24-hour basis
- the Department of Health through its machinery for promoting clinical excellence and imposing accountability, using NICE, the propagation of protocols such as PRODIGY, and the implementation of clinical governance
- the Department of Health through the MIQUEST and other data collection schemes that have been developed for use by health planners, health managers, and epidemiological and operational research agencies
- HAs and PCG+Ts through audit of practice referral, prescribing and investigative procedures
- community health services, Social Services and Community Mental Health Services, through the linkages between their databases and general practice records
- the patient in pursuit of the rights of data access under the DPA
- the legal system in pursuit of evidence for or against the medical profession
- commercial data collection agencies
- commercial sponsors of computer hardware or software, such as communication agencies or pharmaceutical companies
- Pan European developments such as the Good European Health Record, which seeks to evolve a basic architecture for a medical record that can cross the boundaries between primary and secondary care, can be used in all clinical domains and can be translated into nine different languages. The Centre for the Advancement of Electronic Health Records (CAER) organizes conferences for promoting Pan European EHRs
- global organizations that now exist to promote the development of electronic health records. The TEPR (Toward an Electronic Patient Record) Conference and Exhibition is held annually at rotational venues around the world.

16.8 SCANNERS

Introduction

A scanner is a device that converts a visual image into digital signals that can be processed by computers. Using a mechanism that has much in common with fax machines, photocopiers and laser printers, the image's details are transferred via a scan head and a system of lenses and mirrors to a bank of sensors from which commensurate electronic signals are triggered. When transferred from computer memory to computer storage, the scanned files must be labelled, and slotted into a database to permit systematic retrieval.

Scanners vary considerably, both in price and efficiency, so that it is important to specify one's requirements accurately before purchasing. Scanners require, and are provided by the makers with, attendant software packages that upload the scanner's signals into the host computer. The combined scanner package must be fully compatible with the host system, both in terms of the structure of the files to be transferred, and with regard to the hardware interface.

Scanners may read:

- black and white only
- black, white and various shades of grey (greyscales), or
- colours

and can re-present:
- diagrams, drawings and photographs, and
- text.

Competitive development in recent years has meant that most new scanners now offer all five possibilities. Practices that merely intend to scan hospital reports, guidelines and patient instruction leaflets will not require colour or graphics reproduction, whereas those wishing to construct practice brochures that incorporate logos, drawings or photographs may need all options.

There are three basic types of scanner:

- 'Hand-held', in which either the reading head or the whole unit is held in the hand and passed across the image. The width of the strip of image scanned is determined by the width of the reading head, but seldom exceeds 7.5–10 cm.
- 'Sheet-fed', in which single pages are fed through an intake slot. Stacked single documents may also be accommodated.
- 'Flatbed', in which individual image-bearing documents are inverted on to a flat glass plate, below which the reading head passes. As with photocopying, thick documents and books can be accommodated by flatbed scanners.

Text processing

Although a sheet of text could be stored as a picture, this would involve extravagant and wasteful use of hard disk space. Moreover, in this format the data stored could not be accessed by computerized word searches. Optical character recognition (OCR) software allows scanned text to be recognized character by character, and presented to computer memory as ASCII code. Some products provide for conversion to the text files of major word processing formats, and this allows the word processor's spelling and grammar checking programs to assist in amending the small number of errors inherent in the OCR process. OCR-processed text must always be edited by eye and corrected using the keyboard. When OCR software cannot identify a character, it inserts a 'spaceholder' symbol, such as an ampersand, in order to draw the user's attention to the need for correction.

It is essential that practices consult their GP system suppliers before purchasing a scanning package, in order to ensure compatibility with the host system. Integrated scanning solutions are available for all the major GP systems, either from the system suppliers themselves, or from specialist firms such as PCTI.

Graphic image processing

Scanned graphic images are read as either:

- line art (black and white only)

- greyscales (the range of greyscales on offer varies between 16, 64 and 256, the latter providing the smoothest gradation between tones), or
- colour (which requires a system with 24-bit capability).

Graphic image software should let you preview the image you want to scan. It should also let you enlarge or reduce the image size prior to processing and storage, and for this purpose a rough outline is shown on screen, which can be tailored to size, following which adjustments are made by the system to ensure that the correct density of pixels is recorded to conform with a given degree of definition.

It is essential that the graphic image formats provided by the scanning software should be supported by the host system, and in cases of doubt it should be possible to check conformity by requesting sample output files on diskette from the vendor before purchase. Different scanners export in GIF, TIFF, PCX, TGA, TARGA, EPS, MPNT, PIC, IMG, BMP, GEM, MSP, and SIM formats as single or multiple options. Moreover, some TIFF formats are compressed, a file structure that not all computer systems can accept.

Some scanning packages handle text and graphic images simultaneously and display both, with provision for OCR text processing as and when required. Other refinements are the facility to display response curves, which can be adjusted to harmonize scanner and printer function, and filters, which can produce

Fig. 16.1 Text (relating to staff instructions on prescribing) scanned in to practice computer with two areas selected for optical character recognition (OCR) processing. (Scan Agent 2000, reproduced by courtesy of PCTI Solutions, tel. 01977 690977)

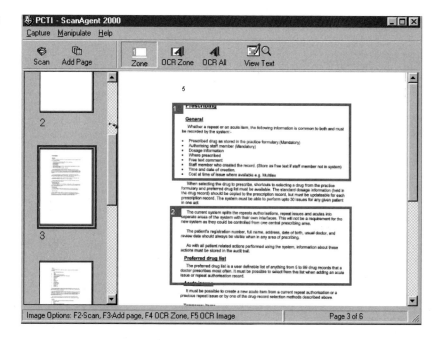

Fig. 16.2 Hospital report
scanned in to Vision system and
integrated with patient record
(In-Practice Systems)

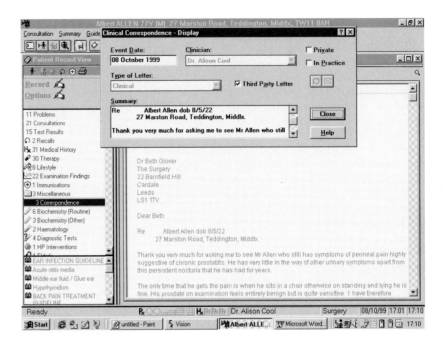

special effects such as the sharpening or softening of
focus. Scanners vary in the degree of resolution which
they can achieve, and also as regards the maximum
image size that they can process.

Scanners may link with the PC through the latter's
serial, parallel or SCSI port, and may require an interface card. A graphics card is also required. While a
standard VGA card can be used, this will limit reproduction to 16 colours or greyscales. Full-colour scanning requires a sophisticated graphics card that incorporates at least 1 Mb of memory; in addition, a high-
grade monitor and a fast host processor with liberal
hard disk space will be needed. A small mono picture
takes up to 250 Kb of storage, but a colour image may
need 1–2 Mb. Most scanner packages run on Windows.

Composite machines, which combine the
functions of scanner, copier, fax and laser printer are
marketed by Hewlett Packard, Canon, Oki, Samsung,
Xerox and Brother.

16.9   VOICE RECOGNITION

When computers were first introduced, one of the
main obstacles to their acceptance by the medical
profession was the need to use a keyboard. The first
converts were those who were already *au fait* with
typewriters or who had bought home PCs for their
families. Resistance to the new technology was
further undermined by the introduction of the GUI,
which enabled much of the data generated at

consultation to be entered using a mouse. Finally,
during the 1990s, voice recognition emerged, and with
it the prospect that the keyboard would eventually be
outmoded altogether.

But despite the fact that many voice recognition
(VR) packages are now well within reach of the GP's
budget, there has been little general enthusiasm for
their use. The reasons given for this are that:

- the headset microphone is interposed between the
  doctor and patient, and may be distracting
- many doctors feel diffident about dictating notes in
  the presence of a patient; on the other hand if the
  procedure is deferred until the patient has left the
  room, the total time required for consultations is
  increased
- there is a general awareness that VR development
  is still being refined, as evidenced by the frequency
  with which upgrades are brought to market. No
  single product as yet possesses the sum of the
  advantages of all its competitors.

OCR and VR are both methods of streamlining data
input to the practice computer. OCR facilitates the
entry of hospital-originated data, whereas VR facilitates the entry of data from general practice.
Inevitably, the need for OCR will disappear when
hospital e-mail outmodes paper mail. By contrast, the
enthusiasm accorded to VR by those who have overcome its inaugural difficulties suggests that this technology is here to stay. Undoubtedly it will improve
further with time.

OCR recognizes characters; VR recognizes sounds and thereby words. Both OCR and VR have an error rate which, though small in experienced hands, nevertheless needs correction by the user.

The principal features of VR systems are as follows:

- Hardware comprises a headset whose gantry suspends a prelabial microphone designed so as to exclude most extraneous noise. Depending upon the package chosen, either a VR card will be provided, or a 16-bit sound card will need to be added.
- Host hardware requirements are a fast processor – usually minimally a 133 MHz Pentium with 32 Mb of memory, 60 Mb of available hard disk space and a CD-ROM drive. (Earlier VR packages were less demanding, but offered less functionality.)
- VR software is based on, and must link with, Windows 95 or NT (OS/2 and Windows 3.1 packages have been marketed but are obsolescent). Software is provided on a CD-ROM disk and installation is usually straightforward. Modern packages allow dictation directly into Windows applications such as Word 97 and other word processing products (for example, WordPerfect and Lotus Notes). If GP systems import word processing files integrally, then it should be possible to dictate directly into patient records, but the system supplier must be consulted to ensure that this can be done. Clinical systems that cannot accept direct dictation may be able to import data from word processors with cut-and-paste routines.
- Early VR systems required that the enunciator should clearly separate contiguous words, but modern systems accept a continuous flow of speech at rates of up to 120 words per minute.
- VR databases are provided with common word vocabularies, in preference to which a field-specific database such as the IBM HealthCare vocabulary may be used. An expandable, custom-built vocabulary may also be accumulated by the user. The size of common-word, field specific, and expandable vocabularies varies between packages – vocabulary size is one measure of a package's competence.
- As dictation proceeds, text appears in a dictation box on the screen. There are 44 different sounds in English speech, which the system assembles in combination as words, using validation from spelling and contextual dictionaries. Given a homophonic word, which might, for example, prove to be 'to', 'too' or 'two', the system checks the frequency with which immediately adjacent words usually appear, in order to make the necessary distinction.
- If errors occur, they must be corrected either by voice command or by use of the keyboard. Early VR systems were only able to correct the last word in a text string by means of voice command, but modern systems allow total voice command correction. Error rates vary between packages but reduce as experience teaches both the user and the system to make adjustments. Long-term error rates should be carefully assessed before purchase of a package, preferably by checking at demonstration, or through consultation with an existing user. Long-term error rates that exceed 4% should be regarded as unacceptable.
- There is a two-way learning process. The new user learns to operate a VR system with the assistance of training software, manuals and experience, and the system becomes acquainted with each user's pronunciation to form an individual 'voice print'. At the outset, a process of enrolment is required whereby the new user reads 200 or more specimen sentences, which the system then digests over a period of several hours. Further autoadjustments are made by the system as error correction proceeds during system use. Voiceprints, like fingerprints, are of course specific to an individual and are summoned into memory after a user logs on with his/her password.
- Navigational commands are also voice-mediated. The dictation process operates within delimiter commands such as 'begin dictating' and 'stop dictating', outside which commands like 'start Word' and 'file save' will be distinguishable by, and obeyed by, the system.
- Templates can be constructed for storage on the system, which will enable the voice completion of standard format documents – the equivalent of preprinting the background architecture for paper proformas. An 'address book' and other organizer functions may be integral with the package.
- Networked VR solutions are available using Windows NT. These will require extra RAM (up to 48 Mb), extra hard disk space, extra headsets and the purchase of additional licences.
- Macros can be custom built for commonly used routines.
- Help texts and manuals are provided, and tutorial software may be available.
- Additional facilities may be offered in relation to VR packages and should be costed at the time when the main package is purchased. These include formal training, the provision of future upgrades, a

text-to-speech function (which requires speakers) and helpdesk support.

VR system manufacturers

The principal VR packages are those produced by IBM, Philips and Dragon:

- Dragon Naturally Speaking and Dragon Dictate (Personal, Classic and Power versions, Dictate Solo Pro and Point and Speak ranges): Endeavour Technologies Ltd, Colette House, 234 Station Road, Addlestone, Surrey KT15 2PH, tel: 01932 827324
- IBM (Simply Speaking Voice Type Dictation and Via Voice ranges) IBM software enquiry desk: 01329 242728
- Philips Speech Processing, The Crescent, Colchester Business Park, Colchester, Essex CD4 4YQ
- Other packages are Angloss Voice, Kolvox Office Talk (incorporating Kurzweil Technology), the Voice Pad-Voice Max range and Voice Xpress.

SUMMARY

- Practice applications should be computerized step by step, but at some point in this process the practice will decide to discontinue using paper documents altogether for its own patient management procedures. The greater the proportion of extraneous data which is received electronically by the practice, the fewer the interim data procedures that the practice will require to implement while awaiting the eventual conversion of all hospitals to computer use. Unfortunately, hospitals are likely to go on providing reports on paper as long as GPs seem prepared to accept them.
- Total conversion to electronic record use saves labour, time, space, raw materials, physical deterioration of records, and costs. It increases data accuracy, accessibility, legibility and security, and enhances staff job satisfaction. The Department of Health has estimated that £100 million per annum would be saved by total data conversion within the NHS.
- The status of electronic records as legally binding vectors depends upon the use of valid audit trails, stringent password discipline and automatic back-up routines, and the total use of the electronic format by all staff. Notes must also be made at or immediately after consultation, and must contain a similar amount of information to that which was previously recorded on paper. Patients' electronic records should be retained by the practice in perpetuity.
- The process of converting GP records to computer use has brought to light a significant degree of inaccuracy and omission, the correction of which will require the future use of computerized data entry protocols and opportunistic reminders.
- Administrative reforms and new legislation have considerably increased the GP's accountability as record keeper. For better or worse, we are entering an era in which many and various third parties plan to influence and access the GP patient record for their own purposes.
- Scanners enable the storage of images on computer and, when accompanied by optical character recognition software, can convert printed text digitally into ASCII code, dovetail with word processing packages, and use word processor spell checking and grammar checking facilities to help correct the small number of errors that inevitably accompany the OCR process. Marketed scanners vary considerably in price, functionality and efficiency. They may be hand-held, or else may accept either single or multiple printed sheets as originals. It is vital that a scanner and its software should be compatible in every way with its host system. Scanners are used in practice principally as a means of converting paper-based hospital data to GP computer storage, a process that will no longer be required once all hospital data are transmitted to general practice through e-mail.
- GPs have been slow to implement voice recognition, despite the fact that it is well within their means and that it has reached an acceptable level of refinement. This reluctance is due in part to the difficulty of dictating notes in the presence of the patient, but the enthusiasm of those who have successfully implemented VR suggests that overall attitudes are set to change. Like OCR, VR carries a small error rate, which must be carefully assessed before purchase. A VR medical vocabulary is needed. Practices should decide whether the extra costs of networking VR are justified.

REFERENCES

Johnson N, Mant D, Jones L, Randall T 1991 Use of computerised general practice data for population surveillance: comparative study of influenza data. British Medical Journal 302: 763–765

Pringle M, Ward P, Chilvers C 1995 Assessment of the completeness and accuracy of computer medical records in four practices committed to recording data on computer. British Journal of General Practice 45: 537–541

Roscoe T 1997 Summaries unearth treasures. Medical Monitor 19 March: 12

Ward P, Morton-Jones A, Pringle M, Chilvers C 1994 Generating social class data in primary care. Public Health 108: 279–287

17 Locality commissioning

17.1 OVERVIEW

When the National Health Service was first introduced in 1948, it removed the irksome need for GPs
to keep daily service accounts and to bill patients periodically 'for professional services rendered'. At last
there would be no further need for the doctor to cost
and invoice each item of care, and Bernard Shaw's jibe
that it paid a surgeon to cut off a man's leg would be
laid to rest.

In 1991, at a time when recessionary factors placed
the governments of all developed countries under
increasing pressure to contain the escalating costs of
their state health care systems, the UK Conservative
government resurrected professional medical com-
mercialism by introducing the General Practice
Funding Initiative (GPFI). On a voluntary basis,
practices could administer notional budgets, exert
pressure on providers by creating an 'internal market',
and use some of the savings achieved through
economies in referral and prescribing to fund
enhanced services within the practice.

Fundholding was neither an unqualified success
nor was it universally popular. The option to fundhold
was only accepted by around half of UK practices.
Rural GPs usually had little choice of provider with
whom to negotiate contracts, and the internal market
was therefore a half-hearted affair. Accusations were
soon rife that fundholders were receiving preferential
treatment from hospitals as regards the quality of service meted out to their patients and from government in
the form of generous levels of funding for the
enhancement of premises and computer systems.

The disparity between fundholding and non-fund-
holding practices led to the coining of the term 'a two-
tiered health service', an epithet so politically evoca-
tive that it became a rallying cry for the New Labour
Party. In the subsequent election campaign that
brought them victory in 1997, the new administration
paid its debt to the electorate by ritually abolishing

fundholding, but it immediately set about introducing
an alternative, though in many ways remarkably similar, system for applying bureaucratic constraint to the
medical profession. The new system was based loosely
on the administrative patterns of several experimental
alternative schemes, which had existed side by side
with fundholding and which included 'commissioning', from which the new scheme took its name. As
with fundholding, the purpose of commissioning is
primarily to make health professionals accountable to
government for the costs of the services they provide.
Although it will take several years for commissioning
to mature, it is clear from government white papers of
1998 and 1999, and other official statements, that the
intention is not merely to contain expenditure, but
also to exert a considerable degree of control over
professional standards.

The introduction of the new controls involved the
establishment of Primary Care Groups and Trusts
(PCG+Ts), interposed between general practices and
the health authorities that administer them and
designed to be the fulcrum upon which the controlling levers would act. As a new link in the chain of
administration, the PCG+T must have its own remit,
its own office, its own staff, its own budget and its
own computer intranet.

The success of the PCG+T is utterly dependent
upon the quality of its information technology and
the information fed to it by its member practices.
Design principles for PCG+T computer systems are
slowly emerging and will continue to be refined over
the next 5–10 years, provided that commissioning
matures in accordance with the plans laid for it. The
long-term success of commissioning will be determined not only by its administrative practicality, but
by the level of funding accorded to it, and by the
degree of antagonism it generates within and without
the profession.

As the PCG+T is an intermediary between the HA
and general practice, the question of who should be

responsible for the design of its computer technology inevitably arises. GP system suppliers are being actively encouraged to rise to the challenge, and most of them are building or have already built, PCG+T modules that will dovetail with the practice systems they market. Like the Duke of Plaza Toro ('because he found it less exciting'), this leaves the NHSE to lead its troops from behind and approve design specifications as and when the latter have been demonstrated to work effectively, much as they did with the RFA scheme.

PCG+T office systems have to provide a wide range of complex and sophisticated facilities in order to function effectively. Primarily they must address the need to replicate, for the most part, the contractual and accounting procedures that were used by fundholding, and to add to these the panoply of trappings called into being by the dictates of clinical governance. Critically, they will depend upon data extraction software that can be applied to disparate GP systems and upon the establishment of highly efficient data communications.

Delays in NHSnet implementation, and doubts over its future, have prompted several HAs to set up their own locality intranets, linking practices, providers and community health services. Such linkages can readily be slotted in to a wider communication architecture when it becomes available.

17.2 THE GENERAL PRACTICE FUNDHOLDING INITIATIVE (GPFI)

In order to understand the rationale, principles and design of locality commissioning it is necessary to take note of the main features of its immediate precursor, the General Practice Fundholding Initiative (GPFI), many of whose administrative, invoicing and accounting routines were retained when the later scheme was introduced.

The GPFI, an exercise in accounting and accountability launched in 1991, provided NHS management with administrative and expenditure data with which to control the service – data that could only realistically be obtained at the point at which care was commissioned. It put commercial pressure on hospital services in large urban areas where there was a choice of provision, and imposed upon GPs the burden of drug budgeting, data collection, financial audit, and reporting.

There were two forms of incentive for GPs to join the scheme. In the first place, a proportion of any economies they achieved could be ploughed back and used to fund improved and innovative practice services. Secondly, it was perceived that hospitals might well be tempted to discriminate in favour of patients from fundholding practices by virtue of the pressures of the internal market. The penalty for being a fundholder was to have to deal with the considerable amount of extra data processing, which made a rod of audit for the practice's own back.

The potential value of statistical data abstracted from multiple GP computers has never been underestimated. For several years before the GPFI, prescribing data had been collected by agencies for resale to the pharmaceutical industry, albeit with limited success. The GPFI was the first serious government attempt to harvest electronic GP data. It was also the first GP computer application whose development was prompted by requirements outside the practice.

The financial support for the GPFI was, of necessity, generous. Originally confined to large practices, or consortia of smaller ones, the extra payments committed to fundholders in management fees and computer reimbursement would have been enough to fund an extra partner. This inevitably raised doubts about value for money.

The scheme ostensibly placed Regional Health Authority (RHA) funds in GPs' hands to enable them to pay for hospital services, drugs, practice staff and NHS community services. Savings made by underspending the allocated budget could be used to improve premises, buy equipment or employ auxiliaries, but could not be translated into profit. In effect, doctors never saw the fund money because payments were made on their behalf by the health authority (HA) – reimbursement of pharmacies, hospitals, NHS community services, and the practice itself in relation to its staff pay. The practice fundholding system was used to keep track of all income and expenditure switched between the relevant health care agencies. Referrals of patients to hospital, with associated costs, were logged as they were made by the practice. End-of-month bills for drugs and community nursing were superimposed on the accounts by the HA, and part reimbursement due for practice staff wages was calculated by the practice, but was subject to ratification by the HA.

Fund holding software

Touche Ross & Co. (management consultants) specified the minimum standard for GPFI software functionality, in conjunction with the Department of Health, and were responsible for running conformance tests on all packages before they were marketed.

As, to begin with, drugs, practice staff costs and NHS community services continued to be paid as they were before the fund's launch, fundholding software was primarily concerned with the contracting, commissioning and payment of hospital services. Elective surgery, all outpatient attendances, all diagnostic investigations commissioned from practice, physiotherapy, speech therapy and occupational therapy were included. Later, community nursing, health visiting, chiropody and dietetics were added.

Figure 17.1 shows how the fundholding database derived the data it required for referral support and ledger updating (the data requirements for automated referral letter construction are described in Chapter 14).

Subsequently, bills from the hospital for completed, incomplete or cancelled services were received by the practice and data from these were entered manually by practice staff on to the fundholding system. These bills also formed the basis of HA payments to the provider.

Accounts were prepared at the month and year end that included drug, practice staff and NHS community costs and analysed all fund income, expenditure and savings. Savings could be carried forward and spent during the following 3 years. The calendar of fundholding events is shown in Table 17.1.

17.3   CONCLUSIONS DRAWN AT THE END OF THE FUNDHOLDING INITIATIVE

- The initiative ran for 7 years and involved just over half of UK practices.
- Fundholding practices effectively controlled 90% of NHS expenditure for the patients on their lists.
- Although it was claimed that fundholding had achieved economies, both in secondary care and

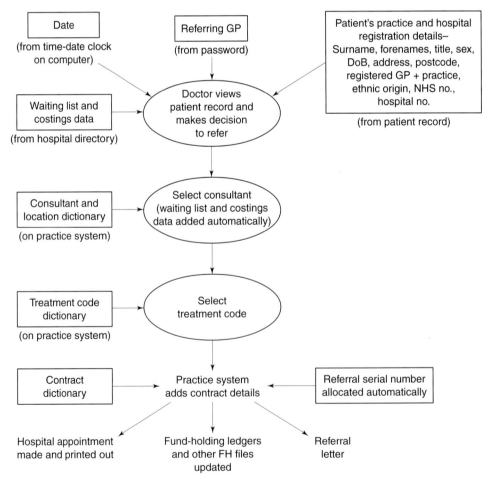

Fig. 17.1 Assembly of data during the referral process

Table 17.1 Calendar of fundholding events

	Daily	Weekly	Monthly	Annually
Input	Referral data entry	Hospital invoice data entered in batches	HA provides data on prescribing costs, practice staff wages reimbursement, and NHS community payments, for entry on the practice computer	HA budget allocated and entered onto practice computer
Output			Monthly returns to HA	Fund savings calculated and carried forward Annual returns to HA

prescribing costs, these were difficult to quantify. Official figures, quoted after the first year of the scheme's operation, suggested that savings in fundholding practices had averaged £44 000. On the other hand, allegations were made that fundholders' notional budgets had been set at unrealistically high levels at the outset, so skewing results. In 1996 the Audit Commission concluded that after 5 years of operation the GPFI had realized £206 million in savings but disbursed £230 million in management costs.

- If fundholding practices overspent their budgets, the deficit was made good by the HA.
- Fundholding practices used savings to improve patient services. In-house counselling services saved money on psychiatric referrals. Physiotherapy and outreach consultant clinics were set up, and further GP specialization allowed colposcopy, vasectomy, dermatology and ophthalmology to be practised in house.
- Hospital waiting lists were reduced.
- Sudden shifts made by large fundholding practices in their choice of provider could destabilize hospital administrative arrangements.
- In 1993 evidence was presented by the Joint Consultants Committee and Association of Community Health Councils for England and Wales that showed that preferential treatment was sometimes given to fundholders' patients, and that 'fast tracking' of hospital services for fundholders' patients was 'extensive and deliberate'.
- Although fundholding savings could not overtly be translated into partners' profits, upgrading of partner-owned premises had the effect of enhancing their property values.
- No large-scale evaluation of fundholding was ever commissioned, presumably because its results might well have jeopardized the success of subsequent plans.

17.4 LOCALITY COMMISSIONING PILOTS

Even though more practices than not had opted for fundholding by the time of its demise, its implementation could not always be taken to imply approval. The controversies that had plagued the GPFI throughout its 7 years spawned a number of alternative schemes, each of which experimented with the way in which the NHS was administered within a locality.

'Multifunds' were conglomerates of fundholding practices that banded together to administer a unified budget. 'Total purchasing' made a practice responsible for virtually all local NHS expenditure. 'Practice commissioning' confined itself, on an *à la carte* basis, to implementing selected items from the fundholding menu, but linked all participants politically under the banner of the National Association of Commissioning General Practices (NACGP). The lessons learnt from all these schemes, from fundholding itself, and from the activities of US Health Service Management initiatives, laid the foundations for the design of locality commissioning, introduced by the new Labour administration in 1998.

Health Action Zones, whose purpose was to gear up local health services in deprived areas, and Primary Care Act pilots, which allowed restructuring of local NHS service provision contracts, were also introduced but were not directly related to the commissioning principle.

39 pilot schemes for locality commissioning were launched in April 1998 to run over a 2-year period. Each pilot was responsible for not less than 50 000 patients. Methodology varied to a minor extent between pilots, but the following general principles emerged.

- Prescribing budgets were held by each pilot and devolved to constituent practices. A special allowance for expensive drugs was provided. No overspend was allowed. Indicative budgets for hospital and community health services were allocated and administered. The HA organized a 1.5% 'holdback' for contingencies. No management allowance was guaranteed to participants. 'Red Book' and Community Fundholding regulations were operative.

- Constituent practices' data were collated on a pilot central server, usually through locality intranets.
- If the overall pilot achieved savings, then a proportion, which varied between pilots, accrued to individual practices to fund service improvements.
- Monthly meetings of participants were organized. Pilot intranet communications enabled feedback to be obtained from practices, and allowed the transmission of progress bulletins, together with directories of hospital services and waiting list data. Health trends were observed, the effects of interventions were measured, and locality audits were carried out.
- E-mail was used to transmit GP–Provider referral and discharge data, and to communicate with the social services.
- PACT data were shared across the pilot and discussed at monthly meetings. Pilot-wide formularies were instituted, generically proportionate prescribing targets were set, and protocols were used for the prescribing of especially expensive drugs. Pharmaceutical advisers visited high spenders to suggest prescribing reforms.
- Some innovative pilot-based facilities were introduced, such as the employment of a diabetic specialist nurse.

In April 1999, although the locality commissioning pilots had only run half their appointed course, locality commissioning was compulsorily extended to all English general practices, with regional modifications of the scheme being applied to Scotland, Wales and Northern Ireland.

17.5 LOCALITY COMMISSIONING COMPUTER SYSTEMS

Because locality commissioning computer systems must of necessity map to the structure and function of Primary Care Groups and Trusts in minutest detail, a clear understanding of a PCG+T's architecture is an essential prerequisite for the analysis of its IT requirements. Figure 17.2 summarizes the main roles of PCG+Ts and their relationships with practices and HAs.

Although the principles of locality commissioning are derived from those of its precursor schemes, its remit has been expanded well beyond theirs to include provision for local health planning, clinical governance, education and training, and communication with the social services and mental health services. Its ambit is now enormous, and it will take several years for proficiency of PCG+T function and PCG+T IT function to be achieved in all intended respects. If it does mature as planned, the PCG+T will become the prime tool through which the government runs the health service.

PCG+T computer systems do not act in isolation. Their interdependence with a host of other agencies is absolute. In particular, they have immediate and close relationships with individual practice and HA systems. GP system suppliers who had already been involved in providing integrated systems for fundholding, multifunding, total purchasing and practice commissioning were at a distinct advantage when they embarked on the design of systems for locality commissioning, because of the similarities all share.

While individual differences in IT design will exist between different PCG+Ts, overall system architecture is dictated by the government specification of PCG+T function, and will be common to all PCG+T modules.

17.6 ORGANIZATION OF THE PCG+T – A SUMMARY

- The PCG+T's primary task is to control the expenditure of funds for hospital and investigatory services, community health services, GP prescribing, and cash-limited GMS funds (now called the Primary Care Investment Fund) from a unified budget.
- The PCG+T has a board to determine its policies, and an executive body to carry out those policies.
- The PCG+T board must include a chairman, a chief officer, a clinical governance officer, GPs, nurses, lay representation, social services representation and Health Authority representation.
- The Locality Commissioning Scheme offers four levels of devolved responsibility. Levels 1 and 2 are Primary Care Groups (PCGs), levels 3 and 4 are Primary Care Trusts (PCTs).
  - Level 1 requires implementation of indicative prescribing budgets, and the operation of Savings Incentive Schemes in relation to them. Shortfalls must be made good from other components of the unified budget allocated to it by the HA (but not from Primary Care Investment

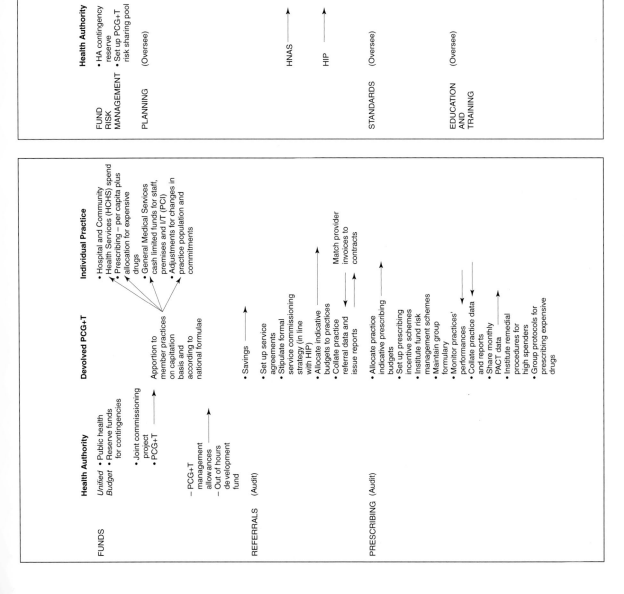

Fig. 17.2 The architecture of locality commissioning

Funds (PCIF) unless these exceed an agreed basic minimum provision).

- Level 2 requirements are as for Level 1, but add the responsibility for commissioning 40% of provider services and for managing the PCG budget allocated to it by the HA.
- Level 3 confers Trust status. All provider care is now commissioned, and the unified budget, which is allocated by the HA, is administered. The Trust cooperates with social services to provide a managed 'package of care'.
- Level 4 requirements are as for Level 3, but additionally impose responsibility for the provision of community health services (midwives, health visitors, district nurses).

- The typical unit size of a PCG+T will be one that encompasses 50 GPs in 20 practices, with a total patient population of 100 000 and a staff of 180. The typical budget size will be £60 million.
- The PCG+T's budget allocation is compiled as a capitation calculation, with weightings for age, sex, long-term sickness, disability, and dependence without full-time care. Justifiably higher provider costs may also be taken into account.
- The PCG+T administers eight main accounts:
  - Elective admissions to hospital
  - Emergency admissions to hospital
  - Referrals to OP clinics
  - Attendances at A&E
  - GP prescribing costs
  - Primary Care Investment Funds (previously cash-limited GMS)
  - Community health services
  - Diagnostic investigations.

The PCG+T sets individual practice budgets in a manner that should reflect the way its own budget has been calculated. In the Total Purchasing Pilots of the 1990s, the problem of individual practice budget allocation proved to be one of considerable difficulty.

72 randomly chosen PCGs will be surveyed annually for 5 years by the National Primary Care Research and Development Centre, Manchester, using performance indicators. All PCTs are subject as Trusts to periodic review by the CHI.

17.7 LOCALITY COMMISSIONING: PRACTICE INFORMATION TECHNOLOGY REQUIREMENTS

In locality commissioning, the administrative tasks formerly undertaken at a single site located at the fundholding practice are now split between the PCG+T office and its client practice sites. The split sites are connected by dial-up telecommunications. The apportionment of functionality between server and client varies between PCG+Ts.

At practice level, locality commissioning calls for the implementation of a commissioning software module, which is grafted on to the practice clinical system for the purposes of data extraction and practice budgetary control. While Level 1 practices have the basic task of implementing indicative prescribing budgets and savings incentive schemes, they must still be able to review actual against indicative costs for the other components of the unified PCG budget, and report actual prescribing and PCI data to the PCG office. They will also be progressing towards higher levels of commissioning, and will need to make appropriate technological preparation to do so.

Levels 2, 3 and 4 practices need *commissioning modules*, which offer the following features:

- Basic system features
  - Compliance with year 2000 requirements, RFA 4 and 5, and Windows
  - PRODIGY compliance and the ability to implement other e-based guidelines
  - Compliance with MIQUEST and other PCG+T-based data extraction software
- Connectivity
  - Access to the PCG+T intranet, compatibility with PCG+T netware, and two-way interactive dovetailing with PCG+T group management software
  - Access to NHSnet and ISDN, use of the Windows Explorer browser, compliance with EDIFACT and NHSnet e-mail requirements
- Database
  - A database to store provider service agreements
- Functionality
  - Software to log practice encounter, morbidity, prescribing and referral data in relation to an identifiable patient, patient post code, doctor and practice
  - Software to acquire, validate, monitor and analyse provider data
  - Software to check provider activity data against practice referral data, and allocate provider data, classified according to PCG+T budget subcategories and costs, and to service agreements
  - Software to log computed costs for prescribing, referrals, PCI and community health services, and compare actual with indicative
  - Software to provide regular reports to the PCG+T on all relevant practice activities, and to interrogate PCG+T bulletins, protocol library,

Table 17.2 Data and staff appointment requirements for a PCG+T member practice

Field of activity	Action	Title
1. Finance	Prepare practice annual business plan Indent to PCG+T for PCI funds (wages, IT and improvements) Prepare annual report on expenditure	Finance Director
2. Commissioning	Receive indicative referrals, investigations and prescribing budget levels from PCG+T Log, monitor, collate and submit to PCG+T records for all above transactions Compare referral, investigative and prescribing levels with indicative budgets Wind up fundholding arrangements Submit practice E-PACT to PCG+T Implement PCG+T formulary	Commissioning Manager
3. Clinical governance	Participate in PCG+T health improvement schemes Implement guidelines recommended by NICE and use PRODIGY Implement MIQUEST to allow data extraction by PCG+T for reports to CHI	Clinical Governance Coordinator
4. Information management and technology	Implement linkages with PCG+T, HA, providers, community health services, mental health services and social services using EDIFACT and e-mail through NHSnet Formulate practice IT strategy Implement audit trails Set up commissioning, PCG+T finances and clinical governance intranets with PCG+T Load PCG+T formulary and protocol library on to practice system Incorporate NICE guidelines in practice system and enable PRODIGY Enable MIQUEST for extraction of practice data by PCG+T Implement educational e-packages supplied by PCG+T Implement printout of PCG+T-based patient information leaflets Formulate practice annual reports to PCG+T	Computer Manager

group formulary, and local provider services data
- The ability to receive interactive educational e-packages and upload responses
• Status
- Notify for registration with the Data Protection Commissioner for medical administrative purposes.

17.8 LOCALITY COMMISSIONING SYSTEMS FOR THE PCG+T OFFICE

The incipient PCG+T must list the current level of practice computerization, hold appropriate discussions with the HA and providers, and formulate an IT strategy. All necessary upgrade plans must be included. PCG+Ts may be able to obtain assistance from the NHS modernization fund. As the data processing tasks required of the PCG+T are many, sophisticated and complex, an IT manager with a high level of skills must be appointed.

PCG Level 1 office IT strategy should be regarded as a preparatory phase whose task is to lay the foundations for Level 2 functionality and above. PCG+T Levels 2, 3 and 4 *office systems* must incorporate the following features:

• Basic system features
- Year 2000, ISDN, NHSnet, EDIFACT and NHSnet e-mail compatibility
- PCG+T server, PCG+T intranet, netware, group management and antivirus software,

---

Box 17.1   PCG+T office staff appointments

1. The duties of a PCG+T Office IT Manager
- Ensure that all PCG+T member practices are compliant with requirements quoted in section 17:7
- Set up and maintain PCG+T IT system, linked to HA, member practices, providers, pathology and radiology departments, community health and mental health services, and social services using NHSnet, EDIFACT and e-mail
- Formulate local IM&T strategy
- Set up commissioning intranet
- Set up contract management software
- Set up PCG+T finances intranet
- Set up clinical governance intranet, using PRODIGY and MIQUEST, with provision of periodic reports to HA and CHI
- Computerize and distribute PCG+T formulary
- Computerize and distribute PCG+T protocol library
- Define minimum data set for the PCG+T's EPR (in conjunction with recommendations of CHDGP)
- Publicize practices' E-PACT data throughout PCG+T
- Issue PCG+T monthly bulletins
- Design and implement Health Needs Assessment Surveys
- Computerize and distribute interactive educational packages
- Enable printing of PCG+T-based patient information leaflets
- Monitor data quality in member practice records
- Provide HA with all required reports

Other Key PCG+T Appointments
2. Chief Executive Officer (overall PCG+T management)
3. Finance Officer
4. Commissioning Manager
5. Health Improvement Coordinator
6. Clinical Governance Supervisor
7. Education Lead Officer
8. Pharmaceutical Adviser (in co-operation with PCG+T Prescribing Subcommittee)

Fig. 17.3   PCG+T office system: data collation and analysis (ITS Safe HCS system's Data Warehouse for PCG+T)

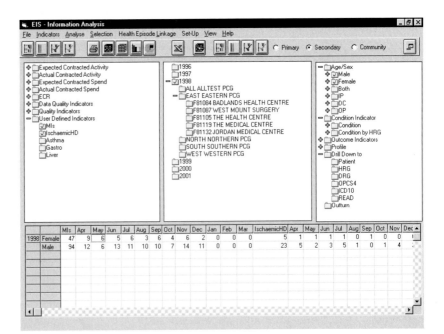

Fig. 17.4 PCG+T office system: prescribing analysis using practice MIQUEST data (ITS Safe HCS system)

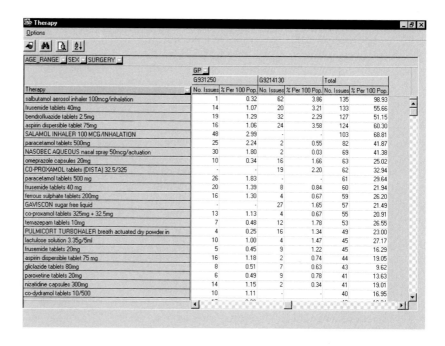

Fig. 17.5 PCG+T office system: morbidity report mapped to postcodes (ITS Safe HCS system)

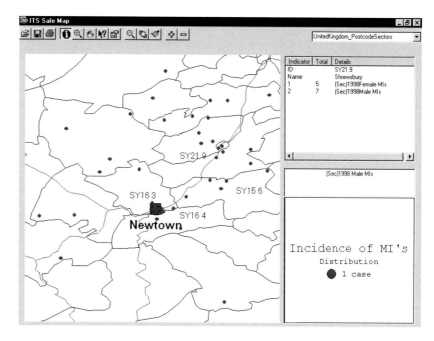

Microsoft Internet Explorer browser interfacing
- Connectivity
  - Intranet interconnectivity with member practice and HA systems
  - Connectivity with providers, laboratory and radiology departments, the CHI, the NICE, the PPA, community health services, social services, mental health services, the LMC and the local health group
- Databases
  - Databases for: practice population data with budget weighting factors, all activity data, performance comparison data, PCG+T manage-

ment data, service agreements, protocol library, group formulary, historical reports, government directives, educational packages, Health Improvement Programmes, PCG+T-wide screening programmes and needs assessment surveys; set up bulletin board facilities for PCG+T forum

- Functionality
  - MIQUEST compliant and other appropriate data extraction software to acquire, validate, monitor and analyse practice activity and costings data classified by encounter, morbidity, prescription and referral, linked to patient identity, post code, doctor and practice
  - Software to acquire, validate, monitor and analyse provider activity and costings data, classified according to the main components of the PCG+T budget
  - Software to link provider data to service agreements and investigate queries
  - Functionality to access all results either by practice or by PCG+T, and to report them to practices, to the HA and to the CHI
  - Software to download e-PACT data and publicize them throughout the PCG+T, with analyses by practice and doctor; software to manage savings incentive schemes and weight indicative practice prescribing budgets with especially expensive drug exceptions
  - Commissioning accounting and reporting software, with ability to allocate indicative budgets using national formulae and to compare actual with indicative costs, both at PCG+T and practice level
  - Software to manage PCG+T budget contingency reserves and practices' risk sharing pool
- Status
  - Notification for registration with DPC for medical administrative purposes.

17.9 ACCOUNTING PROCEDURES FOR LOCALITY COMMISSIONING

Detailed official protocols and templates regulate the implementation of the accounting procedures and reports required of locality commissioning. There is little doubt that, as with the fundholding initiative, these directives will undergo a number of further modifications with time and experience, but it is important for PCG+T boards, IT managers and member practices to be familiar with the basic architecture upon which these procedures are constructed. They may be summarized thus.

- The unified budget is provided annually, calculated in line with national formulae, which must cover the expenditure of all member practices for all health service purposes.
- Budget sub categories:
  - Referrals and investigations – elective admissions to hospital, emergency admissions to hospital, referrals to OP clinics, attendances at A&E, diagnostic investigations
  - Drugs and appliances
  - Primary Care Investment fund (staff, premises, computers)
  - Community health services.
- Accounting:
  (a) Current income and expenditure laid out as:
  - Current month's indicative budget amount
  - Current month's actual expenditure
  - Current month's variance (profit or loss)
  - Current year to date indicative budget amount
  - Current year to date actual spend
  - Current year to date variance (profit or loss)
  - Historical comparisons (see also Table 17.3)
  (b) Balance sheet of PCG+T assets, liabilities, income and expenditure.
- Book-keeping:
  - Referrals ledger – tracks referral administrative and costings data from admission to completion or cancellation
  - Purchase ledger – logs receipt of, and payment of, providers' and investigators' invoices
  - Cash book – lists all payments from bank accounts for staff, premises, and computers
  - Savings (or losses) and amount available for reinvestment, subject to approval, plus details of reinvestment.
- Output:
  (a) Forecasting takes historical data, upgrades costs in line with current budget spending and adds further anticipated enhancement factors in line with inflation and changes in practice activity and population
  (b) Returns
  - Listed patients, referrals, investigations, provider activities by hospital, department, consultant and contract
  - Financial statements, monthly, yearly and for current year to date.
- All accounts, book keeping and output should be available on a per PCG+T, per practice and per doctor basis. A PCG+T management allowance is added, at a level set by the HA.
- Audit trails must be incorporated, and all data must be retained for 3–5 years.

Table 17.3 Use of the spreadsheet to monitor income and expenditure per unit time

| | Month of July 2000 | | | | | Year to date (4 months) followed by estimated annual out-turn | | | | |
	Actual spend £	Budget income £	Variances Better (or worse) Actual £	% Budget	Last year £	Actual spend £	Budget income £	Variances Better (or worse) Actual £	% Budget	Last year £
Purchase of hospital services	90000	100000	10000	10	95000					
Drugs and Appliances						200000	150000	(50000)	(33.33)	140000
						600000	450000	(150000)	(33.33)	420000
Primary Care										
Investment Funds										
Community Health										
Services										
Subtotal of above C/F										

Hospital costs may be further analysed by hospital, by department, by consultant, by procedure, by patient, etc.
Hospital referrals may be analysed by rate, by type, by actual waiting periods, by stage of processing, by treatment, by contract type, by patient, etc.

SUMMARY

- Locality commissioning derives its main design features from the GP fundholding and other similar initiatives that immediately preceded it. The GPFI became regarded as politically unsound.
- The purpose of fundholding and locality commissioning has been to put downward pressure on health-care costs and increase the accountability of health-care professionals. Additionally, locality commissioning carries the responsibility of monitoring and improving professional standards.
- Locality commissioning requires adjacent practices to form groups for the purpose of administering allocated notional budgets. Each group comprises about 20 practices, 50 doctors and 100 000 patients. The group's finances are administered by a PCG+T chairman and board from a PCG+T office.
- The PCG+T board must include a chairman, a chief officer, a clinical governance officer, GPs, nurses, lay representation, social services representation and health authority representation.
- There are four levels of responsibility for PCG+Ts. Level 1 administers a prescribing budget, and takes part in savings incentive schemes. Level 2 additionally commissions 40% of provider services and manages a budget allocated by the HA. Level 3

confers Trust status, and adds the responsibility of commissioning all provider services and of liaising with the social services to produce 'a package of care'. Level 4 additionally requires the Trust to be responsible for the provision of community health services.
- PCG +T budgets are set annually and apportioned between member practices, in line with national formulae. They must cover all the NHS expenditure incurred by all member practices – referrals and investigations; drugs and appliances; staff, premises and computers; community health services. A PCG+T management allowance is determined by the HA.
- A PCG+T's functionality and efficiency is heavily dependent upon its IT services and IT manager. A PCG+T intranet is required to communicate with member practices, the HA, community health services, social services, the LMC and mental health services. Communication must also be established with providers, the PPA, the NICE, and the CHI.
- The procedures for accounting, book-keeping and forecasting, and the provision of returns in relation to locality commissioning, are specified in detail in official directives, and these will doubtless be further modified in the light of experience.
- PCG+T and member practice systems must be year 2000, RFA 4 and 5, Windows, PRODIGY,

MIQUEST, ISDN, NHSnet, Microsoft Internet Explorer browser and DPA compliant, and must use common netware and group management software. A suite of sophisticated data logging, extraction, analytical and collation software modules is required, and feedback on progress must be provided by the PCG+T to member practices.

- 39 locality commissioning pilots were set up in April 1998 and were due to run for 2 years, but in April 1999 locality commissioning was compulsorily extended throughout the whole of the UK, with regional modifications applying to Scotland, Wales and Northern Ireland.

FURTHER READING

Department of Health 1990 General practice funding initiative. Requirements specification for general practice systems, produced in conjunction with Touche Ross & Co. HMSO, London

Department of Health 1993 General practice funding initiative. Specification version 2.1 produced in conjunction with Hoskyns Group PLC. HMSO, London

Department of Health 1998 Health improvement programmes. Health service circular HSC 1998/167: LAC (98) 23 (NHSE)

Elkan R, Robinson J 1998 The use of targets to improve the performance of health care providers: a discussion of government policy. British Journal of General Practice 48: 1515–1518

ITS Wales 1998 New generation GP clinical systems for PCGs. Health Service Computing, Winter: 29–32

Maxwell M, Howie J G R, Pry de C J 1998 A comparison of three methods of setting prescribing budgets, using data derived from defined daily dose analyses of historic patterns of use. British Journal of General Practice 48: 1467–1472

National Association of Primary Care 1998 PCG constitutions. Pamphlet No. 1. http://www.primarycare.co.uk, tel: (020) 7636 7228

NHSE 1998 The new NHS: modern and dependable. Health Service Circulars HSC 1998/171 and 1998/065

NHS Primary Care Alliance (fly. NACGP) website http://www.ncl.ac.uk/nphcare/GPUK/comiss/nacgp. htm, tel: 01788 555008

Primary Care Group Advice Line tel. 01932 826565 e-mail 100574.3401@compuserv.com

Primary Healthcare Development Consultancy 1998 Simple guide to primary care group (published in association with Doctor Magazine)

Scottish Needs Assessment Programme. Primary care network needs assessment in primary care – a rough guide (contact Clare Sharp, tel: 0141 330 5607)

Secretary of State for Health 1997 The new NHS: modern, dependable. Government White Paper. Stationery Office, London

18 Networks

18.1 INTRODUCTION

An impasse was reached in the early days of Australian railway development when individual states built tracks with differing gauges, and rolling stock could not proceed beyond state boundaries. To this day, a journey on the Trans-Siberian railway involves a delay at the Sino-Mongolian border while the carriages' bogies are changed to those of another width. Problems of compatibility have also dogged computer development since its beginning. Earliest software was hardware dependent and, although application software is still heavily dependent upon its operating system, communications standards have at last been introduced that allow computers using different operating systems to talk to each other. The most important of these standards from the standpoint of the GP system are EDIFACT (electronic data interchange for administration, commerce and transport), X400 and SMTP (simple mail transport protocol). These standards dictate the file structure, format and logistics of electronic message transmission that will be used within the NHS. Standards, like computer functionality, are upgraded periodically in the light of continuing development.

LANs and WANs

Although there is increasing overlap between them as computer communications develop apace, there are basically two types of network, local area networks (LANs) and wide area networks (WANs). Familiar examples of LANs are the systems found in most GP surgeries. WANs are exemplified by NHSnet or the Internet. Most networks operate through wire or fibreoptic data-telecommunication channels, but computers in close proximity can be linked by infrared signals, and radio or satellite can be used to establish distant connections. Special communication and network management software, and added communication circuitry within each processor are required. Unless the line of communication used transmits digital data, then a modem to convert and deconvert signals from digital to analogue will also be needed.

18.2 LANS

A LAN shares local data and computer facilities between users. It:

- links compatible hardware components
- links compatible software modules housed on component computers
- uses in-house cabling (or infrared connection)
- uses communications software and networking software
- requires the provision of network interface cards for each component processor
- does not need a modem
- does not provide opportunities for hacking, because it is a closed circuit.

UK general practices began to compute with single-user configurations. Most then graduated to so-called 'multiuser' configurations, which employed a central processor and 'dumb' terminals (ironically also known as Wyse terminals after a prominent manufacturer) that offered no peripheral processing power. The advent of graphical user interfaces, image reproduction and the NHSnet during the 1990s sounded the death knell for dumb terminals because of the requirements these innovations have for distributed processing. Instead, intelligent workstations (effectively personal computers in their own right) began to be employed as terminals and the LAN was born. If all computers in a LAN had equal functionality, the configuration was described as 'peer-to-peer'. If one unit took overall control of the LAN, it was known as the fileserver and its relationship with its outstations was described as 'client–server'.

The cost of upgrading to workstations prompted the development of a cheaper compromise terminal in 1995, in which all the processing required of an outstation was carried out on circuit boards, and the costs of relatively expensive components such as hard disks were avoided. This compromise solution was termed the 'network computer' (NC) or network station. The NC copes with graphics, Windows 95 or NT, Internet access and e-mail, and has low maintenance costs (the 'set-top box' used domestically in conjunction with a television set uses a variant of the same principle). As the lion's share of processing tasks on an NC network are undertaken by the fileserver, the latter must have correspondingly enhanced functionality.

LANs can be accessed remotely by use of a 'laptop' or 'palmtop' computer linked to a conventional or radio telephone, in which case the portable computer makes distant contact with the fileserver and behaves to all intents and purposes as if it were an outstation on the network (*terminal emulation*).

18.3 LAN ARCHITECTURE

Without going into too much technical detail, it is as well that LAN users should have a nodding acquaintance with terms with which they will be bombarded by system engineers and manuals.

The 'bus' or 'daisy-chain' configuration is the simplest relationship between PCs, in which the only exterior link is a length of cable plugged into the back of each. This arrangement is only adequate for small peer-to-peer networks.

The 'star' network copes with more PCs, and links each by cable to a 'central hub' – a piece of dedicated hardware installed to manage the distribution of messages between the components of the network.

'Routers' and 'switches' are also hardware components that may be involved in the distribution process.

A 'token ring' is a configuration usually reserved for mini computers and mainframes.

Cables for networks must be designed so that they obviate electromagnetic interference from their surroundings. Coaxial ('thin wire') cabling has a central metallic core surrounded by an insulating sheath and, outside this, a metallic lattice shield. The geometry of unshielded twisted-pair (UTP) cabling cancels out interference. The cabling most resistant to interference is fibreoptic, but this is also the most expensive (Table 18.1).

In practice, UTP is the commonest type of cabling used in LANs and, as cabling engineers charge high prices for their work, a few technocratic practices have undertaken their own cable installation and maintenance (a knowledge of the intermediary relay hardware is an essential prerequisite). DIY supplies of UTP cable, connectors and crimpers can be obtained from Wadsworth Electronics (tel: (020) 8941 4710).

A suite of LAN software must not only act as a coordinating operating system (e.g. Novell Netware, Windows NT), but must also provide network application programmes ('Groupware', e.g. Team Office, WordPerfect Office 3.1). 'Network management software' offers a third dimension in providing network managers with feedback on data traffic and problem areas, so that appropriate adjustments can be made.

18.4 WANS

WANs link distant computer hardware and software platforms that might not otherwise be compatible, but that conform to common data communication standards.

Examples of WANs are the NHSnet, HealthLink and the Internet.

Table 18.1 Three types of cable used for local area networks

Type of cable	Data transmission rates (bits/s)*	Approx. cost per metre (£)	Minimum cost of network card (£)	Is hub required?	Comments
Coaxial	Up to 10 Mbits/s	3	15	No	Jointing difficult
VTP category 5	10 Mbits to 1 Gbits/s	1	15	Yes	Robust and easily installed
Fibreoptic	100 Mbits to 127 Gbits/s	3	150	Yes	

* The term 'baud', coined after telegraphic pioneer Baudot, goes back to Morse code days, and 'baud rate' is usually accepted as synonymous with bits/s, despite the fact that this does not fit its exact definition. The baud width of a cable is the range of frequencies that it is capable of conveying, although this term is also misused and may be understood to mean transmission volume capacity as well as range.

To access a WAN, a user will require:

- enrolment with a *service provider*. GP system suppliers act as contractors to NHSnet on behalf of their clients. Internet service providers such as FreeServe or Tesconet provide computer users specifically with access to the Internet. On-line service agencies provide access to the Internet, remote databases, bulletin boards and various other computer-related facilities. All types of service provider can and do provide e-mail.
- a modem and public service telephone network (PSTN) line, or a codec (also known as a terminal adapter) and an integrated services digital network (ISDN) line, in order to connect the user's computer with the service provider's WAN gateway
- a communications card, installed in the processor
- software to communicate across the WAN to access remote computers and to search for, download and process data obtained from those computers. Processing will include displaying, printing, and storing data.

WANs are potentially vulnerable to unwanted access from hackers and remote distributors of viruses, and stringent measures must be taken to protect the confidentiality of sensitive data that are being transmitted across them. These measures include access control through passwords and PINs, 'firewalls' and encryption.

18.5 HEALTHLINK

The Family Health Service Data Communications Network (HealthLink) was set up in 1991. It is owned and managed by Racal on behalf of, and with responsibility to, the Department of Health. It made electronic networking facilities available to health service agencies throughout England and Wales, interconnecting all health authorities, the Southport Central NHS Registry, the FHS Computer Unit (NHS Computer Agency, Exeter), hospitals, radiology departments, pathology laboratories, general medical practices, general dental practices, the Dental Practice Board, Community Health Units, pharmacists, the PPA, opticians, the Paymaster General's Office, the

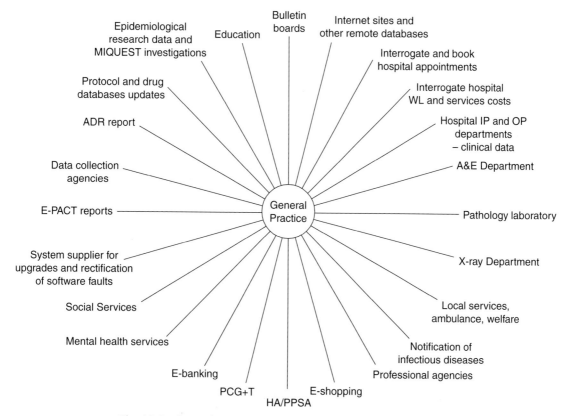

Fig. 18.1 External connections established by the practice computer

National Breast Screening Centre Project and specialist and private health organizations. Cross-linkage with the Social Services Network was planned, and service agencies supplying the NHS were scheduled to be allowed access, subject to approval.

Racal is a highly successful carrier, which set up what was to become the largest private network in Europe when it was commissioned to provide and manage the UK government's own administrative data network, linking 41 government departments. Racal was also given the task of providing the National Lottery network. Racal leases its lines from BT and Mercury, conforms to NHS data communication standards and uses mainframe computers to store client messages on a central hub. The software needed to access its hub can be used on widely disparate client systems.

HealthLink offers two different types of connection:

- direct dialogue, which allows real time 'conversations' between computers and access to remote databases, and provides for NHS banking transactions
- 'mailbox' facilities, in which a dedicated storage area in the Racal central hub is earmarked to accommodate data for an individual recipient. Mail 'posted' to this mailbox by various senders is collated, and accumulates until such time as the recipient 'empties' his mailbox by an electronic download (which is usually an autodial transaction taking place overnight). Mailbox messages may be structured or free-style e-mail. Images may also be transmitted.

The two types of connection are analogous, respectively, to the conventional telephone and postal services. In each case, electronic data transmission has the clear advantage over its older counterpart of providing legible text, rapidity, audited message integrity, confidentiality, accurate recipient targeting, convenience, economies in labour, postage fees and resources.

Network security is obtained by controlling user access through passwords and addresses (12-character codes), by issuing protected mailboxes, by date and time stamping all transactions, and by logging and monitoring all network usage and erroneously attempted access.

System access requirements for joining HealthLink are:

- a modem and PSTN line, or a terminal adapter and ISDN line

- a communications interface, located in the processor
- communications software.

NHS practices intending to join HealthLink for the purpose of setting up GP–HA Links should approach their HA. HealthLink fees, payable either through the HA or directly to Racal, cover registration and an annual subscription. On signing Racal's enrolment contract, practices are issued with an identity code.

BT line charges are levied at local call rates, except in a few very remote sites. Most access from general practices will be by dial-up, although large units such as PCG+Ts and cooperatives may find it economical to hire a permanently leased line. A proportion of the costs of using HealthLink should qualify for reimbursement.

Racal and BT Syntegra reached a reciprocal agreement for jointly handling NHS data, but the prospects for the ultimate survival of HealthLink as a separate entity are uncertain. Racal's contract for services ends in 2001, and even if HealthLink's functions are subsumed into NHSnet after that date, the experience gained from its 10 years of operation will not have been wasted.

18.6 THE NHSNET

After the demonstrable success of Racal's HealthLink in the early 1990s, it came as a surprise to many that BT Syntegra and Mercury Communications (a subsidiary of Cable & Wireless) won contracts in 1995 to implement and market a rival and more powerful secure national electronic network for the NHS. NHSnet development has been expensive and protracted, sign-up and hook-up both seem unnecessarily complex operations, and optimal use of the net's facility requires ISDN; nevertheless the government's commitment to the new network has been unequivocally spelt out in a series of white papers over the last decade. In *The New NHS – Modern – Dependable*, issued in November 1997, it was proposed that all computerized practices should be connected to NHSnet. The target date of 2000 was revised in the light of slippage to 2002.

Whereas HA and GP take-up of HealthLink was almost universal, hospitals, with their higher volume data requirements, began to sign up for NHSnet in preference to HealthLink, a bias reinforced by the mandatory requirement that they should use NHSnet for all Clearing Services transactions. It seemed to be no coincidence that at one point all senior NHS executives were issued with NHSnet-based e-mail facilities.

NHSnet is a secure electronic national network for both voice and data traffic. Its data services provide:

- a message handling service using mailboxes for the transmission of standard messages such as pathology and radiology reports or provider discharge data
- dial-up access for interrogation of remote databases such as those containing waiting list information; dial-up access to facilities for booking outpatient appointments or requesting patient transport
- monitored carriage for the transmission of all NHS-wide Clearing Services traffic
- two-way e-mail for all users
- an outbound (unidirectional) link to the Internet.

In addition to these five main tasks, NHSnet will, in due course, enable:

- access to PPA data (e-PACT)
- transmission of urgent communications to NHS staff from the Chief Medical Officer ('Cascade')
- transmission of research information
- telemedicine
- News Groups for NHS staff
- transmission of patient records on change of practice
- access to sources such as NHSweb (the secure NHS national intranet within the Internet), the National Electronic Library of Health (NELH) and the NHS Information Zone.

In tandem with these enhancements in data communications, government white papers require the rationalization of NHS voice communications and radio facilities through an integrated management structure that will oversee all types of NHS networking.

The requirements for data, file and transmission standards used by NHSnet are now built into GP system accreditation (RFA4).

Connections to NHSnet

NHSnet offers four alternative methods of connection, each having its own tariff. In summary these are:

1. messaging only (replaces existing HealthLink mailbox facilities)
2. stand alone dial-up/dial-up with message store, which offers mailbox and Internet service-provider-type facilities with browsing and single e-mail access (browsing encompasses both the Internet and the NHS Information Zone) – this option requires the use of a stand alone computer

3. integrated e-mail and web browsing (the 'remote user agency solution'), which provides similar facilities to those detailed under (2) but allows integration with a host clinical system, although with data deliverable at one point only
4. integrated desktop e-mail and web browsing (the 'Message Transport Agent' MTA solution), which provides an integrated solution for networked desktop PCs, with all facilities deliverable at all workstations.

While options (1) and (2) can be used with modems and a PSTN line, they would seem to offer little advantage over the use of existing joint HealthLink and ISP facilities. Option (3) may also be used with PSTN and integrates with the clinical system, but is only available on one terminal.

Option (4) is clearly optimal and is probably the only solution that many networked practices are likely to consider, as long as HealthLink facilities remain available. It cannot be used with dumb terminals and requires ISDN, which may be either:

- installed as a dial-up facility
- used with a permanently leased line – a provision that may be suitable for larger combines such as PCG+Ts.

Signing up to NHSnet

Connections (1) and (2) may be purchased from BT or Mercury, but because options (3) and (4) are integrated they are usually purchased through the GP system supplier. There are no fewer than five documents involved in the signing up process. In summary these are:

- the Memorandum of Arrangement (between practice and NHS supplier authority), which allows the practice to purchase net access
- a Code of Connection, which spells out the type of connection selected and the facilities it provides – protocols for implementing strict security procedures have to be formally accepted
- a WAN Access Agreement, made between the practice and BT or Mercury.

When completed, these three documents must be sent to the local NHS Telecommunications Branch before the net provider will agree to sell services to a practice. After the application has been processed, a WAN access number is issued, which must be included in:

- a WAN order form, which, on completion, is dispatched to BT or Mercury
- a registration form, which is endorsed by the carrier to allocate an NHSnet account, practice identification details on the net, and an e-mail address.

Security

The code of connection is a contract signed by the practice, which commits it to implement specified strict security procedures. One nominated individual must accept overall responsibility for ensuring that these are carried out.

A secure identity card can be used to protect access. This displays a numeral, which changes every minute in synchrony with its equivalent stored in the computer. In order to log on to the network, the user must enter this number, adding his/her own password and a four-character PIN number. Access levels correlate with password and type of user.

ISDN access incorporates additional security measures. The challenge handshake authentication protocol (CHAPS) uses an exchange of password identification, and each computer challenges the other in turn. Caller line identification (CLI) provides a display of the caller's number to the recipient, and this can be validated automatically by reference to a list of approved accessing computers.

Various types of encryption are available, which can either be entered from smart cards or built in to the system.

Funding

Taking into account the cost of upgrading dumb terminal configurations to fileserver-driven networked workstations, of installing ISDN lines, of buying into NHSnet carriage access, and of purchasing access software and additional GP supplier services, many practices will have difficulty in funding an upgrade to NHSnet without substantial subsidies. (In mid 1999, for instance, Ulster practices announced that they could not afford to make the necessary changes.) Selective reimbursement, sometimes of an order of 100%, was used successfully in helping to promote the uptake of GP-HA Links. Similar inducements will catalyse migration to NHSnet.

As regards carriage charges, both central and peripheral linkages will now be paid for by the government, the latter payment being made from the NHS modernization funds.

Clearly, the greater the proportion of overall NHSnet expenses that can be paid from central funds, the more will be the benefits obtained from economy of scale.

BT Syntegra has proposed plans to involve private sector investment in a scheme that places remotely managed desktop computing facilities in doctors' surgeries. The scheme, entitled 'Healthnet Plus+' would support, and be supported by, commercially based initiatives.

18.7 INTRANETS AND EXTRANETS

An intranet harnesses Internet and World Wide Web technology in order to use it on an internal network. Just as the Internet connects remote computers around the world, so an intranet can make accessible, to all authorized users, all the information housed on separate computers within a discrete organization. To do this, an intranet borrows the proven techniques of the Internet's global configuration – a graphical user interface, browsers, Internet-style navigation routines and hypertext links. Individual computers on intranets are even referred to as 'websites', and individual screens on them are known as 'web pages'.

Intranets can not only use Internet type technology within a closed local area network but can also impose their selectivity upon the Internet itself, so forming a closed wide area network and getting the best of both worlds. Intranets are therefore ideal conduits through which multinational companies can communicate privately and worldwide, and disparate hardware platforms can be linked together, provided that they have Internet access. To preserve privacy, intranets that communicate through the Internet are usually provided with encryption and protective 'firewalls', and the resulting secure configuration is sometimes known as an extranet, or virtual private network. Intranet access and navigational routines closely resemble those of the Internet. Initial logon, which includes user name and password, may involve additional steps introduced to protect sensitive data. These superadded routines may be telescoped by use of a macro, invoked by clicking on a dedicated company logo button. In turn, this summons the company home page, from which further navigation proceeds.

The intranet toolbar either accommodates Netscape-style icons – back, forward, home, images, open, print, find and stop – or alternatively Microsoft Internet Explorer icons – back, forward, open start page, refresh, open favorites, open print, stop, and send. 'Helper applications' are available that expand browser functions to include graphics and multimedia.

Intranet technology provides for e-mail and is potentially transferable to wide area networks other than the Internet, although this would be a more expensive option.

Intranet technology is appropriate for PCG+T and cooperative use, and in the configuration of NHSweb will be useful for disseminating training and educational facilities throughout the NHS. It is already being used in some hospital environments and in large local multidisciplinary combines within the NHS.

Software packages for constructing intranets, extranets and intranet home pages are all commercially available.

18.8 ON-LINE SERVICES

Prior to the widespread uptake of Internet access through Internet Service Providers (ISPs), several international companies (notably CompuServe and CIX) offered data communication facilities for company and home computing, using their own wide area networks (WANs), accessed through modems and telephone line dial-in. Fees were levied on subscription time or data volume, or a mixture of these components. Telephone line charges were not always available at local call rates.

The Internet revolution, with its industry-standard software, cheap access and massive coverage, has to a very large extent outmoded the services of the older on-line agencies, although there is still a place for more modern ones which target their activities at communities with a special common interest.

If we except ISPs, whose role is basically limited to the provision of Internet access, web space and e-mail, the functions that may or may not be obtainable from on-line service providers (OLSPs), are:

- Internet access
- OLS home pages
- client web space
- e-mail
- access to remote databases
- bulletin boards with notice boards, news groups, conferencing, freeware and shareware
- on-line sales of data CD-ROMs or medical equipment
- a fax gateway
- a helpline.

A number of short lived attempts to harness the GP OLS market with user or pharmaceutical funding were made during the 1990s, but the following projects survived and matured.

Network Medical On line (NEMO)

NEMO offers free membership to approved GPs and is accessed via the PSTN at standard call rates. It uses its own secure WAN to provide a closed user group, and offers a wide range of information of use to GPs, which includes MeReC bulletins, patient leaflets that can be printed out, a library of medical literature including access to Medline, a magazine-type information service with press releases, a bulletin board with news groups, and a sales service for medical equipment and other items of use to GPs.

NEMO is funded by pharmaceutical companies, who sponsor data within their therapeutic areas of interest. Software is provided. Minimum hardware requirements are a 386 processor running Windows 3.1, and a modem.

Contact: Network Medical Services Ltd, Ocean House, Hazelwick Avenue, Crawley, West Sussex, tel: 01293 534411.

Healix (the Health Information Exchange)

Healix uses its own secure WAN, which is accessed via the PSTN at standard rates. Membership of Healix costs £90 per annum. Healix supports evidence-based medicine by focusing on protocols, guidelines, and systematic reviews from major medical journals. Reviews are summarized and referenced so as to enable the user to follow up those likely to be of interest, although the full article must then be accessed by recourse to its original publication. Patient advice leaflets are available on many subjects, as is up-to-date travel medicine advice.

Healix can provide users with gateways to both the Internet and NHSnet, but cannot access NHSweb. It can allow e-mail to be sent and received by users over its secure WAN. Healix's website is at http://www.healix.co.uk. Minimum requirements are a PC and modem running Windows 3.11 with 15 Mb available hard disk space.

Contact: World Health Network, Portland House, Aldermaston Park, Aldermaston, Reading RG7 4HP, tel: 01734 816666.

Doctor's Desk

The most interesting medical OLSP is, perhaps, that set up by the Department of General Practice of St George's Hospital, London, which uses NHSnet operationally through ISDN 2, but also offers a demonstration version on the Internet. 'Doctor's Desk' (DD) plays a prominent role in the practices in which it has been installed, replacing the GP clinical system's front end 'desktop' screen with its own from which the host clinical system itself can be opened, external communications can be initiated, or a wealth of electronic information sources can be accessed. The front end screen takes the term 'desktop' literally, and represents the doctor's desk pictorially. Clicking on the various items associated with the consulting room desk triggers the various software linkages. Thus EMIS, In Practice, and AAH Meditel systems, with which DD can be integrated, are opened by clicking on the desk itself, the telephone is the icon for e-mail, the pill box for drug information, the books on the desk for electronic references, the top drawer for journals, the bottom drawer for information on the business of general practice, and the patient's chair for patient-orientated information.

DD initiates the following communications:

- NHSnet enrolment is enabled on subscribing to DD, and an NHSnet address is allocated
- ISDN 2 enrolment is enabled on subscribing to DD
- Linkage is established with the local hospital trust, if the latter's computer allows access
- Two-way e-mail is provided (up to five e-mail addresses per practice)
- News groups are available
- Video and telemedicine are supported
- An outbound Internet gateway is available through NHSnet
- A 5 Mb personal website is provided.

DD offers access to the following electronic information:

- E-journals: *British Medical Journal, The Lancet, New England Journal of Medicine, Bandolier*
- Search engines: Medline (through PubMed and Artemis), BIDS, OMNI
- E-books: *Merck Manual, Oxford Handbook of Clinical Medicine – updates, ABC of Medical Computing*
- E-BNF and e-Red Book (for which licences must be purchased)
- E-newspapers
- Timetables for radio and TV
- 'What's on' pages: noticeboard, education, research, institutional and topical sections
- Information on evidence-based medicine, the business of general practice, the use of DD
- Patients' information sites
- Access to NHSnet websites.

DD requires a Pentium PC with 16 Mb of RAM. Installation costs are quoted as upwards of £2400, with ongoing monthly fees of £40. To these must be added ISDN and NHSnet charges, the latter including the costs of a router and firewall. DD provides half a day of training, on-site hardware support for one year and a helpline. View:

Internet – http://drsdesk.sghms.ac.uk
NHSnet – http://drs.desk.sthomas.nhs.uk

18.9 GP–SOCIAL SERVICES NETWORK LINKAGE

The Department of Health strategy document *Information for Health* presages local linkage between medical and social services throughout the UK. Social services reforms now anticipate unified local health and social services budgets.

In 1994, Dr Andrew Herd's practice in Co. Durham set up a trial link with the local social services information database to allow him to inspect the database and to provide e-mail interchange. In 1995 Lancashire FHSA completed a 4-month trial under the code name 'Office Power', managed by ICL, which linked the social services network to a three-doctor practice in Preston. The doctors used their terminal to replicate a request form, either for an initial patient assessment or for a follow-up visit by the social services, and the completed 'form' was e-mailed to local social services officers, who emptied their mailboxes several times a day. After case assessment and action, a freestyle report was e-mailed back to the doctor.

The linkage proved to save time and paperwork and avoided the need for telephone trawls in pursuit of social services personnel.

18.10 THE PUBLIC HEALTH LINK AND CASCADE

The Public Health Link was set up in 1994 by the Department of Health to ensure that all doctors were able to receive urgent national health information promptly from the Chief Medical Officer (CMO). The measure was introduced following complaints that postal missives from the CMO were not delivered quickly enough to enable clinicians to deal with the flood of patient enquiries that were sometimes triggered by media hyperbole on health topics.

A communicable disease network employing the commercial carrier Epinet was already accessed by the Public Health Laboratory Service, and this was at first used to pass on ('cascade') messages to those FHSAs which had suitable terminals. Unfortunately, even FHSAs equipped with Epinet links experienced difficulty in relaying their messages to GPs, who had to be contacted either by fax, e-mail or courier if these facilities were available. When this relay proved to be impracticable, which it often did, the FHSA had to revert to conventional postage, which vitiated the whole point of the exercise.

In the end, past deficiencies will be forgotten as NHSnet enables all practices to be contacted within

24 hours. Data from general practice will also be transmittable to the Communicable Disease Surveillance Centre in Colindale, to which all Public Health and all 350 NHS laboratories are now networked. If communicable disease surveillance were to be coupled with data on microbe sensitivity, such as are provided by Glaxo's powerful MicrobeBase, regional control of infectious disease would be greatly enhanced.

A PHLS website giving advice on locality treatment of infection is now accessible at http:// www.phls.co.uk.

18.11 JANET AND SUPERJANET

In 1979 JANET, the universities' Joint Academic Network, was set up to link UK universities and Research Councils. The network is centrally funded and no use-related charges are levied on the open access that is afforded to all accredited users. JANET uses CCITT (telecommunications industry) standards, but responsibility for security over the network is placed squarely on the shoulders of its users, since potential abusers would be most likely to be drawn from the ranks of the academic institutions themselves.

The network's offspring, SUPERJANET, became the UK's largest ATM-based WAN in 1995, connecting 60 universities and research laboratories around the country. SUPERJANET spawned a number of innovative applications, which included making rare books available electronically, promoting remote medical education supported by videoclips (such as for surgical operations), and creating advanced data visualization.

18.12 BULLETIN BOARDS

A bulletin board is remote computer storage that offers users access to notices, messaging, vending and conferencing in an orderly way. The equipment needed by users is much the same as that which accesses remote databases, but the accent is on two-way data traffic. As with Prestel, there are some closed user groups, but most datafiles are available to all users.

In the public domain there are hundreds of UK bulletin boards, devoted to such topics as finance, company information, legal affairs, travel, astronomy, gardening, medicine, and general and selective news. As bulletin boards were originally set up by enthusi-

astic amateurs, computer-related information occupies a prominent place in the list of contents, and technical assistance and advice is exchanged, shareware is marketed, freeware may be on offer, and software upgrades for a number of frequently used modules are made available. Well known trade names, such as Borland, and most of the computer magazines participate.

Bulletin boards may be accessible through the PSTN, other BT WANs, the Internet or NHSnet, and while use of them is usually free, apart from line charges, others must be paid for.

Prominent public bulletin boards are offered by the older OLSPs CIX (the Compulink Information Exchange based in London), and CompuServe, which, although based in Philadelphia, has a European network that can be accessed for the cost of a local call. The CIX messaging facility is both cheaper and quicker to use than the BT Telecom Gold Network, and conferencing between as many as 500 users on up to 15 topics can take place at a time. Charges levied, in addition to the line charge, are for on-line enquiry time.

One bulletin board of particular interest to UK practices is that operated by Dr Paul Bromley at Congleton in Cheshire under the title *PRY-MARIE CARE*. PMC has been set up to encourage interactive support between user practices, and although access requires the cost of a telephone call to Cheshire, no subscription nor interrogation fee is charged. Access may be from computers accommodating MS-DOS or using a number of other operating systems, but prospective users should consult their suppliers if they intend to communicate from their practice system.

The contents of PMC include patient management protocols, specimen employment contracts and job descriptions, patient instruction sheets, patient questionnaires, and software packages. Notices of meetings, courses and locum availability are featured. One program on offer is a mail-packing and off-line reading facility that enables users to download data for perusal on to their own computer and, in consequence, save line time. PMC can be accessed on 01260 299782 and users must present their credentials on first contact.

Bulletin boards are also operated by the Primary Health Care Specialist Group of the British Computer Society, the Doctor's Independent Network and the major GP system suppliers.

Although many operators of bulletin boards screen incoming data files for viruses by running checks on them with antivirus programs, boards must be regarded as a potential source of infection.

It must be remembered that messages published on bulletin boards are subject to the same laws of libel as apply to printed text.

18.13 TELEMEDICINE

Overview

Telemedicine is the practice of medicine on a remote patient, using intermediary data transmission. In the past many of us have dragged our weary limbs out of bed for a home visit in the early hours, having already made a diagnosis of croup, asthma or pertussis by overhearing their telltale sounds in the background when the patient's relative phoned. However, the term *telemedicine* is used to imply that sophisticated purpose-built hardware devices are being used as intermediaries in the flow of data between doctor and patient. Telemedicine hardware may enable patients to be diagnosed, monitored or treated remotely, and the methods used may provide spin-offs in the form of medical audit or education.

Although the application of telemedicine may employ transmission of voice and textual data, the main innovation of the method has been to incorporate and exploit the use of still and video images, which enable the expert to inspect the patient in one way or another. Methods do not yet exist that will allow the clinician to use palpation, percussion or auscultation. Fields of application are therefore those in which the patient's skin, diagnostic images, injuries, body language and retina can be photographed, or in which histological slides can be visualized. Apart from its use of digital image transmission, telemedicine has also been employed in a few highly specialized applications that focus on cardiovascular and obstetric parameters such as pulse or fetal heart rate and uterine contractility.

18.14 AREAS OF APPLICATION OF TELEMEDICINE

In summary, the areas of application of telemedicine so far implemented have been:

- Dermatology, in which GPs or trained nurses periodically transmit still images, together with textual histories, to dermatologists
- Imaging, in which X-rays or ultrasound signals are digitalized, thus enabling:
  - orthopaedic or trauma cases to be referred from GPs to orthopaedic consultants
  - abdominal or other ultrasound scans to be referred to surgeons or obstetricians
  - the staff of mammography or osteoporosis scanners to communicate with consultants
- Minor trauma clinics, from which nurse practitioners communicate with their local A&E departments
- Distributed diabetic clinics, from which retinal photographs are transmitted to an ophthalmologist
- Distributed pathology services, from which microscope slides or other pathological images are transmitted to a consultant
- Situations calling for the use of a specialized 'CAM' headset, which incorporates a miniature video camera, a miniature computer screen, a microphone and earphones. This headset transmits radio signals to a remote specialist who responds with advice. Appropriate situations for the use of this equipment include paramedical attendance at traffic accidents, battlefields, remote locations such as islands, oil-rigs or ships, and thinly populated or underprivileged communities for whom on-site medical support cannot be provided.
- Specialized monitoring of specific diseases in the home environment. These include 12-lead portable ECG tracings for postmyocardial infarction or cardiac arrhythmias, and combined blood pressure, fetal heart rate and uterine tone readings in pre-eclamptic toxaemia.
- Video recording of GP consultations with patients suffering from psychiatric problems, where the manner in which the patient responds to the live situation may be more revealing than the text of a written report. This method has the particular advantage of avoiding the stigma associated in many patients' minds with a visit to a hospital psychiatrist.
- Remotely instigated surgical procedures have been performed, both using video camera and 'talk through' methods, and by on-line manipulation of machine-mounted surgical instruments using a video camera and a remote command procedure. Open access video sigmoidoscopy clinics have been performed by nurse practitioners supervised remotely.
- The general monitoring of elderly frail patients at home or of neonates (sometimes referred to as 'telecare'). Dial-up access is required using PSTN, ISDN, mobile phones, the Internet, cable TV or satellite networks. Dial-up is triggered by locally sited monitoring equipment if signals beyond normal range are created. Functions monitored include accidents, gas leaks, low temperature, air pollution, incontinence, nocturnal wandering,

drug compliance, hypertension, cardiac arrhythmia, epilepsy, asthma, rehabilitation after surgery, and day-to-day routine activities. Telecare may be coordinated through networks linked by mobile phones and laptop computers, and may employ PCG+T-based care assistants. Telecare in the USA frequently uses video telephones.

- In time, cumulative telemedical records become an invaluable data bank, which can be used for medical research or medical education, and as a vehicle for those learning to use the technology. For these purposes, it is important that a patient's informed prior consent is obtained and noted when the recording is taken. A further consideration is that telemedical recordings rank as medical records under the provisions of the Data Protection Act, so that patients have the right of access to them.
- Because of the demonstrable, unequivocal and permanent evidence they generate, telemedical records are ideal tools for supporting 'before and after' outcome audit, with all the implications this has for the construction of evidence based medical protocols. In the same way, professional performance can be audited.

18.15 SYSTEM CONFIGURATIONS FOR TELEMEDICINE

The technological requirements of telemedicine depend upon whether text, audio, still photographs, video, one-way or two-way communication are required. Depending upon the application, the configuration will either be e-mail based or video conferencing based. There are five alternative strategies:

- E-mail-type store and forward facilities, whereby, for instance, still dermatological photographs accompanied by a textual history can be stored in a dermatologist's mailbox pending an e-mail report
- One-way video recordings, for example of a psychiatric interview, can be stored in a psychiatrist's mailbox pending an e-mail response
- One-way live on-line video transmission, in which images from, say, a minor injuries clinic may be transmitted to an A&E consultant, with on-line responses being supplied through the conventional telephone
- Two-way e-data transmissions, such as are used with the CAM headset, in which text, audio, still images and video can be transmitted in both directions
- Applications in which digital signals are generated by purpose-built patient monitoring equipment

other than cameras, and transmitted continuously or periodically to a remote overseer (e.g. for supervision of remote domiciliary cardiac care or pre-eclamptic toxaemia).

18.16 EQUIPMENT NEEDED FOR TELEMEDICINE

The application to be implemented will determine the degree of sophistication, and therefore the cost, of the equipment required.

Still images

High resolution digital still cameras are required for teledermatology and telemicroscopy, with the provision of specialized light units to ensure standard lighting conditions. Scanners have been used to transmit photographic plates both for teledermatology and still X-ray teleradiology. Although still image transmission is basically an e-mail application, it requires a high-grade Pentium processor, a modem and an ISDN 2 line.

Smith (1998) reported using laptop computers with high-resolution cameras and a specially designed light source to enable nurse practitioners to undertake teledermatology.

Video images

The basic tools needed to record and transmit commentary-supported video images are a digital video camera, a microphone and speakers, a video capture card, a fast Pentium processor with generous memory and storage, a fast modem and an ISDN 2 line.

Digital camcorders have been used, but specially designed 'web cam' cameras are now the norm, and it is important that the length of cable attaching either the camera or the microphone to the computer should not be restrictive. The Peterhead community hospital reported using two video cameras, one focused on the doctor and the other on the patient, during consultation (Leslie 1998).

Specialized telemedicine terminals are now available that incorporate all functions, together with the necessary processing power. Peterhead reported using an HS2000 Healthstation supplied by VTEL (http://www.ccs-uk.co.uk). Aberystwyth University used BT telemedical workstations (TNWS) for teleconsulting (Wynn-Jones, 1994). Imagine Medical Systems A/S (Copenhagen) markets a teleradiology workstation that handles both still and video images (Imagine I).

Satellite telecommunication has been used in the medical context from ships and oil rigs.

18.17 THE BENEFITS OF TELEMEDICINE

These are:

- Reduction in the delays to treatment inherent in the hospital waiting list system
- Savings in patient time and expense, increased patient convenience
- Abolition of missed hospital appointments
- Condensation of consultant workload, reduction in consultant appointment rates, and thereby more efficient overall use of specialist services. Smith (1998) estimated that between 7% and 12% of all GP consultations were dermatological, and that of these, 80% could be dealt with at a general practice level. He inferred that telemedicine would greatly assist in this process.
- Improved prioritization of cases, and direct booking for subsequent hospital treatment if such proves to be needed
- Levels of patient satisfaction with telemedicine have been high. Psychiatric patients are spared the stigma of a psychiatric hospital visit.
- Increased delegation to nurse practitioners reduces consultant and GP workload (as demonstrated by remote video-sigmoidoscopy, remote minor trauma clinics, teledermatology and mammography). Increased use of home monitoring equipment will reduce GP and nurse workload.
- Spin-offs, such as support for protocol construction, medical education and audit.

18.18 COSTS OF TELEMEDICINE

Pilot telemedicine projects at Peterhead (Leslie 1998), Manchester (Smith 1998), Belfast (Steele 1996), Portsmouth (Tyrrell 1998), Aberystwyth (Wynn-Jones 1994), Bristol (Murthy & Rees 1998), Plymouth (Jones 1998), Truro (Steward 1998) and St Mary's Paddington (Wan & Darzi 1998) have all benefited from special funding structures. At the time of writing, no framework exists to enable health authorities to assist in this work, and no cost benefit studies are yet available. The cost of equipment has so far been at a level that would be regarded as prohibitive by most practices, but costs are falling dramatically and will reach a point where telemedicine becomes a practical proposition, both for large practices and for PCG+Ts.

18.19 REDISTRIBUTION OF SKILLS AND RESPONSIBILITIES

Telemedicine requires the enhancement of nurse practitioners' skills in order to enable nurses to run the various types of clinic that telemedicine now brings within their reach. Like nurse triage and nurse prescribing, telemedicine should ultimately have the effect of lightening the GP's workload, and will sometimes mean that the GP is circumvented altogether. Both GPs and consultants need, mutually, to readjust their skills and procedures, particularly in remotely populated areas where telemedicine offers outstanding advantages.

When GPs seek consultant opinion using telemedicine they are effectively making a referral and have the responsibility of ensuring that all relevant information has been made available. A copy of the referral letter should be stored in the GP system. Presumably, responsibility then passes to the consultant. Members of the legal profession and the Medical Defence Union are reported to have expressed provisional approval for the methodology of telemedicine (Jones 1998), although it may take several years and several test cases for the exact boundaries of responsibility to be defined. Where nurse practitioners run telemedicine clinics, strict protocols must be set in place, as for nurse prescribing.

Government approval for the principles of telemedicine and telecare, as expressed in its strategy document *Information for Health*, is likely to accelerate acceptance of the method's legality.

18.20 MODEMS AND TERMINAL ADAPTERS (CODECS)

Public service telephone network (PSTN) telephone lines were designed for the transmission of voice frequencies and, if they are to be used to carry computer data, then a preliminary conversion from digital to analogue signal will be necessary. Deconversion takes place on receipt. The conversion is performed by a modem (an abbreviation of **mo**dulator–**dem**odulator). Modems transmit and receive data, and some may do both simultaneously.

Modems may take the form of a circuit board housed inside the processor, in relation to the latter's output port, or it may be a piece of freestanding equipment interposed between the output port and the telephone circuit. External modems have the advantage that a small LED signal emitted from them confirms that they are functioning.

A modem has to be 'installed' by a processor in order for its functionality to dovetail with the system's communication routines, and the software to do this is provided as part of the processor's operating system. Modems may additionally incorporate fax or voice capabilities.

The efficiency of a modem is determined by two principal factors, conversion speed and compaction (compaction allows some types of data to be compressed as much as sixfold, thereby enabling them to be transmitted in a shorter time). Both factors combine to determine the speed at which data can be actually transmitted, which has a direct bearing on line time and therefore on transmission costs (Herd 1993). Transmission speeds will also be affected by processor power and communications software.

Standards for modem efficiency were originally set up with category labels such as V, X, Y, Z, Hayes compatibility and 'Kermit'. The V label was further divided into a number of subcategories, each of which equated with a different conversion speed. To simplify matters, we now refer to modems solely by their conversion speeds. Modem conversion speeds suitable for PSTN line use are 14.4 K, 28.8 K, 33.6 K and 56 K (the K symbol here represents 1000 bits per second, kb/s). Some modems are capable of checking each block of data before allowing the transmission of the next, of slowing the speed of transmission if background line noise threatens data integrity, and of resuming data transfer at the point of an interruption rather than requiring total retransmission.

Some carriers have operated tariffs based on volume of data rather than line time, but it is economically important for the NHS to insist on time rental, so that efficient modems can play their part in reducing costs. Dial-up procedures should be programmed to take place during 'cheap rate' hours wherever possible.

ISDN lines are conveyors of digital data and merely require that computer data are converted into communication code rather than into analogue signals. The piece of equipment that performs this task was originally termed a **cod**er–**dec**oder (codec), but is now known more commonly as a terminal adapter (TA).

Modems and TAs must meet the standards required by carriers such as BT or by ISPs (Internet service providers) with whom they are to dovetail.

SUMMARY

- A LAN enables the sharing of data and compatible computer facilities, characteristically between users at a single site. Interconnecting cables, communications cards, and communications and networking software must be installed. A LAN's isolation is its safeguard against hacking. LANs use workstations or networkstations as terminals; processing is distributed to a greater or lesser degree but the responsibility for overall coordination is vested in the fileserver.

- WANs link remote computers, which may be disparate provided that they all adopt the same communication standards. To access a WAN, a computer must possess a communications card, communications software, a modem and PSTN line or a terminal adapter and ISDN line, and must enrol with a WAN service provider. WANs are vulnerable to hacking, so it is imperative that adequate security measures are employed.

- HealthLink and the NHSnet are protected WANs provided for NHS personnel, which can only be used under contract and with the undertaking that specified strict security measures are observed. User passwords and access protocols are issued, fees are charged for enrolment and on-going service provision, a mailbox is allocated for dial-up messaging, and facilities for real time 'conversational' style data interchange and e-mail are also provided. The user is liable for his own telephone line charges. NHSnet provides an outbound Internet connection.

- Whereas HealthLink has proved to be commercially and operationally successful over the 10 years of its existence, the development and implementation of NHSnet has been slow and expensive. Nevertheless the UK government's commitment to NHSnet and the latter's penetration of key areas such as hospitals should ensure its ultimate viability. Widespread uptake of NHSnet by GPs is likely to depend upon inducements.

- Intranets are able to use private and public WANs in secure mode, and as such constitute closed user groups. They are therefore suitable configurations for locality commissioning units (PCG+Ts), hospital trust groupings, or networks within which all locality NHS and social services agencies are integrated.

- Older on-line service providers (OLSPs) have been outmoded for the most part by the advent of Internet technology, although there is still a place for more up-to-date OLSPs that target their activities at communities with a special common interest.

- Bulletin boards offer users access to notices, messaging, vending and conferencing in an orderly way and in interactive mode. They may operate through the Internet or the telephone networks, and are a potential source of virus infection.

- Telemedicine uses electronic communication to enable health-care professionals to practise medicine remotely. The method may employ e-mail for the transmission of photographs or one-way video recordings, and real time for the exchange of one-way or two-way video. Audio messages may accompany any of these options. Most of the applications are used by the medical disciplines in which inspection and imaging are dominant, but monitoring devices to record pulse, blood pressure and uterine contractility also use telemedicine technology.

- Modems convert the computer's digital signals into their analogue equivalents for transmission through the public service telephone network. The message must be de-converted by the receiving computer's modem. Modems may be housed inside the processor or may be external to it. A modem's power is now expressed in terms of its speed of data conversion. ISDN telephone lines do not need a modem as they carry digital data. Instead, a terminal adapter is used to convert signals into communication code during transmission.

FURTHER READING

Bromley P 1992 Pry-Marie Care – a new way to communicate. Practice Computing, November: 6

Bradley S 1992 Electronic links to break the paper chain. Practice Computing, November: 24

BT 1977 Press release BB/355: 2

Crichton C, Macdonald S, Potts S et al 1995 Teledermatology in Scotland. Journal of Telemedicine and Telecare 1: 185

Darkins A, Dearden C H, Rocke L G et al 1996 An evaluation of telemedical support for a minor treatment centre. Journal of Telemedicine and Telecare 2: 93–99

Evans K 1991 How Kent GPs learned to love the micro. Practice Computing, April: 12

Family Health Services Computer Unit 1990 GP systems specification – communications and financial. Family Health Services Computer Unit, Exeter

Herd A 1991 Bulletin board bonanza. Practice Computing, September: 4

Herd A 1993 Modems. Practice Computing, February: 24–27

House A M 1981 Telecommunications in health and education. Canadian Medical Association Journal 124: 667–668

Jones R 1998 Practice innovations: teledermatology. GP 4 December: 34

Leslie A 1998 Peterhead video link lets GPs take consultant advice. Rx April: 14

Maclean J R, Naji S A, Grant A M et al 1996 Teleradiology education in Scotland. Journal of Telemedicine and Telecare 2: 60

Murthy M S N, Rees J 1998 Switched on outreach clinic gets the picture. Rx, June (http://www.rad.bris.ac.uk)

NHS Executive (Information Management Group) 1994 A strategy for NHS-wide networking

PC User 1990 The PC user guide to networking and communications. PC User, November: 27–42

Stafford K 1991 A new national grid for the health service? Practice Computing, June: 7

Steele K 1996 GPs fear telemedicine plan may threaten patient safety. Screen stars of the dermatology world. Doctor 19 September: 74

Steward A 1998 GP 4 September: 18

Smith N 1998 Diagnostic telemedicine service beats dermatology waiting lists. Rx, September: 15

Trower C 1990 Organising for quality. Wycombe primary care computing. Practice Computing, September: 13

Tyrrell G 1998 Video links provide a diagnosis in minutes. Doctor 18 June: 38–41

Wallace P 1998 GPs put video link-up to test. Doctor 2 April: 18

Wan A, Darzi A 1998 Primary care shapes a role for medicine at a distance. Rx, April: 22

Wynn-Jones J 1994 Video link GPs glimpse the future. GP 1 July: 39

19 Some remote and locally held sources of information – the Internet, e-mail and CD-ROM

19.1 INTRODUCTION

There are four important advantages of reference information on the computer:

- One of the minor irritations in life is to lend a book (especially a reference book) to a friend who fails to return it. This situation does not arise with computer-stored reference data, because the same source material is available simultaneously to as many users as there are linked terminals.
- Another big advantage that computer reference data have over books is the method of access. It is no longer necessary to hunt through shelves of books, indices, pages and paragraphs, because a brief command keyed in with the name of the data required will suffice to bring them on to the display. If users of the system are uncertain as to the exact description of the block of data they require, they can be led to their choice through a succession of lists of options, each of which narrows the field of search. Computer searches can be made for blocks of data that contain a single specified term, or multiple specified terms with or without the provisos 'and', 'or' and 'not' linking them. Searches can also be made for sources containing longer specified strings of text. Articles and their references, timetables, calendars of events, whole books, catalogues, dictionaries, directories and encyclopaedias are all rapidly available electronically through the computer terminal.
- A third significant advantage that computer reference data enjoy is the speed and facility with which the data may be electronically changed in order to bring them up to date. Whole reference sections can be altered at will without the need to buy expensive new books and discard old ones.
- Finally, the computer's potential capacity for storing information is virtually limitless.

19.2 TWO WAYS IN WHICH REFERENCE DATA CAN BE INTERROGATED BY COMPUTERS

The practice computer may access reference data in two ways. It may act as a communicating terminal to interrogate, via the telephone line, data held on a second, remote computer. In this case an excerpt is usually taken from the remote database and may be downloaded for examination on the user's computer, a provision for which royalties may or may not be charged. Data downloaded in this way may subsequently be stored or printed out locally.

By contrast, reference data may be sourced from local storage media. Data may already be 'saved' to the hard disk, in which case the computer can open a specified electronic 'file' stacked within a 'folder', or else can search its own database, either for specified terms or by using specified criteria. Alternatively, reference data may have been stored on diskettes or CD-ROM disks, in which case these must be loaded into their respective drives for interrogation by the computer. Diskettes contain 1.44 Mb of data, which it is practicable to copy to the system's hard disk before use. CD-ROM disks contain 640 Mb and are not, as a rule therefore, fully downloaded. Instead, most of the data will be left on the original and accessed on an *ad hoc* basis.

19.3 REMOTE SOURCES OF REFERENCE DATA

A considerable amount of reference data housed on remote computers may be accessed free of charge through the Internet. Other remote database operators will charge for access, and tariffs may be applied to data accessed either through the Internet, through conventional telephone line direct dial-up, or through the gateway of an OLSP. Access to some remote data-

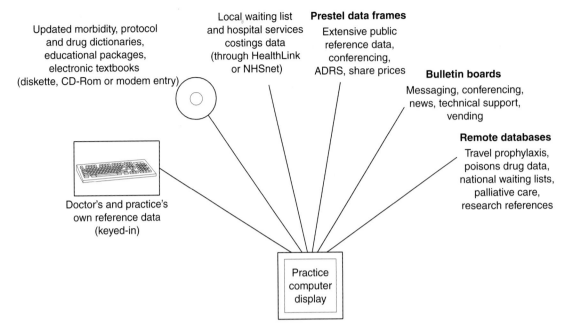

Fig. 19.1 Local and remote sources of reference data for the practice computer

bases can only be obtained if one or more specified gateways are used, an arrangement which tends to inflate charges.

19.4 AN INTRODUCTION TO THE INTERNET

The Internet must take pride of place as the most astonishingly successful technical development that has resulted from international cooperation in modern times. The number of its users runs into nine figures and doubles every year or two, and traffic volume doubles every 100 days. It originated in the 1960s as the Advanced Research Projects Agency Network (ARPAnet) whose original purpose, according to its chairman Charles Narzfeld, was to link university computers and researchers in the USA (an equivalent of JANET in the UK). Later, research projects at the US Department of Defense participated, and this put the network's robustness and standard protocols at a premium. Fuelled by the need and desire for all computer users to intercommunicate, further development spread across the globe.

The Internet is essentially a giant wide area network that links PCs, Macintoshes, minis, mainframes or supercomputers, of whatever type, often using widely disparate operating systems. It conveys infinitely varied types of information, with text expressed in a variety of languages, through telecommunication wires, radio waves or satellites, provided always that Internet protocols are used for the conveyance of data. All countries of the world own a piece of the network jigsaw, but none has outright ownership. Users pay telephone line costs and may have to pay tolls of one sort or another for the facilities they access, but economy of scale has minimized these charges, and brought the Internet within reach of all computer owners. Advertising revenue also plays its part, as is the case with the provision of access services and search engines. The whole thing hangs together because it is supremely useful to all concerned.

19.5 INTERNET FACILITIES

The following facilities are available to Internet users:

- Access to remote databases to browse for, search for, download, view, print and store data
- Provision of Web space to make a user's data available to others
- An e-mailbox and the ability to send and receive e-mail as text and images, with or without added colour and sound, plus the ability to search for an e-mail address
- News groups – like bulletin boards, the Internet offers like-minded participants a platform on which to discuss topics of mutual interest

Table 19.1 Results of a survey of GP requirements for reference data to be provided on the practice computer – figures refer to votes recorded by individual RCGP faculties (Davies 1995)

Data category	Votes*
Trust waiting list duration, inpatient and outpatient	21
DoH statements of fees and allowances	18
Other regulations, e.g. Health and Safety, DPA; guidelines for data provision to agencies; requirements for GP research; requirements for audit	16
Template contracts for employment, partnership, fundholding, etc.	17
Template for practice annual report, practice brochure design, etc.	16
Patient instruction leaflets for disease management	24
Poisons, constituents, symptoms and treatment	22
Travel prophylaxis, including malaria	21
Locums available	17
Practice nurses available	14
Hospital and residential nursing homes; self-help agencies	14
Yellow Pages directory of all professional agencies	14
OTC guide to products and prices	14
Drug tariff	20
Professional guidelines and protocols for chronic disease management such as the RCGP clinical series	20
Special situation prescribing (e.g. pregnancy, lactation, childhood, old age, hepatic and renal failure)	26
National and regional distribution of incidence and prevalence	17
Gateway access to remote databases such as GP Lit and Medline	20
Antibiotic sensitivity and resistance patterns	20
PGEA courses and conference diary	19
PGEA tuition packages for on-site use such as the PEP program	23
Pathology services – costings, sample requirements, normal values	21
Palliative care	16
Sports medicine	13
Current legal information – employment law, complaints management, etc.	13
Insurance advice – requirements for each area, list of agencies, etc.	5
Personal financial management – requirements, agencies, etc.	3
Electronic banking services facilities and conditions	10
Health education for patients	20

* Total number of votes for 'essential' and 'desirable' responses

- Chat channels (IRC – Internet relay chat) – live discussions carried out with a series of typed messages on-line
- Voice and video conferencing (surgical operations have been watched live on the Internet)
- E-shopping and marketing
- E-education
- Games – downloaded or on-line
- E-publishing.

19.6 INTERNET TERMINOLOGY

The development of the Internet has prompted the coining of a plethora of terms, some of which are legitimately necessary and many that are merely flippant. A dozen or more of the former are here to stay and must be accommodated in this chapter, because they embody concepts that are fundamental to the understanding of the Internet. They include:

- *Browser.* User software that locates a specified remote computer and makes the latter's data available.
- *Search engine* ('search tool'). User software that searches one or more remote computer directories in order to identify the specification of an individual remote computer and its contents, so that the browser can then be brought to bear on them.
- *Downloader.* User software that copies files from a remote computer to a user's computer.
- *Server.* A computer which makes its database available to interrogation by remote users, or *clients.*
- *Client programs.* There are four basic types of 'client program' that provide the user with Internet functionality. These are *client browser, e-mail client, newsreader* and *voice and video.* Most 'browser packages' bundle these four components, which are supplied to a new user by the Internet Service Provider together with other ISP software.
- *Internet communications software.* User transmission software that conforms to the TCP/IP (transport control protocol/internet protocol) standards that all must use to send ASCII data over the Internet. The FTP (file transfer protocol) standard likewise governs the way files must be handled.
- *World Wide Web* (www). The www is really a network within a network. It uses the Internet's existing communication channels but has introduced improved design features into its navigational procedures. As a result, it has become by far the most commonly used Internet conduit. Web technology was invented by Tim Berners-Lee, a British atomic scientist.
- *Frames* and *panes.* A screenful of data is referred to as a frame, and is the customary unit of information used in data communications. If the screen is subdivided into two or more subsections, each subsection is known as a pane. A pane may be subjected to independent navigational commands provided that, as a preliminary, the cursor has been 'clicked' within the pane's margins.
- *Hypertext links* are nodes within a frame of data which, when 'clicked' on by the user, automatically trigger the retrieval of a further screen to which the node refers. The node may be a text term (in which case it is shown in a different colour and underlined), or an image or part of an image.
- *Domain, folder* and *file.* Data on a server, which may relate to text, images or programs, are stored

in a *file.* This in turn may or may not be stored in a *folder* and will be located on the server database or *domain.* Domain, folder and file must all be named when seeking to retrieve a file, e.g. http://www.open.gov.uk/hmis/waitime.htm signifies that the file on patient waiting times is located in the folder 'hmis' housed on the domain (server) 'open.gov.uk', which can be accessed through the World Wide Web using the hypertext transfer protocol. The suffix 'htm' or 'html' shows that the file contains hypertext mark-up conventions. Xhtml is a variant of html that extends its use to mobile phones and large monitors.

E-mail addresses are configured in a different way, the user name being quoted before the domain name, the two being separated by an @ symbol.

The term *website* refers to any Web address from which data can be retrieved.

- *URL (uniform resource locator).* This is a central data source to which several subsidiary data sources are linked. The term URL can therefore be applied to a website from which a number of other related websites can be accessed, a hypertext-linked screenful of data, or a nodal point for news groups.
- *ISP* (internet service provider) The ISP makes a *gateway* (point of access to the Internet) available to the user. The ISP usually supplies sign-up, start-up, dial-up, communication and client software packages bundled together on a CD-ROM. E-mail is therefore customarily part of the deal, and a limited amount of user Web space may also be included. On sign-up, an ISP opens an 'Internet account' giving the user the right of access to the Internet, for which tolls may or may not be charged. Internet accounts may be 'dial-in direct', which most users possess, or 'permanent', which enable large organizations, such as NHSnet, to retain continuous access. Access to the Internet can also be obtained through on-line service providers (see Chapter 18).
- *On-line, off-line.* Time spent accessing remote databases is described as *on-line*, but data downloaded can be processed locally, such as with the use of an off-line mail reader.
- *Web pages* and *home pages.* Frames of data accessible by interrogation on the World Wide Web ('Web') are known as 'Web pages'. 'Home pages' pertain either to servers or users, where the term is used to describe the nodal or 'start-up' page from which further navigation can proceed. Thus when the user initiates the 'start-up' procedure, he is presented with his own home page, and when he

accesses a remote server he will first be shown the server's home page.

19.7 SIGN-UP AND SET-UP WITH AN ISP

For those planning to access the Internet for the first time, the following steps should be taken.

- The reputation of, facilities offered by, and charges levied by alternative ISPs should be carefully considered before a selection is made.
- It is essential that the modem or terminal adapter installed by the user should be compatible with the ISP server – a point on which the ISP should first be consulted.
- The ISP with whom the user proposes to contract will provide him with printed instructions and a CD-ROM disk that contains bundled software packages, to sign up to, set-up and operate Internet access.
- Loading the CD-ROM disk will initiate the sign-up/set-up routine. The user must first agree to observe any stipulations and pay any tolls required by the ISP. All contract details (including those of the user's credit card, if requested) are logged electronically, and up-loaded before installation can proceed. The ISP should offer a secure line for financial transactions.
- The following sign-up/set-up details are then allocated for use on the client's computer:
  - the ISP's telephone or other WAN access number
  - the client's log-on name (chosen by the client)
  - the client's secure password for log-on purposes (chosen by the client)
  - if a dial-up account, whether the PPP or SLIP protocols are to be implemented (SLIP accounts are rare nowadays)
  - the client's e-mail address
  - the client's e-mail user name and password (chosen by the client)
  - all other user and server electronic addresses that are required for all services provided in conformance with Internet protocol (IP; this allocation and implementation is usually performed automatically by the system).
- The set-up software provided by the ISP takes the user through all the steps necessary to incorporate the above details in the client's system. Some of these steps will be performed automatically, but some will call for details to be input by the user. At the end of this procedure, a notice displays the fact that installation is complete, and new Internet icons are positioned tactically on user system screens so that, when these are clicked on, future dial-up will be automated. The options for the way in which the user system handles Internet access ('properties') can subsequently be viewed and amended.
- The ISP provides helpline details which include telephone number, hours of availability and call line tariffs.

19.8 WEB ACCESS

The connections now set up will enable future dial-up when the computer and modem are switched on, the telephone line is connected, the appropriate Internet icon is clicked on, and user name and password are given. Although precise details of routines vary between ISPs and computer systems, the following steps are then enabled.

- The client's computer autodials the ISP server, which verifies user name and password, and establishes Internet connection. A connection time window appears temporarily, logging the onset and duration of connection.
- The Web browser is now opened on the screen, together with the home page of either the ISP or the search engine agency. The principal features of this combined screen are, from above downwards:
  - the browser toolbar containing command icons
  - the address box – a one-character-high data entry space that usually occupies the full width of the screen
  - the home page, which offers quick access through hypertext links to news, special user facilities and advertisers' information; embedded somewhere within the home page will be the search box, a one-character-high data entry space, shorter than the address box, that allows the user to begin the hunt for sites for which he does not have an exact address
  - the status bar, which identifies the URL/site currently in view (see Fig. 19.2)
- The destination of the next URL/site the user requires is now typed into the address box. Typing in must be preceded by 'clicking' on the box, and followed by pressing the return/enter key or 'clicking' on an equivalent icon. If a URL/site is already displayed in the address box, 'clicking' once in the box will enable it to be retyped and 'clicking' twice in the box will allow terms to be amended. It is essential that the address entered is exact in every detail, including spacing, punctuation and case, otherwise connection will fail.

- The home page of the URL/site server whose address was specified by the user now appears on the client screen, with text being transmitted more rapidly than images. Hypertext links embedded within the data enable the user to move to other frames. Navigation icons on the browser toolbar enable the user:
  - to move back to a previous frame, or forward again
  - to stop any process under way
  - to list a viewed frame in the user's address book of 'favourites' (or 'book marks') so that he can return to it without retyping
  - to return to the user's own home page
  - to initiate a search.
- Text files may be downloaded and saved for off-line reading or printing. Program files may be downloaded, but great care should first be taken to ascertain their volume, whether they are compressed, and the integrity of their source. If there is considered to be a possibility of virus infection (and there usually is), then virus scanning software should be used; the correct procedure is first to save the file to hard disk for a virus check before opening it. Users seeking to download programs must register with the originator, and will either obtain them free of charge (freeware), as a demonstration sample allowing later full purchase (shareware), or as an outright purchase. Payment may be required either by cheque, direct debit, or credit card but, if the latter applies, the integrity of the data source must be beyond doubt and the transaction undertaken over a secure line.

The distinction between types of file can be made by looking at their suffixes: .exe is a program file; .com is a program file; .doc is a document; .asc is a plain text file; .txt is a plain text file; .zip is an archive containing compressed data that must be decompressed before use. The commonest compression protocol on the Internet is PK Zip, which requires shareware from sources such as http://www.winzip.com. Large selections of shareware can be obtained from both http://shareware.com and http://download.com.

The user's computer usually keeps a log of the sites that have been visited most recently, listed in reverse chronological order, so as to facilitate rapid re-access. The size of the list can be determined by the user.

19.9 BROWSER PACKAGES

There are two browser-bundled packages in general use, and these are available in versions for most oper-

ating systems. Both packages offer closely similar facilities and provide for automatic configuration with the Windows 95 (and above) operating systems.

- Netscape Navigator, release no. 6. This contains:
  - *Navigator browser* (which has multimedia capability)
  - *Messenger:* for e-mail which includes an address book and meetings organizer
  - *Collabra:* a news reader and newsgroups organizer
  - *Conference:* live voice and video conferencing software
  - *Page Composer:* a Web page editing facility for the creation and publication of Web pages
  Navigator can translate from English into seven other languages.
- Microsoft Internet Explorer, release no. 5.5. This contains:
  - *Internet Explorer browser* (which possesses multimedia capability)
  - *Outlook Express:* for combined e-mail and newsgroups
  - *NetMeeting:* for voice and video conferencing
  - *Chat:* typed messages are exchanged on-line.

A 'plug-in' is a piece of software that can be added to a browser in order to extend its functionality.

By January 2000 there were four times as many users of Microsoft Internet Explorer as there were users of Netscape Navigator. A third browser, code-named Opera, is available for download at http://www.opera.com.

19.10 SEARCH ENGINES

There are at least a dozen search engines in general use, and it is common practice for an ISP to offer access to several when a search routine is summoned. If an ISP only offers one search engine, the others can be accessed by keying their Internet addresses into the address box.

Creators of search engines each assemble huge site directories of their own, either by inviting website originators to contact them spontaneously, or by computerized word search trawls. These directories can be interrogated:

- by specifying single words within the Web page title
- by specifying a combination of words in fixed relationship to each other
- by specifying terms in which contained words are searched on separately, in which case results can be

Fig. 19.2 AT+T's home page showing, from above downwards, Microsoft Internet Explorer icons, the address bar, hypertext links to topical items, the search bar and advertising material (Reproduced with permission from Kiley 1999a)

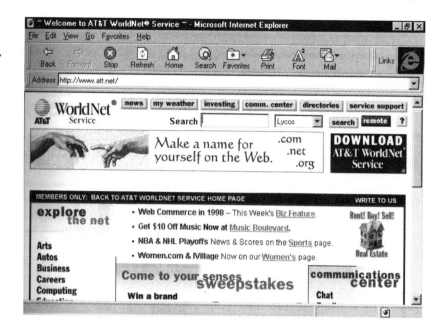

expressed in terms of Boolean logic ('and', 'or', 'not' options).

Searches can also be made by thumbing through the categories into which the directories have been classified. Some search results provide that if the exact target cannot be found, approximations to the term searched are quoted, with the degree of approximation being expressed as a percentage, or results being ranked in the order in which they approximate most nearly to the term searched.

Commonly used search engines are Yahoo!, Alta Vista, ExCite, Lycos, Infoseek, Magellan and Open Text. The user does not pay for the operation of these search engines, which are funded by associated advertising.

Northern Light is a search engine that not only maintains an extensive directory but also offers inspection of the electronic versions of many medical and scientific journals on payment of a fee – see http://www.northernlight.com/.

19.11 INTERNET ACCESS – A CHOICE OF PROVIDER: ISPs, OLSPs AND THE NHSNET

Those who sign up to the NHSnet are provided with a ready-made outbound gateway to the Internet but will still need client software packages. NHSnet has standardized on Microsoft Internet Explorer as a browser.

The role of OLSPs was described in the previous chapter. The facilities that they offer have a broader range than those offered by ISPs, and these include the provision of Internet access. Historically the most widely used commercial OLSPs were CompuServe, CIX and America On-line (AOL). The Microsoft Network (MSN) was a relative latecomer in this field, and offers a variety of enhanced facilities not provided by other OLSPs. A sign-up option for joining MSN is built into the Windows 95 (and later versions) operating system. OLSP access to the Internet has always tended to be more expensive than that available through the more competitive ISPs, but AOL has waived charges in order to stay in the race.

Those who wish to use the Internet but have not signed up to NHSnet will need the type of access best provided by an ISP. As the number of ISPs has recently mushroomed to well over 200, the process of choosing one can be confusing, but should take into account the following factors:

- the client facilities supported – browsers, search facilities, chat lines, conferencing, news groups, e-mail, voice and video. As ISP services can be obtained nowadays at little or no cost other than that for line charges, there seems little point in opting for a partial service.
- the funding structure used – tolls may be by subscription (annual or monthly), by call volume, by time spent on line, or by a combination of all three. An ISP may also be partly funded by high tariff

calls to its helpline. ISPs that do not charge tolls make their money from a rake off on call charges, advertising, and the sale of mailing lists.

- the accessibility of its helpline and the quality of support that this provides
- the speed and reliability of its links to the Internet, and the speed with which disconnection is enforced if the on-line connection is not transmitting
- support for the modem if the user already has one, and whether extra charges are made for particular models (use of some faster modems may attract a higher charge rate). Some ISPs do not yet support ISDN.
- whether access to the ISP server is charged at local call rates (this is now nearly always the case)
- provision of Web space and Web page editing, and arrangements for Web publishing.

Demon Internet has enjoyed a reputation for economy and reliability for many years, and has been the UK's largest independent ISP (tel: (020) 8371 1000; Internet http://www.demon.net). More recently, BT has established itself as an ISP (BT Click), but at the time of writing was adding a penny to all user calls. (tel: 0800 515585; Internet http://www.btclickplus. com, or http://www.bt.com/internet/index.htm).

One of the most attractive newcomers to the ISP frontrunners has been Tesconet, which recently restructured its tolls to make no charge for unlimited access and generous Web space, but instead to charge helpline use at 50p per minute (tel: 0845 7576169; Internet http://www.tesco.net). FreeServe is another ISP offering free access and Web space, though initially it charged £1 per minute (later reduced to 50p) for its technical support helpline (PC World Stores – http://www.freeserve.co.uk).

Virgin net and Line One have also launched, and are offering free interrogation.

Many users change their ISP, and those who do so should be advised to delete their old ISP's access routines from their system, as the opposing sets of routines sometimes conflict. Changes of ISP involve changes of e-mail address.

19.12   HARDWARE REQUIREMENTS FOR INTERNET ACCESS

Although text files and e-mail can be handled by 14.4 Kb/s modems, 640 × 480 displays and older computer models, the volume and complexity of data handling for the Internet are increasing all the time, and correspondingly increase demands on equipment.

Realistic minimum requirements are now a fast 486, 32-bit processor with a 28.8K modem and an 800 × 600 (256 colour) display, but those considering adding animation, multimedia, voice or video conferencing should budget for Pentium 166 MHz machines and 56K modems in addition to the digital cameras or microphones that they may be proposing to buy.

19.13   CREATING A PRACTICE WEB PAGE

Increasingly, practices are constructing Web pages to inform patients of the services they offer – practice brochures in an electronic format. Some practice sites also incorporate hypertext links to other sites that offer further patient health information of which the practice approves. Experimental use has also been made of the practice website as a platform for reordering repeat medication or requesting sickness certificates, for patient enquiry for test results, patient registration and 'cyber' consultation. The Medical Protection Society warns that all medical advice published on a website carries legal liability.

Basically, text entered through a word processing package must be designated in HTML (hypertext mark-up language – the architecture that provides for hypertext linkages). The finished product must configure with both Netscape Navigator and Internet Explorer browsers. With the ISP's cooperation, files are then uploaded to the ISP's server using a file transfer protocol (FTP). Most ISPs include a limited amount of available client Web space in their range of services.

Web authoring is well catered for by commercially available packages such as Microsoft Front Page 2000, Adobe Sitemill, HotDog Professional, or Luckman's Web Editpro. Freeserve offers an on-line package.

19.14   WEB TV

The so called 'set-top box' that connects a television set through a telephone plug with the box supplier's Internet provider, allows Internet access, e-mail, and entry to news, sport, chat and shopping channels.

Although a basic remote control panel is provided with the package, this is inconvenient to use when keying-in text, and it is better to purchase the additional option of an infrared transmitting 'QWERTY' keyboard with roller ball. Internet pages can be downloaded to a printer, which must also be purchased separately.

As compared with Internet access from a computer, the resolution of a TV monitor is inferior to that of a PC, and images and text cannot be used for incorporation in word processing or desktop publishing packages.

NetProducts was the first company in the UK to produce a set-top box, for which it charged £300 with a tariff of £14.95 per month for unlimited Internet access (telephone use at local call rates). JetSet now offers an infrared keyboard, remote control handset and 128 bit 'Secure Socket Layer' secure transmission for e-commerce and e-banking for around £200.

19.15 SHOPPING ON THE INTERNET

Overview

The Internet allows vendors to create electronic catalogues on their websites, exhibiting descriptions, pictures and prices. Being an interactive medium, the customer can then indicate which goods are required and, by quoting bank card details, can pay for them to be delivered by post or courier. Medical equipment, computer equipment, software and consumables, CD-ROMs and office equipment can be bought in this very convenient way. Electronic book-shops, such as amazon.com, display titles with authors, book reviews, author interviews and lists of similar books. It would be helpful if computer CD-ROM vendors showed image samples, just as audio CD vendors include audioclips in their website advertisements. Any commodity may be bought or sold over the Internet, which now also hosts e-investment and e-banking (Chapter 20).

Definitions of terms used

Bank cards may be credit cards, which allow purchases against a loan, or debit cards, which allow purchases up to the total held in a customer's account. 'Virtual wallets' are bank cards that carry limited amounts of electronic funds downloaded from a debit or credit card, or from a bank account. Details from all three types of card are used for Internet shopping.

A 'virtual shopping basket' is the scheme that allows a customer to log a succession of items from an electronic catalogue, compiles an order, and accepts bank card details as payment. Most vendors confirm the order by e-mail.

Regulations

UK consumer laws apply to goods bought through the Internet. Goods must be of satisfactory quality, fit for their purpose and safe, and must correspond with their description.

UK vendors' websites count as advertisements, as regulated by the Advertising Standards Authority, and their content must be legal, decent, honest and truthful.

The IMRG (Interactive Media in Retail Group) is the industry representative body for Internet shopping, whose vendor members are additionally committed to state their full postal address, package and postage costs, and to send a confirmation of order.

The UK banking code, which covers nearly all bank card issuers, has the discretionary effect of limiting customer liability for fraudulent transactions, perpetrated against a bank card identity, to £50, provided always that the card owner has not been negligent. The transmission of card details over the Internet is not regarded as negligent (Consumers' Association 1998).

As with other purchasing venues, credit card issuers are jointly liable with vendors for misrepresentation, breach of contract and consequential loss following sales over the Internet.

Problems

Interception and misuse of card details by unauthorized parties has so far proved to be no more of a risk on the Internet than that associated with disclosure over the telephone. Responsible vendors offer a secure conduit for the transmission of card details, and store those details behind the protection of an electronic 'firewall', issuing a password linked to the user's address for subsequent transactions. Netscape and Microsoft Internet Explorer browsers both have encoders that may be acceptable by vendor sites.

As with postal shopping, Internet customers have occasionally been charged for undelivered goods, and it is wise to request confirmation of all orders.

Good can be purchased from overseas sites using bank cards, though there will be a premium for currency exchange. The Post Office collects import duty and VAT on delivery, and adds a clearance fee (currently £1.20 for Royal Mail and £5.10 for Parcel Force). Downloaded software has so far avoided tax. When importing goods, customers must ensure that these are suitable for use in the UK (as with electrical equipment), and that they are legal (receipt of a pepper spray for use in self-defence could attract heavy penalties). Some prescription drugs are cheaper when obtained from abroad, but their quality cannot always be guaranteed.

A URL with links to most secure UK shopping websites can be found at http://www. enterprisecity.co.uk.

19.16 INTERNET SITES

For a list of interesting sites, see Appendix A.

The number of Internet sites is legion, and is expanding so rapidly that no comprehensive directory exists, nor could ever be fully up-to-date. The search engines taken together provide the closest approximation to a full index of sites that we are likely to achieve but, as with telephone numbers, sites are not only added but may be deleted or retitled without warning.

Considerations that are important in relation to an Internet site are:

- whether the site's files are accessed free, or whether a toll is payable
- when the site was set up and when it was last updated (these dates should be, and nearly always are, quoted)
- whether the site acts as a useful node of access to multiple related sites
- whether the site's files contain data other than text – e.g. still images, video, audio programs – and, if so, whether the interrogating equipment has the necessary power to access and download them; some of the more sophisticated multimedia sites use a language called Java that makes taxing demands of client systems
- the specificity, relevance and reliability of the data on offer; if a single word in common use is employed as the criterion for a site search, an excessive number of 'hits' will be identified, most of which are likely to be irrelevant, and many of which will offer data of dubious validity – a situation that is analogous to an overkill of 'junk' e-mail.

There are two possible approaches to overcoming this problem. They are:

- To evaluate sites oneself in order to be able to compile one's own list of 'favorites' (Internet Explorer) or 'bookmarks' (Netscape Navigator). Silberg et al (1997) suggested that the following criteria should be considered when assessing a site:
  - Are the authors of the website clearly stated, along with details of their affiliations and credentials?
  - Is the owner of the website prominently displayed, along with any sponsorship or advertising details that could constitute a conflict of interest?
  - Are any claims made by the site supported by research findings and, if so, are details given to the original source?
  - Does the Web page contain details of when it was created or last updated? If it does not, the data contents should be disregarded.

The self-selection process is, of course, facilitated by referring to lists of sites that have already been evaluated by sources, such as Kiley 1999.

- To use URLs that display or connect to data sources that have been carefully selected for their validity and relevance. Four sites in particular should be mentioned in this context:
  - OMNI at http://omni.ac.uk
  - Health on the Net, at http://www.hon.ch/ (at this site not all contributions have been vetted, but the distinction between those that have and those that have not is clearly displayed)
  - Medical Matrix (a free US medical site) at http://www.medmatrix.org/index.osp
  - Cliniweb (US medical site) at http://www.chsu.edu/cliniweb/.

19.17 REMOTE DATABASES USING COMMERCIAL WANS

To add to a researcher's problems, there are at least 600 health related electronic databases that are not accessible through the Internet, but to which access must be made through a licensed gateway, a commercial search engine and a commercial WAN, by an intermediary agency on behalf of a client. Royalties and agency fees are payable. Line charges, although variable, are to an increasing extent levied at local call rates.

The BMA, through its library, offers a search service, acting as an intermediary on behalf of its members, and the RCGP extends its intermediary search facilities to all fellows, members and associates, for which modest fees are charged.

Remote research databases may consist of lists such as titles of books or articles, authors' names or drug names, or alternatively may quote full descriptive text. Search of a database may start with any one, or more, of terms such as author's name, keyword, subject or chemical component. Targeted data found by the search are transmitted to the interrogating computer for inspection. Interrogators usually have the option to request a printout of the object of their search, which may be posted to them, or else to print the targeted data on their own computer.

The BMA and RCGP use gateways such as DataStar, Dialog and Blaise, which are capable of interrogating virtually all English language medical databases and many in other languages.

19.18 MEDLINE

Medline, the electronic version of *Index Medicus* prepared by the US National Library of Medicine, is a medical reference source in its own class, both as regards its comprehensiveness and its accessibility. A condensed version of Medline is available free on the Internet at PubMed or at the UK Med W3 server http://www.ncl.ac.uk/~nphcare/gpuk and is accessible commercially through on-line services providers, but the BMA offers access to the unexpurgated version through its library service.

19.19 TOXBASE

The prestigious Scottish databases begun by Dr Alexander Proudfoot in 1982 were originally offered on Viewdata equipment, but they have now become so well established that access to them has been transferred to the Internet and NHSnet as definitive NHS resources.

Toxbase, the poisons database, lists 13 000 items under the headings of pharmaceuticals; industrial, agricultural and domestic chemicals; plants; animals; and veterinary products. Each entry includes details relating to its identification, constituents, symptomatology, laboratory procedures, treatment, and associated references. Interrogation is initiated by keyword, with software assistance if requested, and verbal advice will be offered if required. To request registration, visit the Toxbase website at http://www.show.nhs.scot.uk/spib/ (toll charge details on application). The West Midlands Poisons Unit, City Hospital, Birmingham, uses Toxbase and offers health professionals 24-hour poisons advice. Visit http://www.hsrc.org.uk/links/cci/wmpu.htm or http://www.show.nhs.scot.uk/spib.

19.20 TRAVAX

The Scottish travel prophylaxis data bank is divided into three main sections. The first deals with requirements for both vaccines and malaria prophylaxis,

country by country, with two frames being devoted to each country. The second section gives full details on individual vaccines, and has subsections dealing with such related issues as the use of vaccines in immuno-compromised patients, immunization schedules where several vaccines are involved, and more precise details on dosages, treatment packs and side effects. The third main section is a bulletin board called 'current notes', which gives up-to-the-minute new and amended data on vaccines and policies (see also Chapter 22).

19.21 HEALTH DATA ACCESSIBLE THROUGH PRESTEL, TELETEXT, CABLETEXT AND TELEVISION

Both Prestel (telephone line transmission) and Teletext (radio wave transmission) were designed to be mounted on colour television apparatus, but Prestel can be used on computer colour screens. Both presentations allow pages of reference text to be selected, either from menu options or by keying in the page reference number from a keypad. A wide choice of display subjects is available, particularly with Prestel.

Prestel was developed, and is marketed by, British Telecom. Prestel pages number over 50 000, supplied by over 200 different organizations, which include the Health Education Council, the Department of Health and the Consumer Association.

Meditel Ltd. has the responsibility of managing and delivering, through the Prestel network, publicly accessible health information in the UK. It also organizes a wide range of displays of interest to the medical profession. Although most Prestel pages are available for general enquiry, access to some is limited by extended password, and this enables closed user groups to be set up. Meshtel is one such closed group which enables general practitioners, in a number of postgraduate medical centres throughout the country, to combine in their consideration and discussion of clinical problems at prearranged sessions. Meshtel is a joint enterprise of the Royal College of General Practitioners and the Wellcome Foundation.

The Committee on Safety of Medicines maintains an information service on drug reactions on Prestel, and this database can be interrogated by drug name or by reaction. Prestel, unlike radio propagated displays, allows two-way transmission so that user response can be received by the central computer. In this way, a Prestel screen can be used to report an adverse drug reaction to the CSM. A database for poisons information is another interesting application of Prestel.

Fig. 19.3a, b and c Medline search (as accessed through Reuter's Health Information gateway)

Fig. 19.3a

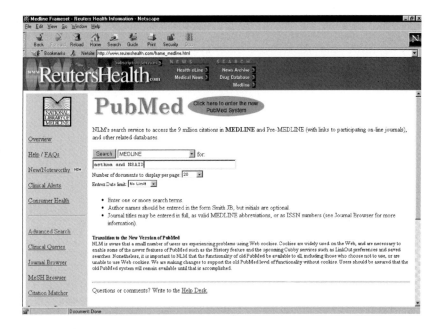

Fig. 19.3b

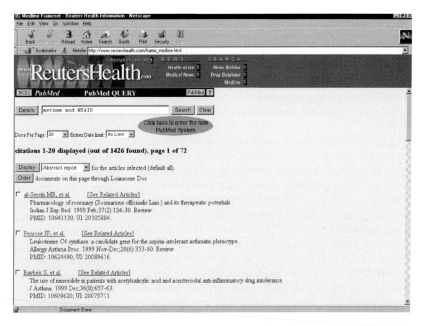

Teletext, the broadcast form of database enquiry, has three outlets – Ceefax (BBC), Oracle (ITV), and 4-TEL (Channel 4). A keypad enables users to select the radio-wave signal appropriate to the page they wish to view. A certain amount of Health Education Council material is transmitted through Teletext. The number of available pages is far fewer than with Prestel, and access cannot be limited by password.

Cabletext combines primary transmission by broadcast with local distribution by cable.

The term *videotex* is a generic one that encompasses Prestel, Teletext and Cabletext. A television receiver accepting videotex has the potential to add sound and mobile graphics. If electronic storage is added to videotex receivers, then further reference can be made to pages without the need for remote access.

Sky Digital has launched 'The Medical Channel' and provides free satellite dishes and digital receivers at selected health centres. The signal is encrypted and topics covered are medical news, current affairs, med-

Fig. 19.3c

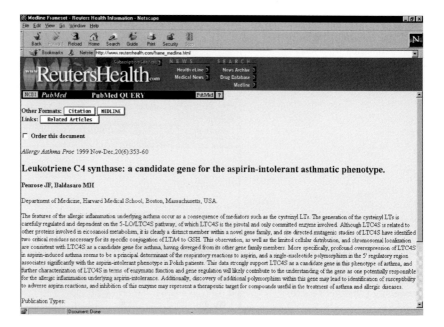

ical advances and further education. The facility is regulated by the ABPI.

19.22 E-MAIL

Although electronic mail (e-mail) is demonstrably faster, cheaper, more accurately targeted and more convenient than conventional mail, it may be many years before a final transition is made from one to the other. In the meantime, we are obliged to operate both postal systems in parallel, and cope with voice mail and fax traffic as well – a logistical nightmare. There is an urgent need to collate and process all incoming messages, other than conventional telephone conversations, on the practice computer from whatever source. Until this happens, many people will look upon the daily checking of e-mail as an unwelcome added chore.

The term e-mail is sometimes used to describe the way in which memoranda are passed between terminals in a local area network – LAN messaging. However, e-mail, as it is usually understood to be, has the potential to communicate globally, and for this the following are required:

- a modem and PSTN line, or a terminal adapter and ISDN line
- a communications interface card
- E-mail software
- the use of a wide area network (WAN) such as the Internet or NHSnet (or an intranet within a WAN)

- access to the WAN through an e-mail 'domain provider', who allocates the user a personal e-mail address and mailbox, and manages e-mail services.

The last three requisite categories may be provided separately or as a package.

There are six alternative ways in which e-mail services can be obtained:

- through the NHSnet or HealthLink, usually by arrangement with the GP system supplier
- through on-line service providers, who may or may not provide their own software and who offer 'gateways' to the Internet
- through internet service providers in conjunction with Internet access provision
- through the Microsoft Network (MSN)
- through a private domain provider using the Internet, and e-mail software such as Microsoft Exchange (a component of Windows 95) or Eudora (a free version of which can be downloaded from the Internet)
- through an enhanced BT terrestrial telephone that possesses a small display and slide-out keyboard in addition to its touch-tone keypad (Easicom 2000), or as an enhanced cellular phone with integral display and keypad using WAP technology.
- Doctors.net.uk (Freepost SCE 6579, Abingdon, Oxon OX14 4YG) is an executive e-mail domain provider for the UK medical profession which monitors customer specified Medline bibliography and job opportunities. The RCGP offers a web-

Fig. 19.4 Sending e-mail using Netscape Navigator (Reproduced with permission from Kiley 1999a)

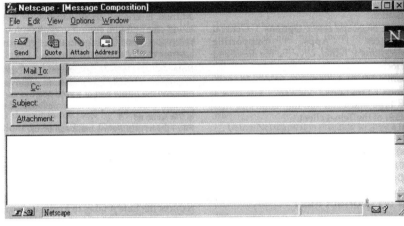

Fig. 19.5 Receiving e-mail using Simeon, Signet and JANET (Courtesy of Southampton University Computer services)

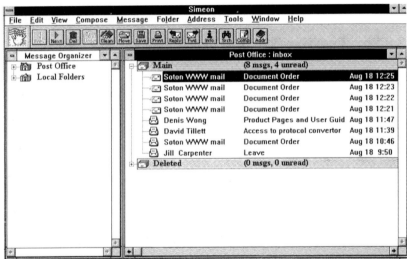

based e-mail domain service through its internet site (http://www.rcgp.org.uk).

Historically, e-mail has been a method of exchanging electronic text in its simplest form as ASCII characters, with formatting restricted to the provision of a few basic data fields and the use of line and paragraph spacing in the main body of the message. As the highly structured electronic messages used for NHS hospital reports employed different and stricter protocols, they have in the past been referred to as a separate entity from e-mail, though the basic principle of 'store and forward' used by both is the same.

Further enhancement in e-mail design has enabled more refined packages, such as those transmitted on the MSN, to incorporate font options, bullet points, colours, images and spreadsheets, and to bundle incoming data from multiple sources such as other OLSPs or fax input. It is likely, therefore, that the technologies used for NHS e-mail and structured messages will merge in future.

E-mail receiving software first selects the sources of mail to be accessed, then downloads it and processes it. There are usually two options for doing this:

- An *ad hoc* dial-up instigated by the user, which permits inspection of the subject headings of waiting messages; these the recipient must choose either to accept or reject. Those that are selected are then downloaded for processing.
- At pre-determined intervals, the recipient's computer autodials and empties the mailbox while at the same time uploading any new messages that are to be posted. Here, messages are transferred in their entirety.

Incoming messages are received into an 'in box' on the recipient's system and will be read, discarded, stored, printed, or replied to, in which case there is an option to return both original and reply. Comments may be added to incoming messages and, when outdated messages have been deleted from hard disk, compaction programs are available to rationalize storage space.

E-mail addresses consist of two data components separated by the symbol @. The first component is the addressee's name and the second component is the domain name.

Outward messages are prefaced by the addressee's e-mail address, which can be obtained from the sender's stored 'address book' or entered anew. Date, time and sender will be appended by the system. The subject heading and the body of the message then follow. Copies can be scheduled for other recipients, the message can be saved and printed, priority can be allocated, encryption can be imposed, and delivery may be instituted immediately or delayed until the next scheduled transmission. Some e-mail packages record the fact that a message has been delivered. If the recipient cannot be located, the message is 'returned to sender'.

All retained messages are stored in a user's personal files in the computer's e-mail database. Thence, inward messages can be searched according to sender, subject or date received, and outward messages can be searched according to addressee, subject or date sent. Other components of the e-mail database are the address book and a log of all e-mail transactions.

A specialized e-mail software package for transmission of out-of-hours data from NHS Direct outstations to general practices has been developed by Dr Paul Cundy of Wimbledon and trialled successfully in 40 practices.

The potential for e-mail to become virus-infected must be born in mind. Even e-mail transmitted over the NHSnet is potentially vulnerable, and it is wise to install antivirus software for all e-mail use.

Whether we like it or not, e-mail is here to stay and will become increasingly important as a means of communication between health professionals. We must adapt to it and blend it with our intake of data from other sources on the practice computer. In this respect, the approach adopted by the Microsoft Network could well be emulated.

19.23 CD-ROM

Compact disk (CD) technology uses a laser beam to write to and read the face of the storage disk, unlike the magnetic read/write heads used on hard and floppy disk drives. Reflections from microscopic pits scored on the CD surface spell out whether the signal

is an 0 or a 1 bit in the binary system. Because the reading head does not actually touch the surface of the disk, such little wear and tear as occurs is the result of intrusive dust or clumsy handling. With care, a CD should be playable at least 1000 times and have a life expectancy of 100 years. CDs may be used for audio, computer data, or movie making, but the technology for all three is basically the same. The CD-ROM (compact disk read-only memory) is the format most often associated with personal computers, and its 640 Mb capacity provides that in this context it can accommodate textual data, images, video, sound or programs, or a combination of any or all of these. As its name implies, a CD-ROM disk cannot be deleted or amended by the user's computer.

Most CD-ROMs have their reference data and their programs for installation, navigation and interactive education bundled together on the same disk. Although programs are usually downloaded to hard disk during use, reference data are often processed directly from the CD-ROM disk. Brands such as Silver Platter supply programs and reference data on separate disks, which saves replicating the programs each time a new CD-ROM is issued.

Navigational programs on CD-ROM frequently use conventions derived from Internet browsers. The user is able to interrogate reference data by keyword search or index browsing. Interactive tutorial programs may be provided to assist in the assimilation of reference data, and these frequently offer optional MCQs, correct answers, and response assessment. Help screen facilities are usually present.

For a list of interesting CD-ROM disks see Appendix B.

19.24 COMPUTER CD-ROM DRIVES

Computer CD-ROM (CCD-ROM) drives may be:

- mounted internally within the processor housing, or else free standing (external)
- either SCSI or IDE compliant, a distinction it is essential to recognize in order to ensure compatibility with the processor; IDE machines are now much more commonly used
- rated as two-, four-, six-, eight-, 10- or 12-speed models. While two-speed machines are obsolescent, many CCD-ROM multimedia disks are configured to work at quad (four-) speed ratings, and faster rates of spin do not necessarily produce better results. (Other factors involved in this equation are the CPU bandwidth, and software driver functionality.)

(For smaller practices a useful storage box for up to eight CD-ROMs, which fits into empty drive bays in a tower unit, is marketed by the mail order firm Innovations.)

19.25 CCD-ROM CONFIGURATIONS

CCD-ROM has proved so attractive a medium to computer users that the number of available titles is increasing exponentially. New software, textbooks, dictionaries, encyclopaedias, and updates of reference material in constant use in general practice, are now not only obtainable but may be exclusively provided on CCD-ROM. The GP system must of necessity incorporate a CCD-ROM drive in its functionality. There are three options:

- a single disk drive
- a single user multidisk autochanger ('juke box'), which possesses a single reading head but can hold four or more disks in its library. A feed mechanism transports the reading head to the required disk. Disk input is into individual trays, or into a magazine. Currently marketed small autochangers operate at quad speed and cost around £100, but models accommodating a greater number of disks are also available.
- a networked multidisk autochanger.

A practice's choice of drive will depend upon the number of users, the accessible CPU capacity, and the types of data that need to be accessed. The software driver that installs and operates the drive should be included with the purchased product.

Manufacturers

Many companies manufacture CCD-ROM drives, the principal ones being Mitsumi, Pioneer, Teac, Toshiba, Flextor, Sony, Hitachi, Samsung and Aztech.

19.26 OTHER TYPES OF COMPACT DISK

Apart from the CCD-ROM, which is purchased prerecorded and cannot be altered, compact disk technology is used in three other principal formats:

- CD-recordable (CD-R), in which the disk can be written to by the user's disk drive once only. This format can be useful for making copies of working programs.
- CD-rewritable (CD-RW), which uses hybrid technology and allows up to 1000 rewrites. This format is useful for routine system backup.
- Digital video disk (DVD) ROM, which holds from 7.4–17 Gb, depending upon design.

The more sophisticated the storage medium, the greater the functionality required of the drive. However, in general, manufacturers have tried to ensure, when they produce designs with improved functionality, that their new machines retain the ability to accommodate older storage formats.

SUMMARY

- Computerized reference information can be offered simultaneously on all accessing terminals, searched rapidly and updated simply, without the need for re-printing, and may be stored electronically in virtually unlimited quantity.
- Reference data may be held remotely, accessed through WANs either using the Internet, OLSPs or commercial organizations whose data can only be interrogated by using dedicated WANs, gateways and agencies. Remotely accessed data may be inspected, downloaded, stored and printed locally, and to do this the user may or may not have to pay tolls, depending on the source.
- The Internet was an American innovation that has spread throughout the world because of the need and desire of computer users to communicate. It grows so rapidly that it is not feasible to maintain an up-to-date directory of all the information it contains, but search engine operators assemble categorized lists of the sites about which they have been informed, or which they have detected by searches. These lists can be interrogated by users who use the search engine function on the Internet.
- The Internet can be accessed by any computer that conforms to the network's protocols, given that they have at least a fast 486, 32-bit processor, a 14.4 K modem and a 640 × 480 display. ISDN access, and animation, voice or video transmission have more exacting requirements. Access realistically requires the services of an ISP or OLSP, or the use of NHSnet. A service provider may offer set-up, communication, browser, e-mail, news group, voice and video software, although not all do so.
- Facilities made available by Internet access include the interrogation of remote databases, provision of

client Web space, e-mail, news groups, chat channels, voice and video conferencing, e-shopping and marketing, e-education, e-games, e-publishing, e-banking and e-investment.

- The principal browsers used on the Internet are Netscape Navigator and Microsoft Internet Explorer. Each enables the user to enter a site address, to bring the site's data on screen and to 'click' on nodes embedded in these data in order to switch to other related frames, which may or may not be housed on the same computer. The World Wide Web offers the most efficient technology for Internet navigation. Data contained in frames may consist of text images, animation, video, sound, or a mixture of any or all, and colour is frequently used. The reliability of data obtained through the Internet cannot be guaranteed.
- Internet operations are funded from a variety of sources, which include user tolls, line charges, helpline charges, advertising and the sale of mailing lists.
- Web pages are created by some practices as an alternative to printed practice brochures, and the communication platform created has also been used to allow requests for repeat prescribing. The creation of Web pages requires the use of word processing and HTML, configuration with Netscape Navigator and Microsoft Internet Explorer, and transmission to the ISP using file transfer protocol.
- Internet shopping allows the inspection of catalogues, the compilation of orders and payment by bank card, to result in postal or courier delivery. UK consumer laws, advertising regulations and the UK banking code apply to transactions.
- Medline, Toxbase and Travax are important remote medical databases, but all have restricted access. Medically related information is also relayed through Prestel, Teletext and Cabletext.
- E-mail can be sent through HealthLink, the NHSnet, ISPs, OLSPs, the Microsoft Network, private e-mail domain providers and enhanced terrestrial or cellular telephones. It is faster, cheaper, more accurately targeted and more convenient than conventional mail, but its use will constitute an additional chore until virtually all mail, structured messaging, voice mail and fax traffic are received through computers. E-mail is stored remotely in the user's mailbox until downloaded and processed on the user's computer. Outgoing mail is uploaded to the addressee's mailbox by use of an e-mail address, which consists of the addressee's e-mail name, separated from the domain name by the symbol @. E-mail can be infected by viruses.

- Computer CD-ROMs offer 640 Mb of storage and can accommodate textual data, images, video, sound or programs, or a combination of any of these media. CD-ROM drives can be limited to the use of single disks, in which case they may be internal or external to the processor. Multiple disk drives use autochange facilities, and alternative designs are available for use, either with single or with networked computers. CD-ROM drives are rated by their speed, but speeds in excess of ×4 may confer no advantage, as many multimedia disks are configured to run at this speed. It is important to ensure compatibility between the CD-ROM drive and the processor. The number of available computer CD-ROM titles continues to increase exponentially in line with the capacity, reliability, resilience and popularity of the medium.

FURTHER READING

Consumers' Association 1998 Which?, September

Davies T 1995 On-line date for GPs. Practice Computing, Winter: 23

Kemp P 1995 The complete idiot's guide to the Internet with Windows 95. Que, Indianapolis, IN, p. 14

Kiley R 1999a Medical information on the Internet, 2nd edn. Churchill Livingstone, Edinburgh

Kiley R 1999b The doctor's Internet handbook. Royal Society of Medicine Press, London (orders from website http://www.roysocmed.as.uk/handbook.htm)

Lowie A, Duckitt P 1986 Computer based sources of information in medicine. Royal College of Physicians, London

Proudfoot H T, Davidson W S M 1983 A viewdata system for poisons information. British Medical Journal 286: 125

Sanfey J 1996 MSc in general practice can be done over the Internet. British Medical Journal 312: 978

Silberg W M, Lundberg G D, Musacchio R A 1997 Assessing, controlling, and assuring the quality of medical information on the Internet: caveant lector et viewor – let the reader and viewer beware. Journal of the American Medical Association 277: 1244–1245

Snell N 1998 SAMS teach yourself the Internet in 24 hours, 2nd edn. Sams Publishing, Indianapolis, IN

Wentk R 1998 The Which? guide to the Internet. Which? Books, London

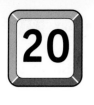

20 Financial packages, e-banking, private practice

20.1 INTRODUCTION

With the introduction of the National Health Service in 1948, the replacement of billing by regular state payments to doctors brought a sense of freedom to the doctor–patient relationship. The quality of mercy was no longer to be strained by 'Shylockian' materialism. It took many years for the profession to learn that considerable sums of money could be forfeited in badly managed practices from failure to optimize services, to submit claims effectively or to check incoming payments. Default in resource and tax planning also caused loss. The income accruing to a well managed practice could prove to be twice as high as that earned by a poorly managed rival, given the same number of hours of work. The need for stricter financial control over practice affairs is also central to the containment of health care expenses that is required by the government.

The earliest financial software packages to become generally available were generic spreadsheets, and some GPs adapted these for NHS practice use, although in the days of multiuser GP system configurations a financial package had to run independently on its own standalone machine. The business community's demand for electronification catalysed elaboration of the spreadsheet principle and spawned a generation of early generic book-keeping and accounting packages, some of which became widely applicable and popular.

At a time when UK GP system development was still focusing almost entirely on the need to produce patient management software, many practices were obliged, of necessity, to purchase generic packages such as those marketed by Sage, Intuit and Maclean McNicholl if they wished to implement financial applications. In this situation, there could, of course, be no data integration between the GP system and the financial package, even if the two packages could be run on the same computer.

During the 1990s, four new factors were introduced into the equation.

- GP suppliers started to develop and market their own financial packages.
- As generic financial software had become more sophisticated, its development had been fragmented by the need for specialization, so that many available commercial packages were no longer suitable for practice use.
- The use of, or compliance with, the Windows operating system was slowly becoming an industry standard requirement, a development that brought with it the prospect of increased data and file transfer fluency between applications.
- In the practice context, the need to process electronic financial data was increasing. It no longer sufficed to provide book-keeping facilities on the practice computer. It was becoming clear that the practice's financial software should, in addition:
  - provide full monthly, quarterly, annual and concurrent practice accounting facilities
  - link with the HA/PPSA claims procedure
  - dovetail with the practice's electronic bank account
  - dovetail with the practice payroll package
  - provide an upgrade path for the storage of new tax tables and new comparative 'national average' statistics
  - provide for the export of data in electronic format to the practice accountant.

20.2 CASH FLOW AND BALANCE STRIKE

Practice profitability is determined by controlling income and expenditure – its positive and negative components. Most NHS practice income is related to data held in the patient record, whereas most practice expenditure is unrelated to patient data.

If the income ledger is brought up to date at the end of each month when the HA cheque is paid to the practice bank account, and at the same time the expenses ledger is updated with reference to cheque stubs, the monthly bank statement, and provision for anticipated tax and large bills, then the computer can strike a balance.

The occasions on which it is appropriate for this balance to be obtained are:

- monthly, to coincide with the monthly division of profits
- quarterly to follow receipt of the quarterly payment statement from the HA
- yearly to provide the data required by the accountant and the Inland Revenue.

Routines for dealing with the end of month financial transactions vary widely between practices. A typical example that illustrates the underlying principles may be quoted:

- A few days before the monthly NHS cheque will be credited, the partnership bank statement is obtained.
- The sums to be credited from HA/PPSA sources are shown in the HA statement and must be entered on to the income ledger. Also entered are the sums from private patients and other cheques received by the partnership during the month, together with cash payments. After ledger entry, these monies are promptly banked.
- Staff pay, PAYE and National Insurance, and all bills that have accrued during the previous month

are paid by cheque and entered on the expenses ledger. Standing orders and direct debits are also recorded.
- Provision for anticipated large bills, subdivided into monthly instalments, are made and entered on the expenses ledger in a manner that demonstrates that they have not yet been paid – these monies are transferred into an investment account.
- Provision for anticipated tax is made in a similar way.
- To the balance shown in the bank statement is added the new income shown in the income ledger. Debits and provisional debits shown in the expenses ledger are subtracted from the total and the resultant profit is subdivided between partners (Fig. 20.1).

Items of income and expense that are individualized will obviously make the computation more involved. Seniority pay, night visits and the use of deputizing services, 'added years' and leave payments may all be subject to special provision between partners, but can be accommodated by a well designed practice financial package.

Accurate control of cash flow avoids bank overdrafts and removes the need for doctors to use their private savings as a buffer against the practice's monetary fluctuations.

The preparation of formal accounts is greatly facilitated by the computer's ability to strike a balance as at any date, and to quote details for a retrospective period of any duration. Monthly, quarterly or annual printouts are all available 'at the touch of a button'.

Annual accounts, which will be used as a permanent practice record and will be submitted to the tax authorities for assessment, are usually prepared by

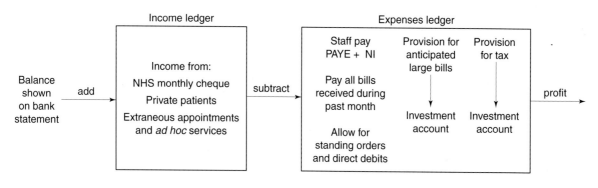

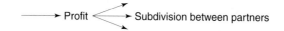

Fig. 20.1 Specimen routine for end-of-month financial transactions

accountants but can be produced by the practice computer. The two main types of formal account are the 'profit and loss statement', which is taken directly from an annual balance strike, and the 'balance sheet', which integrates both income and expenses, and capital assets and liabilities such as premises, equipment, motor cars, overdrafts, loans and mortgages. 'Balance sheet' compilation will therefore require capital data to be stored on the computer.

Figure 20.2 shows the chain of accounts needed to execute and monitor practice finances.

20.3 TWO LEVELS OF SOPHISTICATION OF PRACTICE FINANCIAL PACKAGES

Financial packages suitable for NHS practice use are available at two alternative levels of sophistication.

- *Basic book-keeping packages* provide income and expenditure ledgers, petty cash management, reconciliation between practice ledgers and bank statements, and facilities for apportioning profit between partners. Straightforward generic spreadsheets such as Excel or Lotus 1-2-3 provide adequately for these functions.

- *Accounting and advanced financial management packages*, in addition to basic book-keeping functions, offer a wide range of financial management support, which may include:
  - calculation and monitoring of NHS fee and allowance funds
  - superannuation
  - the handling of multiple bank accounts
  - provision for direct debits and standing orders
  - the recording of items of income and expenditure, with the use of codes and subcodes which allocate them accurately, and to more than one spreadsheet
  - profit and loss accounts, and provision for comparison with previous periods of time
  - a fixed asset register and balance sheet compilation
  - links with payroll

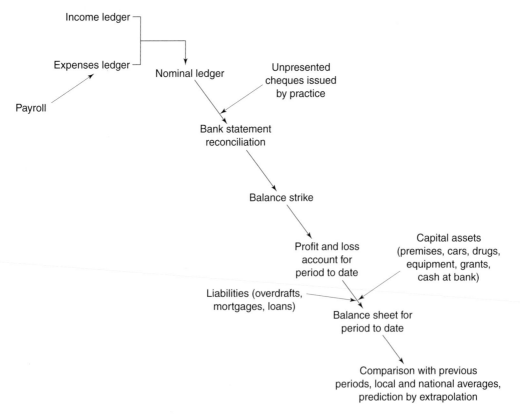

Fig. 20.2 The chain of accounts needed to execute and monitor practice finances: although the last three steps are usually undertaken by accountants, all could be conducted on the practice computer

- forward budgeting and comparison with actual figures
- 'IF–THEN' putations
- comparisons with national average income and expenditure taken from sources such as Medeconomics
- VAT calculations
- reports and charts for monthly, quarterly and annual output
- reconciliation with health authority statements.

An audit trail should be available in advanced financial packages to log the date, time, user identification and category codes for any transaction. The system should be password protected, and have help screens and a phone helpline.

Few accounts packages possess all the above features, and practices need to match requirements against availability. Generally speaking, a product's cost will be proportional to the refinement and range of facilities on offer.

20.4 TWO USEFUL OFF-THE-SHELF FINANCIAL PACKAGES

Two reasonably priced financial packages have proved widely popular in NHS general practice. Both provide basic book-keeping facilities, but each has its own interesting additional features.

Windows-based Quicken Deluxe (2000) (Intuit)

This is a generic financial package, which, in addition to offering a range of straightforward spreadsheet-derived applications, also:

- prints its own cheques
- offers 'IF–THEN' putation
- calculates income tax and VAT
- has a rapid invoice routine for small businesses
- triggers alerts when preset levels are reached
- includes an integrated Web browser that allows direct access from Quicken to its own personal finance website – links from this website lead to a wide range of daily updated financial information, such as the most competitive mortgages, loans, deposit accounts and tables of share prices
- provides an automatic refresh facility, activated each time the user connects to the Quicken website, which provides that all data previously downloaded to the user's computer will be updated automatically; Intuit's products are regularly updated.

The Maclean McNicholl Accounts Package (MMS)

This has been created especially for NHS general practice, and has already been installed in over 2000 sites. Available in DOS or Windows versions, its spreadsheet-type functions are ready-labelled for all NHS fee and allowance categories. It does not calculate targets but, given national average data, will supply comparative results.

MMS dovetails with the Ferguson Payroll Package, and uses simple codes and subcodes for data entry. It provides a comprehensive range of reports, including those required for VAT, but cannot connect electronically with Health Board/Authority linkages.

MMS claims to be the only accounts package that is able to support the complex requirements of dispensing practice expense claims, in which the dispensing and practice elements have to be apportioned. MMS has also worked with the accountancy firm Pannell Kerr Forster to coordinate a data input coding system that enables the firm's GP customers to transfer all practice accountancy details to them on a diskette for processing. Helpline: 0141 942 3446 from 1–4 pm on Mondays, Wednesdays and Fridays.

Other packages

Other commercially available packages are the Sage range, Microsoft Money, Medicalc, Quickbooks Accounting and the Hacker Young Module.

20.5 FINANCIAL PACKAGES MARKETED BY GP SYSTEM SUPPLIERS

All major GP system suppliers now provide financial packages to run beside their clinical software, but the degree of integration achieved between the two software packages, and the range of functionality provided with the financial package, vary considerably between suppliers. If the two software modules do not integrate to a degree that enables data to be shared across files and so to obviate the need to re-key data, then the use of an imported generic financial package may still be a better option. Others factors to be considered are, of course, price (some GP system suppliers' financial software is now much more competitively priced than it was), and the need to apportion software support.

20.6 PAYROLL

The tasks of payroll are:

- to maintain a payroll ledger for each staff member

- to produce a pay slip showing the computation and amount of pay and deductions for each employee on each pay day
- to produce PAYE tax and National Insurance returns
- to update the expenses ledger with the details of payments made
- to formulate a claim for repayment from the HA/PPSA.

The format and arithmetical functions of a spreadsheet are ideally suited to the computer application of payroll. PAYE tax codes and tables must be loaded electronically on to the system each year and are commercially available as floppy disk updates. Special stationery is required for the production of pay slips, and special stationery, or equivalent formatting printout, is needed for tax returns. Employee details on the payroll ledger include name, dates, hours, overtime hours, tax code, rate, gross pay, Statutory Sick Pay, tax, National Insurance, Statutory Maternity Benefit, any other deductions, and net pay. Of these, only dates, hours and overtime hours may need updating at each pay day. Weekly or monthly pay slips may be produced quickly and with minimum effort by an efficient menu-driven system. Electronic banking procedures (such as Autopay) may be used by the system to credit the employee's bank account directly. Global payroll accounts are required.

Standards for pay records are set by law, and there is a wide choice of payroll packages that comply with these standards. Only the formulation of claims to the HA/PPSA needs to be tailor made, and all GP system suppliers market payroll packages that include this requirement.

Payroll packages

- *QTAX* is one of the most competitively priced generic products.
- *Quickbooks Accounts and Payroll* has highly effective functionality.
- *David Ferguson's GP Payroll Package*, which supplies over 3500 sites, gives full NHS pension scheme support, automatically reminds practices to supply dates, and produces all reports required for health authority reimbursement. It maintains and monitors staff holiday schedules, logs grievance procedures and dovetails with the Maclean McNicholl accounts package. Ferguson's Payroll Package is currently undergoing further development as a practice manager support tool and is adapting to the needs of Primary Care Groups (fax: 0141 616 0691).

Bank payroll processing

Some clearing banks operate a computerized payroll processing system on behalf of customers. Given

Specimen print-out of Staff Quarterly Reimbursements:

QUARTERLY SUMMARY OF STAFF PAYMENTS   QUARTER 3

Number	Name	Number of pay days this quarter	Total gross pay (inc SSP)	Statutory sick pay (if any)	Employers NI Contributions	Overtime Paid (Included in totals)	Cash Adjusts
2	RECEPTIONIST 1	3	2168.36	0.00	226.55	0.00	60.92
3	RECEPTIONIST 2	3	540.34	0.00	27.10	0.00	29.64
4	RECEPTIONIST 3	3	1004.64	0.00	70.28	0.00	29.12
5	RECEPTIONIST 4	3	302.91	0.00	0.00	0.00	18.20
6	RECEPTIONIST 5	3	521.82	0.00	26.20	84.25	17.16
7	RECEPTIONIST 6	2	288.00	0.00	10.00	0.00	0.00
8	RECEPTIONIST 7	3	626.35	0.00	31.30	0.00	20.97
9	RECEPTIONIST 8	3	440.95	0.00	8.00	0.00	13.86
10	RECEPTIONIST 9	3	606.31	0.00	30.30	0.00	19.06
11	RECEPTIONIST 10	3	688.99	0.00	39.44	0.00	21.66
12	RECEPTIONIST 11	2	257.23	0.00	0.00	0.00	0.00
13	RECEPTIONIST 12	2	329.52	0.00	11.40	0.00	0.00
	TOTALS		7775.61	0.00	480.57		
	ESTIMATE OF REIMBURSMENT		5923.50				

Fig. 20.3 Specimen printout to support quarterly staff reimbursement claim (Courtesy of AMC Systems)

faxed particulars of pay rates, hours, bonuses and overtime, the bank works out tax and NI rates and pays net salaries direct to employees' bank accounts.

20.7 OTHER FINANCIAL PACKAGES

Tax returns

Generic tax calculation packages (e.g. QuickTAX, from Intuit) provide interactive programs that enable the entry on screen of all data necessary for the completion of a personal tax return form. These data can then be printed out on a facsimile form approved for the purpose by the Inland Revenue. Other packages are QTAX and TaxCalc.

Partners' tax returns will be supported by practice profit and loss, and balance sheet reports, as prepared by practice financial software.

Personal financial management

One of the most effective generic packages for personal financial management is Quicken Deluxe (Intuit).

20.8 ELECTRONIC BANKING – AN OVERVIEW

When *Punch* magazine commissioned a survey of the bin bags left for disposal outside a series of high street banks in 1998, it did not find a shred of evidence of customers' personal details. This was because the evidence hadn't been shredded. Explicit salary and account information, and phone numbers, were all in the trawl.

Even shredded paper documentation can be reassembled with enough patience, much to the embarrassment of embassies hastily vacated in times of surrounding turmoil. By contrast, the security of electronic data transfer is becoming increasingly refined. A double-layered encryption process, in which the two layers are related by a randomly allocated linkage, can now be used to enable banking transactions to take place over the Internet.

Migration away from paper has had far-reaching effects upon the banking industry. In successive steps, postal, voice, touch-tone telephone, PC-based, interactive-TV-based and Internet-based banking have been introduced. Building societies have become banks; supermarkets, Marks & Spencer, Virgin and overseas banks have joined the competition, and the clearing banks' high street branches are in demise. Insurance quotes and implementation, share dealing,

foreign currency and travellers' cheques, and pensions have been added to the bank service's portfolio. The customer benefits from the new competitive edge offered by the market, no longer makes the weekly pilgrimage to queue for the bank teller, writes fewer cheques, does little or no manual ledgering, and keeps all spare cash on high-interest deposit until it is needed.

General practitioners, having dependable and relatively generous incomes, are valued bank customers and the main clearing banks each put together a package of services for them (Table 20.1). The Royal Bank of Scotland has even set up four distributed Medical Finance Units to focus on the profession.

20.9 VOICE TELEPHONE BANKING

Voice telephone banking is now offered by all the major financial services providers, and is secured by the ability of the customer to replicate a sequence of personal identification details that have been recorded previously with the agency. As telephone and postal accounts incur lower overheads, they usually give better rates of interest. As a rule, money has to be input by cheque or direct debit. Access is provided at local call rates. The facilities offered by voice telephone banking are included in Table 20.2.

20.10 PC BANKING

Before most households possessed computers, the TSB launched an intriguing system whereby the account holder used the buttons on a touch-tone phone to converse with a hierarchy of recorded voice messages at the bank in order to make financial transactions. At this time, the Bank of Scotland also provided dedicated 'HOBS' terminals, each approximately the size of four reams of A4, with which the customer could access the bank server via the PSTN.

As a high proportion of households and businesses now use PCs, all major clearing banks currently offer PC banking, using a modem to access the bank server. Access is established either through the bank's own dedicated telecom network (WAN) at local call rates, or through the Internet. Specialized software is required both on the server and peripherally.

Unlike voice telephone banking, the computer screen allows rapid appraisal of bank statements, and is a very convenient platform for decision making and interaction. The medium also allows the bank to billboard its range of services.

Table 20.1 Specialized banking facilities for general practice

Standard banking services targeted at general practitioners	Electronic banking services
Cost-rent scheme and surgery improvement package	Check balance
Business loans	Order statement (delivery by post or fax)
Surgery protection insurance, including cover against computer breakdown	View statement on VDU screen (print-out if required)
	Free practice cashflow forecast sheet
Financial and tax advice	Order cheque book
Loans to medical students	Transfer payment (electronic cheque)
Medical 'help desk' (telephone hotline)	Account switching
	Payroll
	View standing orders
	Reconciliation facility
	Send messages to bank (maximum 10 lines)
	User manual
	On-line help facility and telephone advice facility
	Password protection at two levels – view and pay
	Additional software support on floppy for remote location
	Software supports for remote printer

Table 20.2 Comparison of facilities offered by voice telephone, PC bank WAN and PC Internet banking

Facility offered by most electronic banking providers (January 1999)	Voice telephone	PC and modem via bank WAN	PC and modem via Internet
Check balance	+	+	+
Request statement	+	+	+
Pay bills	+	+	+
Transfer cash between accounts	+	+	+
Post account holder a cheque	+		
Set up standing order	+	+	
Amend standing order	+	+	+
Amend but not set up direct debits	+	+	+
Request new cheque or paying in book	+	+	+
Arrange loans	+		
Arrange foreign currency and travellers' cheques	+		
Provide electronic cards for cash withdrawals	+		
Stop a cheque	+	+	
Report missing cash cards	+	+	
Insurance quotation and policy implementation		+	
Arrange overdraft	+		
Share dealing	+		
24 hour service		+	+

The facilities on offer through the Internet are currently fewer than those obtained through bank WAN banking (Table 20.2).

PC access to the bank's own WAN

Peripheral software is usually provided by the bank free of charge, either on CD-ROM or a sequence of floppy disks, and this enables the entry, validation, protection and communication of customer data. Access is password protected and the customer is required to notify the system of the identity of all authorized users. Passwords have to be changed at regular intervals. As transmission is provided by the bank's own network, it shares the same adequate level of security.

PC bank WAN access is provided by the Bank of Scotland, Barclay's, the Clydesdale, the Co-operative Bank, Lloyds-TSB, HSBC, the National Westminster, the Nationwide Building Society and the Royal Bank of Scotland. Other financial institutions such as the Alliance & Leicester Building Society are set to follow.

In an interesting joint development between VAMP (now In Practice Systems) and the National Westminster Bank, using on-line banking, the VAMP Business System was enabled to produce automatic reconciliation between the practice ledger and the practice bank statement.

20.11   INTERNET BANKING

Globally, the first on-line banking network services were launched by the Wells Fargo Bank in the USA in 1989. The same bank initiated its Internet-based operation in 1995, and by 1998 had succeeded in opening 200 000 screen-based customer accounts.

The first financial agencies to launch Internet banking services in the UK have been the Nationwide Building Society (http://www.nationwide.co.uk), the Royal Bank of Scotland (http://www.rbs.co.uk) and the Co-operative Bank (http://www.co-operativebank.co.uk) which has named its Internet venture 'smile'. First-e was the first independent Internet bank in the UK and insures its customer against computer failure – an example which other banks will have to follow. The Prudential's Internet bank trades under the name 'egg'. Several other Internet banks are now being launched.

Customers are issued with a four-digit security number, which is subject to periodic change, and they must submit a range of personal identification data for security checks each time they log on. The two-layered interleaving levels of encryption previously described are required to conform with European information technology security evaluation criteria. Contact with the bank's server is made through a standard Web browser.

Other methods of access

Interactive television, using cable or BT connections, has been used for banking as well as shopping purposes, and the introduction of digital television will accelerate the uptake of this form of access. Cellular phones using the Smart Messaging Service or WAP technology can access some bank accounts.

20.12   PRIVATE PRACTICE SYSTEMS

Overview

Although private practice systems use patient files as their hub, most of them otherwise differ fundamentally from NHS-based systems in that they record only those clinical details required for billing. Private practice software focuses on the administrative control of charges, invoices and payments, appointments and accounts. Codes relating to insured procedures are used in place of Read codes.

Principal features of typical private practice systems

- Patient file details usually include a record code number; name; address and post code; business and home phone numbers; date of birth; usual general practitioner and referring practitioner; insuring agency; solicitor; religion; next of kin; diagnosis or diagnostic procedure with insurer's code reference; and medication. If the MEDICS Security Group is involved, some additional clinical details are required.
- For each patient, the charges associated with services given and invoices and payments received (all per specified time period) are administered. Reminder letters for unpaid bills are automated. Debtors may be patients, insurance companies or solicitors.
- An electronic appointment system, with sessions per listholder and slots per session, allows printed appointment slips to be issued and reminder letters in advance of appointments to be posted to patients.
- Accounts are prepared monthly and annually, which will incorporate expenditure items as well as income from services (it would be useful to append a payroll package to this facility).

- Reports include lists of charges, invoices and payments per patient or per doctor, lists of unpaid invoices, times taken for debtors to settle, and lists of appointments.
- Directories may be set up to give reference to the codes and costs per procedure for each insurer, and to list the contact details of GPs, consultants, insurers and solicitors. Templates will be created for standard letters, invoices and appointment slips.
- Security features will include password control over access levels to the system, encryption for the storage of data, and automated backup.
- A maintenance contract, which includes the provision for a helpline, should be obtained. On-site assistance should be available when appropriate.

Marketed software

Generic business software packages, such as those offered by Quicken or Sage, can be adapted to the requirements of private practice.

The IMPRESS system is custom-designed for private practice and is marketed by Medical Information Technologies. The system has many refinements, is Windows-based and is available in a network version. Its minimum requirements are a 486 processor with 8 Mb of RAM. Installation is from, and backup is to, floppy disk. (MIT, The Manor Lodge Consulting Centre, Mill Lane, Cheadle, Cheshire SK8 2NT, tel: 01565 830890.)

Miriam Healthcare markets two packages suitable for private practice, Private Fee Monitor and its more powerful sibling Maximise. (Miriam Healthcare Ltd, 384 Laird Street, Birkenhead L41 7AL, tel: 0151 670 1660.)

SUMMARY

- The ideal practice financial management package should:
  - record income and expenditure
  - provide for periodic balance strikes
  - provide easy reconciliation with bank statements
  - facilitate division of profit between partners
  - dovetail with, and utilize, electronic banking, and this should allow provision of both a current account and a high-interest account (which will act as a reservoir for future scheduled outgoings); it should be possible to switch money between current and high-interest accounts on demand
  - provide and dovetail with a payroll module
  - calculate and facilitate the payment of tax, and allow yearly upgrades to dictionaries containing tax tables and national average statistics
  - dovetail with the HA/PPSA Links claim procedure and enable payments to be checked
  - possess appropriate linkages with the locality commissioning system
  - provide a billing module for private work
  - generate a full set of formal 'profit and loss' and 'balance sheet' accounts, and provide monthly, quarterly, annual and concurrent reports as required
  - allow statistical analysis for audit and forecasting
  - provide for export of data in electronic format to the practice accountant
- Financial management software packages are obtainable generically, in which case they may offer either basic book-keeping functions (ledgering, petty cash management, reconciliation with bank statements, and subdivision of profits) or, alternatively, may provide a wide range of more sophisticated functions, which include those needed to produce a full set of accounts.
- Financial management packages are also marketed by GP system suppliers, and these have the advantage that data can be shared between the clinical and financial management systems. GP supplier financial software varies considerably between brands, both as regards functionality and cost.
- Payroll packages should maintain a payroll ledger for each staff member, produce detailed pay slips each pay day, generate tax and NI returns, update the expenses ledger, and formulate a claim for HA/PPSA repayment.
- Electronic banking is now available from a user's computer terminal and is channelled either through the bank's secure network or through the Internet. Peripheral software is provided by the bank and this enables the entry, validation, protection and communication of customer data. Passwords have to be changed at regular intervals. Internet access also requires that additional personal identification data shall be provided and that encryption shall be used. Balances can be checked, statements requested, bills paid, transfers made between accounts, standing orders and direct debits amended, and new cheque books or paying-in books requested.
- Private practice systems differ from NHS clinical systems in that they focus primarily on billing and accounting. Appointment systems are also incorporated. Codes used relate to procedures and are

those specified by the insurance industry. Debtors may be patients, insurance companies or solicitors. Templates enable the creation of standard letters and appointment slips.

FURTHER READING

Anderson R 1981 The business side of general practice. Pulse 11 July: 28

Bowles R 1987 GP Finance. 24 April: 43

British Medical Association GMSC 1989 Report to a special conference of representatives of local medical committees on 27 April 1989. British Medical Association, London

Doyle L 1985 Compare your earnings with doctor average. Medeconomics, January: 20

Financial Pulse 1991 Quarterly statements. Financial Pulse 16 July: 10

Department of Health and Welsh Office 1989 General practice in the National Health Service. A new contract. Department of Health and the Welsh Office, London

Higson N 1990 Can you calculate your own targets? GP 16 March: 66

Millward P 1982 Keeping control of the practice cash. Medeconomics, May: 44

National Health Service Review 1989 Working Papers 2, 3 and 4. HMSO, London

NHS Statements of Fees and Allowances

Pearson A 1991 How to figure out your finances with a spreadsheet. Practice Computing, September: 14

Rural Practice Payments Scheme Section 43 NHS FPN Statements of Fees and Allowances

Steel R, Anderson R 1981 How to balance your practice books. General Practitioners (Supplement 11) 13 November: 37

Research – audit – near-patient testing – patient-held monitors – dispensing practice

21.1 THE SEARCH PROCESS

Computers, like old soldiers, live on their memories. It is a twist of fate for humanity that the memory fails in old age. Without being too precise about the term memory (as applied to computers this is, by common usage, taken to mean the space available for processing data as opposed to storing it), it is true to say that the computer's potential for storage and retrieval of data is virtually limitless. Users have the option to buy as much or as little data storage and handling capacity as they want. Often, they have the choice of adding further units of capacity to their original system.

The subject of computer searches is a fascinating one. Computers have the power to search their records for specified attributes and can do so with impressive rapidity. Their speed of action allows them to inspect huge volumes of data in order to identity their target, and finding the proverbial needle in its haystack becomes straightforward. In its simplest form, the computer will search for a given symbol, word or statement. If the search is for a unique symbol the computer will recognize it. A large block of text will require identifiable symbols (delimiter symbols) to have been placed at the beginning and end to make the target stand out.

When successive entries of text are preceded by dates (as in consultation records), the dates themselves can act as delimiters. Where a term or statement of fixed length (such as a six-figure date of birth) always occupies the same position in a record, there is no problem in locating and defining it. More sophisticated searches will allow a short string of text to be recognized by using a matching technique akin to Cinderella's slipper.

The computer can search for one item and print the name of the records in which it occurs, or it can search for multiple items and list or count those records in which all occur. The several terms used as criteria for a search can be related to each other by conjunctions such as 'and', 'or' and 'not'. The computer can likewise print out multiple predetermined areas of records selected on the basis of one or more attributes. The computer is not limited to naming, counting or printing out sections of record. It can detect records with set attributes, tabulate those attributes, and produce graphs or bar charts to show the mathematical relationships between them.

21.2 DATA INPUT DISCIPLINE AND THE USE OF INTERNAL COMPUTER DICTIONARIES

The vitally important distinction that users have to make when considering future search programs concerns their data input. If, at a later date, they may wish to display or print out a statement *en bloc*, then it can be written in free style, but its limits must be defined. If they are likely to want to carry out word searches, then they must avoid, or allow for, all synonyms and avoid all ambiguities and mis-spelling.

The ultimate step that users can take in avoiding synonyms, ambiguities and mis-spelling is to adopt symbols or codes as a paraphrase for their statements. It is not possible for the human memory to store large numbers of coded equivalents for terms, and we are all familiar with the confusion caused by the use of non-standard abbreviations within the handwritten records of colleagues. As a component of *exhibited* text, it is therefore essential that all symbols, abbreviations and codes are reserved for a very few common place terms, and that these must be agreed, understood and easily remembered by all users of the system.

Modern GP computer record programs now have large dictionaries of common clinical and pharmaceutical terms within them, with internal codes so that only the codes need to be stored when the terms are entered – a manoeuvre that saves storage space. Taken one step further, if the computer knows that it must only accept into a particular area on the record a term taken from a specified subset held in its internal dictionary, it can reject input that does not conform, and thus weed out synonyms and mis-spellings as they occur. With a strictly defined internal dictionary of this sort, the computer can also complete the word that the user intends to write as input, when sufficient letters have been keyed in to render the word unique to the dictionary.

As an alternative, the user may key in the first three letters of a term, and the internal dictionary will list on display for selection all terms beginning with those three letters. Medical internal dictionaries are based on standard classifications of morbidity (such as Read), drugs (such as Multilex), or occupation (such as the OPCS), so that statistical analysis within and across subgroups used by these classifications becomes possible.

Internal dictionaries to check the spelling of all common language words, and to check grammar (usually by referring to the frequency with which adjacent words are associated) are now included in all major word processing packages. Voice input uses even more sophisticated dictionaries, and begins its reference process by assembling words from permutations of the 44 sounds that are used in English speech.

21.3 GENERAL PRACTICE RESEARCH

Although, in the past, most medical research has been hospital-based, general practice has the great advantage that its basic population is much more nearly representative of the national population than are the selected patients referred to hospital. The NHS general practice record is a 'cradle-to-grave' document, collecting reports from all orthodox medical agencies dealing with the patient. There is a record for every patient in the defined practice population. With this comprehensive database, the potential for research, using computer search techniques, is impressive. But the data must be 'accessible' – the terms sought must be free from ambiguity, synonym and mis-spelling. Validation of entry data by the computer with reference to inbuilt dictionaries of terms helps later computer searches. So does the use of summary records and the allocation of defined areas for allergies, immunizations, medication and pathology results. The arithmetical functions available on the computer may be associated with the search programs to produce and analyse research results, and these results may be further enhanced by the computer's ability to display them as tables, bar charts or graphs.

There have been three significant obstacles to the promotion of research in general practice:

- In contrast with their hospital colleagues, GPs do not have a requirement for research experience built into their career structure. Training in research technique does not therefore constitute part of a GP's education, and the time that needs to be spent on research projects has to be found from what little remains after service requirements have been met.
- The population base of many general practices is too small to allow the differences obtained in many types of survey to attain statistical significance. This difficulty can only be overcome by collating data from groups of practices where the size of the group is related to the expected difference between determinands.
- Underfunding.

In 1997, identifying the considerable potential for research in general practice, the Medical Research Council published recommendations to encourage:

- improved provision of research time and infrastructure
- more research into the ways in which people become patients, and into the interactions between practitioners and patients
- improved descriptive epidemiology of common symptoms, with assessment of how these affect the individual, the health service and society, taking into account quality of life and costs
- increased involvement of lay people in the design of GP research projects
- strengthening of the science base of primary disease prevention and health promotion
- greater emphasis on research into acute disorders.

In response, Department of Health funding of GP research has been increased and is destined to reach £50 million annually by the year 2002. The Scottish Office Research Practitioner Scheme is also offering improved funding levels.

Infrastructure

General practice systems already have adequate functionality to search individual practice clinical record, financial, and appointment files for the data required to support most types of GP research. However, other components of the research infrastructure still need further development:

- The NHSnet
- MIQUEST and other forms of data extraction software to enable information to be obtained from disparate GP systems

- Standardization of GP minimum data sets and file structures. Although Read codes have enabled conformity of term usage, general practice minimum data sets and file structures remain in urgent need of standardization, and these standards should be enshrined in the RFA. The need for this to be done is further strengthened by plans for the introduction of the electronic health record (EHR).
- The implementation of PCG+T office systems and realization of their potential for member practice data collation
- Expansion of the chain of research practices, already initiated by the RCGP, and their linkage by intranet – the Primary Care Research Network seeks to set up at least one cluster of practices per region
- The National Centre for Clinical Audit (NCCA). This body is tasked with reviewing guidelines on clinical intervention and with implementing national clinical audit investigations, some of which will be based in general practice. The NCCA would be well placed to collate data from any other national GP research schemes.

Links with community health, community mental health, and social services databases will serve to increase the range of data that can be interrogated on practice systems.

Networked research in general practice is not new. The commercial data collection agencies, the Public Health Network, and the RCGP Centre for Primary Care Research and Epidemiology have all proved viable and useful in this context, but eventual abandonment of anecdote-based practice in favour of evidence-based medicine requires a volume and quality of feedback from general practice that can only be obtained by building a strong national research infrastructure.

21.4 AUDIT

The controversial concept of medical audit began in the USA as an instrument of governmental control over doctors in the Medicare and Medicaid programmes, where the extra expense involved in auditing is met from government sources. Recertification of the doctor, which is due every 6 years, depends upon a performance review and has the effect of renewing the right to use a higher fee scale. In Canada, continuation of professional collegiate membership depends upon satisfactory 5-yearly reviews.

In the UK, no auditing initiative was taken in general practice during the first 30 years of the National Health Service. There followed a prolonged phase in which fears were widely voiced that the government would impose audit on the medical profession if the profession did not impose it on itself. This view was equally balanced by fears that, if the profession introduced audit, then the government would take over the process for its own purposes. Further equivocation was ended in 1990 by the introduction of practice annual reports and MAAGs.

Government grip on clinical standards was extended in 1999 by the creation of a cumbersome superstructure that imposed patient management guidelines, enforced their use by audit, made revalidation mandatory and beat a path to the GMC's door that any complainant could follow. The device that enabled the government to exert its now considerable influence on the point of care was, of course, the practice computer.

The adoption of American-style control procedures was probably inevitable. As Dr D. Lawrence wrote in 1998, our society is now more consumer orientated, it demands better services, is better informed, and better equipped to challenge professionals, to complain and receive compensation. A giant electronic audit trail is being created throughout the NHS from which there is no escape. If they get their hands on it, litigation lawyers trawling for new business could have a field day.

21.5 CLINICAL GOVERNANCE

The term 'clinical governance' was coined to describe the system of controls introduced in 1999, the components of which are illustrated in Figure 21.1.

Briefly, the National Centre for Clinical Audit researches guidelines for medical intervention, which are propagated by the National Institute for Clinical Excellence in a number of ways, among which the protocol database PRODIGY features prominently. (PRODIGY's computerized guidelines are evidence-based and suggest suitable interventions for all common clinical presentations – see Chapter 23.)

Individual practices are responsible for implementing the guidelines and for auditing their results in annual reports submitted to their PCG+T or HA. Individual doctors are responsible for their own revalidation.

All Trusts including PCTs are responsible to the Commission for Health Improvement, which commissions the production of league tables, and conducts periodic reviews of all trusts, providing further support where it identifies defective local clinical governance

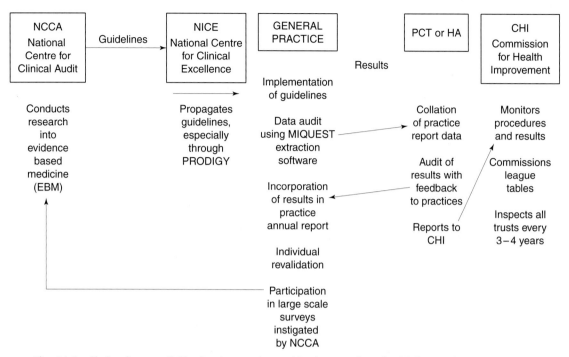

Fig. 21.1 Chain of responsibility for the creation and implementation of guidelines and audit of their use

schemes. The GMC can be involved as a result of action initiated at any point in the chain of control.

The principles of clinical governance were clearly laid down by the Department of Health in its publication *Clinical Governance: Quality in the New NHS*, issued in March 1999, incorporating a 5-year development plan. Key issues were a commitment to standards of quality, learning, research, clearly targeted resources, multidisciplinary team working, accountability to the NHS Trust board, cooperation with the public, planning, access to relevant information, and dealing with poor performance (DOH Health Circular HSC 1999/065).

A performance assessment framework document must be used by PCG+Ts to audit and report on the implementation of clinical governance. Performance indicators used will be responsive to NICE guidelines and will include cost-effective prescribing, generic pre-scribing rates, the incidence of conception before the age of 16, accident and suicide rates, emergency hospital admission rates for patients over 75, the volume of prescribed benzodiazepines, the standard of manage-ment of chronic diseases such as asthma, diabetes and epilepsy, and the standard of acute care for conditions such as ENT or urinary infection, and heart failure. Facility of patient access to primary care, standards of record-keeping, and immunization and screening rates

will also be taken into account. Bonus payments to practices for quality of service will be determined by some of these criteria used as benchmarks.

The thrust of policies on which clinical governance is attendant is largely determined by local Health Improvement Plans and National Service Frame-works (of which the first three have targeted cardio-vascular disease, mental health and elderly care).

General practices will themselves be invited to take part in large-scale audit of those intervention proce-dures for which they are responsible. Organization may be through research orientated subnetworks, as envisaged by the RCGP, or may be under the direc-tion of the National Centre for Clinical Audit.

21.6 AUDIT INITIATED BY THE PRACTICE

Externally imposed clinical governance is not, of course, the only form of audit with which practices will be concerned. For many years, those with an interest in research, or in monitoring their activities with a view to improving efficiency, have set up their own audit procedures.

There are nine main areas of investigation:

- The *structure of healthcare resources* – premises, equipment and staff

- *Procedural audit* (also known as audit of the process of care or practice workload) examines all those practice activities that are undertaken for patients. In most cases this is simply a question of logging each activity as it occurs, as will be done automatically where a full computer record system operates, and expressing results as actual totals or as rates (e.g. referrals per thousand patients or percentage uptake of child immunization). Procedural audit can also examine activities in terms of the time spent, the cost of the procedure, the income accruing from it, or the benefit to the patient, but for these enquiries additional types of data will need to be entered by the user. Activities studied may include administration, consultations, home visiting, referrals to hospital, immunization, screening, surveillance, or letters and reports.

There is no doubt that the results of some activity studies and the discipline involved in carrying them out have had beneficial effects on practice organization. Examples have been a reduction in the visiting rate, a reduction in the consultation rate, and an increased delegation of practice duties to nurses – all of which reduce the doctor's burden of work. Comparison of their own values with the average from other general practices may have a salutary effect upon individual doctors.

Because procedural audit is an accurate record of the practice workload, it constitutes information that governments need to acquire if they are to ensure value for money and fix a 'rate for the job'.

Experience in the USA shows that government-instigated procedural audit faces a dilemma. If it seeks to secure a minimum standard of care activity below which none fall, then it checks for, expects and thereby comes to impose fixed routines in care management geared to that minimum standard. By contrast, if it tries to impose a higher than average standard of care activity, health costs are forced upwards. In either event, value for money is undermined.

- Audit of the *outcome of care* is fraught with problems. If complete recovery or death occurs, might either outcome not have been the inevitable result of the patient's condition, regardless of all efforts of care? If only partial recovery takes place, is this an indictment upon the doctor, and if so how should the doctor's shortcomings be measured? Every case is different, and it would require a huge discrepancy in the outcome of any one form of illness to achieve statistical significance between two practices, given the number of patients involved.
- *Financial audit* compares income, expenses and profit with those for previous comparable time periods and with local and national averages. Results may be expressed as profit per partner, per nurse or per patient, and earnings per hour for different activities.
- *Prescribing audit* (see Chapter 11)
- *Audit of commissioning activities* (see Chapter 17). A variety of integral accounting procedures is used to monitor locality commissioning.

Fig. 21.2 Practice asthma audit: In-Practice Systems

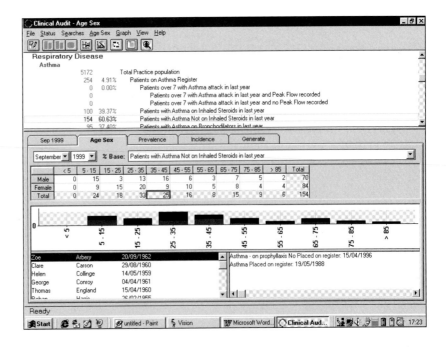

Fig. 21.3 Search and report: Global Clinical System's Audit Manager (Aremis Soft Healthcare)

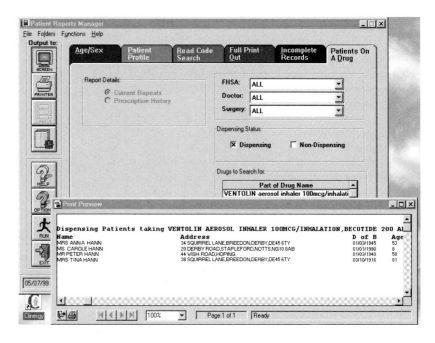

- *Teaching audit*. Three-yearly peer review of clinical and teaching performance is required for the reaccreditation of UK trainers in general practice.
- *Record-keeping audit*. Standards of manual record keeping can be assessed by checking for the presence of important components, structure and legibility on a sampling basis. Automated checks capable of testing all patient records can be run in computerized practices.
- *Appointment system audit* (see also Chapter 13). Appointment systems can be audited by a paper questionnaire given to the patient, by the use of the manual appointment book or by computerized appointment systems. Each method should log the time and date the appointment was requested, the time and date of the appointment, and the time and date that the patient is seen. A grade of perceived urgency should be recorded. If a hiatus occurs between consultations, this should also be noted. Latent intervals should be calculated for all grades of perceived urgency, and changes made in appointed interval and availability to meet standards acceptable to the practice.

Figure 21.4 shows the sequence of events for conducting an audit.

21.7 DEDICATED AUDIT SOFTWARE

MIQUEST data extraction software has already been described in Chapter 11.

Glasgow University and IT Technologies have developed a dedicated software package that can be used to interrogate some of the foremost GP clinical systems and present audited results in formats which are suitable for the clinical governance requirements of practices and PCG+Ts.

The software has been entitled NEMAS (Networked Medical Assessment Systems), is written in Visual Basic and is fully compatible with Windows

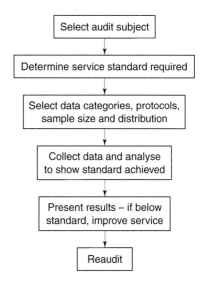

Fig. 21.4 The sequence of events for conducting an audit

95, 98 or NT. Microsoft Access is used for data analysis. Four principal areas of clinical audit are provided:

- Appointment systems
- Chronic disease – initially the diseases investigated have been:
  - Asthma
  - Diabetes
  - Hypertension
  - Epilepsy
  - Coronary heart disease
  - Rheumatoid arthritis
- Significant event analysis
- Pharmacotherapy monitoring – multiple parameters are comonitored and the results are presented as either tables, graphs or charts:
  - Digoxin
  - Lithium
  - Theophylline
  - Thyroxine
  - Vitamin B 12
  - Warfarin.

The package is supplied on CD-ROM and will bolt on the GPASS, In Practice Vision and EMIS systems. NEMAS meets the explicit official standards now required of performance monitoring.

21.8 POINT OF CARE TESTING AND PATIENT-HELD MONITORING DEVICES – INTRODUCTION

Point of care (POC) testing, as its name implies, is carried out by the doctor or nurse when the patient attends the medical centre. Patient-held monitoring (PHM) devices are characteristically used by the patient at home, although in some cases these may also be used in the POC context.

Many POC and PHM assay devices have now developed close relationships with the practice computer, exchanging signals through a cable or infrared connection. The computer may be used to schedule either PHM or POC machines, and in the latter case may entirely control it. Assay devices, especially those used for PHM, are increasingly able to store a series of time/date stamped readings and download these to the practice computer for re-presentation and analysis. As assay device design becomes increasingly refined, so the relationship with the practice computer is strengthened, and a variety of tasks that were formerly carried out by hospitals and pathology laboratories become part and parcel of primary care.

Table 21.1 lists POC tests currently reported as being used in UK general practice. Of the 31 procedures listed, 15 are now capable of integrating with a computer system and are therefore relevant to this book.

21.9 ELECTROCARDIOGRAPHY

Relatively inexpensive software, router and leads have been marketed under the trade names SmartHeart Pro (Harley Street Software of Canada), and the ILEX Interface (IIex Innovations, Philip Harris Medical). The computer (which may be a PC or laptop) polls the leads in turn, and records and prints the traces. Minimum requirements for SmartHeart Pro are a 386 processor running Windows 3.1, and for ILEX a 486 processor running Windows or DOS.

Standalone ECGs are marketed by many companies, and several models now store results which can be downloaded to the practice computer by software supplied with the machine. Depending upon the degree of sophistication of the software, the options for re-presentation are:

- the trace only
- quoted 12-lead measurements including intervals, durations and axis figures
- full interpretation, such as is provided by the Glasgow Interpretive option.

Appropriate adjustments may be provided for age, low or high sensitivity and pacemakers. An alphanumeric keyboard may be integral, which will allow annotation of the trace.

Standalone units are roughly twice as expensive as PC-driven ECGs.

The wave form of an ECG can be transmitted telephonically to a remote recorder/interpreter, and this has enabled GPs using domiciliary ECGs, or paramedics in ambulances or on oil-rigs, to request cardiological advice from hospitals. Responses may be through voice telephone or fax/printer.

In a miniaturized version, using the same principle, a PHM ECG recorder the size of a matchbox can be worn around the neck (NOVACOR R-Test Evolution, Cardiac Services UK), which records signals for up to 8 days. Stored readings can then be transmitted over the patient's telephone to a surgery or hospital ECG department, and this will enable the production of fully configurable reports on a PC and printer.

The Rhythm Card (Lifesign Record), which is roughly the size of a credit card, records a trace lasting 30 seconds on each of three occasions when the patient applies it to his/her chest. The patient then dials up the Lifesign Centre and holds the card to the handset microphone, whereupon the cardiology

Table 21.1 Point of care and patient–held assay devices currently reported as used in UK general practice

Haematology
Haemoglobinometer
Oximeter
Glycosal for glycated Hb

Cardiovascular
C Electrocardiogram
  Defibrillator
C Sphygmomanometer
C Echocardiogram
C Arterial ultrasound

Respiratory
C Spirometer
C Peak flow meter
  Carbon monoxide monitor

Biochemical
C Blood glucose meter
C Urine test multistrip reader
C Blood lipids
C Multichannel autoanalyser
C PT/INR

Auditory
  Audiometer and tympanometer

Ophthalmic
C Baby vision assessment with video camera and flash

Gynaecological and obstetric
  Ultrasound
  In-house hysteroscopy
  First void urine for DNA amplification (*Chlamydia*)

Urological
  Uroflow meter
  Automated peritoneal dialysis
C Ultrasound

Skeletal
  Ultrasound (*os calcis*)
  Osteosal

Digestive
  Helisal for *H. pylori*

Body fat
  Scales with low voltage electric current impedance

General
  C-reactive protein
C Telemedical monitoring of neonates and elderly at home
  Baby movement monitor (radio-linked)

C = potential for interaction with computer

technician downloads the recorded signal, analyses it and faxes a report to the patient's GP. The service is available throughout the UK. The Cardiac Alert organization uses a larger device and a service that operates using similar methods, except that it provides the patient with an interpreted result within minutes. Cardiac Alert offers 24-hour availability.

ECGs as components of defibrillators are not currently able to download to PCs.

21.10 SPHYGMOMANOMETRY

Automated sphygmomanometers, which can be used at the medical centre or by the patient at home, inflate the arm cuff, read pulse rate and systolic and diastolic pressures (usually by the oscillometric method), and record the result. The patient has only to apply the cuff in the first place and press the appropriate button on the machine. The Omron IC is battery-operated, takes up to 350 successive readings, each of which is time/date-stamped, displays each result on an LCD screen, and can

download all results to the doctor's PC at the patient's next surgery attendance. Results can then be analysed and stored within the patient's computer record. Omron provides database software that will store blood pressure records for multiple patients, and thus support the administration of a hypertension clinic.

Cardiacare markets a wrist-worn sphygmomanometer with memory and downloading facilities.

21.11 AMBULATORY BLOOD PRESSURE MEASUREMENTS

In 1992 the British Hypertension Society (BHS) urged caution in the use of ambulatory blood pressure (ABP) assays, pointing out that the method had not then been fully validated as a means of diagnosing and monitoring hypertension. The Society also found at that time that many of the marketed machines were of dubious quality. They observed, however, that there was a place for ABP assay in uncontrolled, and suspected 'white coat', hypertension.

One of the BHS validated models is the AMD TM 2421/2021, marketed by PMS Instruments Ltd. The assay unit is powered by rechargeable batteries, autoinflates the cuff periodically and records blood pressure by a combination of oscillometric and Korotkoff methods. To deliver its results it attaches to its own printer unit, which is also used to program the frequency of day- and night-time readings required. The patient has the option of instigating additional readings. Results can be uploaded to a PC via the serial port. A wide range of statistical routines with graphics is available, and results can be exported to a spreadsheet.

The Omron HEM-705CP has also proved accurate in BHS tests.

21.12 SPIROMETRY

British Thoracic Society guidelines on COPD management suggest that caution should be exercised in the purchase of a spirometer, particularly in the case of cheaper models. Many spirometers now possess electronic memory and display, an option to download to a PC, and spirometry support software. In combination with a PC, a spirometer should ideally provide:

- readings of one-second forced expiratory volume (FEV_1), forced vital capacity (FVC) and the ratio between the two
- a volume–time graph
- trend analysis on successive readings
- pre- and post-bronchodilator comparisons
- an adequate memory for storing multiple tests, categorized by patient
- automatic interpretation
- predictive values for age
- easy recalibration facilities.

Some spirometer software can be customized. The resolution, status and size of the computer display, and the status of the computer's printer, must be suitable for the package purchased.

Peak flow meters with downloads to computers are now available.

21.13 BLOOD GLUCOSE METERS

It is now common policy for many diabetic patients to use pocket-sized blood glucose meters. One drop of blood placed on a test strip or pad is subjected to a similar enzyme reaction as that used by urine test strips, and the degree of colour change produced in an indicator is read on reflectance from an integral light source. Results are time/date-stamped and stored in memory. Often there is an option to record symbolized data such as 'before' or 'after' food, insulin administration or exercise.

Engel et al (1998) surveyed six commonly used blood glucose meters marketed by the manufacturers Boehringer Mannheim, Medisense, Bayer, and National Diagnostic Products, and concluded that their level of accuracy was satisfactory. Most blood glucose meters now have the option to download data to a PC and to process results with dedicated software.

One software support package, Glucom TM for Windows (Paramount Software UK), allows patients to keep their own records on a home computer. There are two principal modes: diary mode allows users, page by page, to enter daily glucose and insulin levels, and events such as a hypoglycaemic attack. Graph mode displays results, either as two-dimensional or three-dimensional ribbon charts over time, or as pie charts. Navigation is by button bar and hypertext links.

Glucom TM for Windows can process data downloaded from several meters. One Touch II, Accutrend, Accutrend DM and Reflolux meters can transfer glucose readings to the package. Accutrend DM can also transfer insulin dosages, and One Touch II and Accutrend meters can transfer event data. Hardware requirement is a PC running Windows.

Blood glucose meter data can also be downloaded to a practice computer via cable, or from the patient's home to hospital through a telephone line and appropriate modem. The method is particularly useful in antenatal, 'brittle' or adolescent diabetics. The receptive computer has software which enables data to be presented in tabular or graphic format, and results can be overlaid so as to produce a typical 24-hour distribution (the 'modal day'), or a typical 7-day distribution (the 'modal week'). Results can be autofiled in a folder within the patient's computer record.

As the number of different parameters which a blood glucose meter can record increases, the device will replace the paper-based diabetic diary that most patients have kept in the past. If all health professionals dealing with the patient access the data that the meter holds, then the records of the GP, diabetologist, diabetic nurse and ophthalmologist will be synchronized, and shared care will be greatly facilitated. Ultimately, the device has the potential to be programmed with guidelines on disease management, which will include insulin dosage related to glucose levels, so that it becomes a diabetic 'personal organizer'.

21.14 BIOCHEMICAL ASSAY

Biochemical autoanalysers are now available for consulting room use in which reagents and samples interact to produce colour changes that can be assayed optically. Results are linked with the assay identity and serial number, and can be exported to a practice computer. Automatic filing of results depends upon the prestorage of the assay serial number in the patient's record. A serial port, and communications and data management software, will also be required.

The tests available on a machine such as the Abbot 'Vision' are listed in Box 21.1.

The tests most commonly used are blood glucose, haemoglobin and cholesterol. To the purchase cost of the equipment must be added the cost of reagents, quality control support (such as that provided by the Wolfson Research Laboratory), machine maintenance, training and labour.

Multichannel autoanalysers with data download to a PC are still too expensive an option for most practices, but enzyme technology is undergoing vigorous development. The recent introduction of the GDS Stat-Site Analyser, using a single drop of blood to assay haemoglobin, glucose, ketones, cholesterol and paracetamol levels within minutes, is an indication of what we must expect (Ivitech, tel: 0191 519 4700, Internet: http://ourworld.compuserve.com/homepages/ivitech/).

21.15 PROTHROMBIN TIME INR

Anticoagulant assay has increased fourfold in recent years, largely because of recognition of the need for its use in atrial fibrillation. The Thrombolytic Assessment System (TAS) from Diagnostic Testing Ltd provides a result from fingerprick blood in 2 minutes. With the use of computer assisted dosing software (such as the package C-Quel RAID, as recommended in British Society of Haematology guidelines), up to 1000 test results may be stored, with data categorized by patient, prothrombin time/International Normalized Ratio (PT-INR), reagent, lot number, date and time of test, and operator. Facilities are also available for checking potential drug interactions.

21.16 ULTRASOUND

Interfaces for most forms of ultrasound scanning are now available for computers, enabling still and video images to be shown on the computer's display, stored on hard disk or transmitted through telecommunication channels. Data thus shared at the time when they are generated enable GPs to have instant discussions with their consultant colleagues with regard to relevant obstetric, gynaecological, renal and prostatic disorders.

21.17 BIOIMPEDANCE ELECTRONIC BODY COMPOSITION MONITORING

It is now possible to assess the relative and absolute amounts of lean and fat tissue in the human body using the principle of electronic bioimpedance.

The TBF-305 is a set of scales with electrodes that make contact with the feet. Body fat is calculated and results can be downloaded to the serial port of a computer.

The Bodystat® 1500 uses two electrodes on the right hand and two on the right foot to pass a current whose impedance value, coupled with age, gender, height and weight, can be used to calculate body fat, lean mass, water level and metabolic rate. Readout is given on a two-line LCD and there is a Windows-compliant software option to enable downloaded data to provide for patient education, trend analysis, weight and activity management, and cardiac risk analysis.

Box 21.1

Albumin
Alkaline phosphatase
Amylase
Calcium
Cholesterol
Creatinine
Glucose
Haemoglobin
HbA_{1c}
HDL
LDL
Potassium
Phenytoin
Prothrombin
SGOT
SGPT
Theophylline
Thyroxine
Total protein
Total bilirubin
Triglycerides
Urea nitrogen
Uric acid

21.18 DISPENSING PRACTICE SYSTEMS – INTRODUCTION

In the days when pharmacists had to count out by hand all the tablets they dispensed, I patented and pilot tested a machine that performed the task automatically, read a bar code on the stock bottle to identify the drug, and was linked to a computer that memorized stock levels and printed out reorder lists. I little realized that, within a few years, the introduction of blister packs would bring an end to direct handling methods and that, instead, pharmacy computing would begin with container label printing. In time, drug identity and quantity data may yet come to be read from packs at the dispensing point, just as merchandise is logged out at the point of sale in supermarkets, or may even be taken directly from an electronic form of prescription that has been fed down line to the pharmacy. Until then, these data must be input from a keyboard, as items either included on the container label in pharmacies or on the prescription in dispensing practices.

Although their continued existence has been under threat, approximately one in 10 practices dispenses, and these practices require both a general practice patient management system and a pharmacy system. The two computer systems must be integrated so as to be able to communicate with each other and share dictionaries, files and data. Because dispensing practices are in a minority, the major GP system suppliers prioritized development in other practice areas during the early years of marketing, leaving pharmacy software houses to fill the vacuum and graft practice patient management facilities on to their dispensing packages. The situation is now changing, and many leading GP suppliers are offering dispensing practice options.

When assessing the suitability of computer systems or drug databases for dispensing practice, it is essential to remember that prescribing and dispensing are discrete and separate processes, despite the fact that they may take place under the same roof. In conventional prescribing, the only link between the two processes is a small piece of paper, with the minimal data it bears. The creation of an electronic prescribing–dispensing axis provides the opportunity to transfer other types of information between prescriber and dispenser. It also provides the opportunity to furnish outside agencies with data to which they are properly entitled (in an immediately processable form).

It is also essential to recognize that, in non-dispensing practice, drug usage data taken from the act of prescribing will be approximately 15% greater in volume than data obtained from prescription redemption at the pharmacy. (Some patients find cheaper alternatives to the prescription charge, others recover before the prescription can be dispensed, or disagree with the prescriber's choice.) This discrepancy necessarily distorts any comparison between prescriptions written and PACT or Indicative Prescribing Scheme statistics. Practices with partial responsibility for dispensing will experience a proportionately smaller discrepancy. Only in a practice, all of whose patients have dispensing status, will prescribing and dispensing data equate.

21.19 REQUIREMENTS OF A DISPENSING PRACTICE SYSTEM

A multiuser or networked system with prescribing and dispensing terminals is needed, which has access to a drug dictionary and which maintains clinical, prescribing and dispensing records. This complex configuration will be compounded if, as may be the case, the practice uses portable terminals for split-site consulting.

The requirements for prescribing are the same as for non-dispensing practices and have been described in Chapter 11. The requirements for dispensing are similar to those for pharmacies except that:

- there are usually no purely cash ('over-the-counter') sales
- small practices in which doctors do their own dispensing often prefer to continue using manual stock control and reorder methods.

Table 21.2 summarizes the prescribing, dispensing and communication requirements of dispensing practice systems.

21.20 DISPENSING SUPPORT

Label printing

Labels are printed automatically by the system for attachment both to the container and to the paper bag into which all containers relating to a prescription are placed to await collection by the patient.

The container label should show: the patient's surname, forename and other initials, and title; the drug name, formulation, strength, dosage and supply; added administrative instructions; date dispensed; partnership name, address and telephone number; and the warning 'Keep out of childrens' reach'.

Table 21.2 Requirements of an integrated prescribing–dispensing system

Prescribing	Dispensing	Communications between prescriber and dispenser
Full drug database with visual look-up and electronic interrogation	Full drug database with label print, prescription endorsement and stock control data	Warn prescriber of impending drug expiry, offer prescriber alternatives to out-of-stock items
Full and summarized medication record with repeat medication subset and link between drug and diagnosis	Container and bag label print	Enter drug batch number and maker on patient record
Prescription writing software that interrogates patient record and drug database during script construction	Script endorsements, reminders 'to pay', etc.	Dispenser can check patient's dispensing and fee payment status on patient record
Streamlined data entry routines to assemble drug statement on script	Stock control and reorder	Fully electronic prescribing requires validation and transmission to dispensary of prescriber's signature by system
Automated checks on suitability of drug for individual patient	New stock check-in; 'owing' item routine	
Automated entry of patient, doctor and HA identity data and date	Shelf stock-take and reconciliation with computer	
Automated drug status warnings – CD, ACBS, etc.	Checks on PPA operations, monthly turnover – costs, script and item totals, prescription charge counts, resolution of PPA script queries	
FP 10 counterfoil printout of patient instructions, etc.	Total stock valuation, yield on capital	
ADR reporting	Pay wholesalers, keep accounts	
	Running comparison with indicative prescribing amount	

Table 21.3 Types of data provided by principal drug databases

Types of data	PPA	Chemist and Druggist	Drug and Therapeutics Bulletin	Read codes	Data Sheet Compendium	e-MIMS	EBNF	Multilex
For dispensing stock control	+	+	+	+				+
For textual reference in prescribing					+	+	+	+
For interactive electronic reference in prescribing								+

The bag label should show the patient's full name as above, the patient's address, the date dispensed and the patient's prescription payment status. It should also carry the warning 'Keep out of childrens' reach'. The proposed introduction of prescription serial numbers for practices will imply that this number also appears on the bag label.

Prescription endorsements

The pharmacist is required to make a number of endorsements on the prescription when dispensing, namely, pack size, broken bulk, zero discount, extemporaneously or aseptically dispensed, measured and fitted, controlled drug, urgent prescription details, generic manufacturer or wholesaler, and number of dispensed items. While some systems provide for endorsements to be made through the computer, there is a legal obligation on the doctor to sign a prescription at the time of issue, which involves printing-out in the consulting room. Overprinting of the prescription at a second print run in the pharmacy hardly seems worth while but, when electronic prescriptions are batched to the PPA, computerized endorsement will be required, at which time the signed paper original will presumably be retained unendorsed as a security copy, or abolished altogether (reliance being placed on the prescriber's password). An alternative approach will be to use an electronic pen and pad with signature recognition. Some endorsements attract additional reimbursement, and dispensing software now includes reminders that promote maximization of income. This principle is even more important in independent pharmacies, where the chemist can be prompted to suggest additional over-the-counter lines.

Stock control

Although stock control policies vary considerably between different dispensing practices (as they do between different pharmacies), the guiding principles followed are that the minimum amount of stock should be held that is compatible with the provision of a reasonable level of service to the patient, and that stock should never be held past its expiry date. If too much stock is held, then the capital 'locked up' loses interest, but if too little is held, then some prescriptions cannot be redeemed. The terms 'minimum stock' and 'reasonable level of service' are very much open to interpretation.

In dispensing practices up to 1000, and in pharmacies up to 3000, lines of stock may be held – a large capital investment that deserves careful servicing. Of these lines, only a small proportion will be stock with a fast turnover; the remainder is of intermediate or very slow turnover, and the stock control requirements of the three types differ.

Fast-turnover drugs have to be reordered so frequently that their expiry date never poses a problem, and their reorder pack size and quantity can be determined by scrutiny of the rate, and change in rate, at which they are dispensed. If demand is increasing, then a computer system can automatically suggest a larger pack, with corresponding economy in unit cost. A fall in demand has the reverse effect.

Intermediate-turnover drugs pose some threat of expiry on the shelf, and a restrictive holding policy is imperative. Practice policy may decree that only the equivalent of a few days' treatment, or enough drugs to redeem one or one and a half average prescriptions will be stocked, and that, when necessary, the patient will be asked to return for the balance. For intermediate-turnover drugs it is essential that expiry dates, as well as pack size and quantity, are noted on the computer system when checking in new stock. Here the computer system must not only control stock levels but also warn when the expiry date of a line is imminent.

Very-slow-turnover drugs should not be stocked unless they are necessary for life-saving emergency care, because the risk of expiry is such that they constitute a loss of profit. These drugs should preferably be ordered as necessary from the wholesaler.

Manual methods of stock reorder

Manual methods of reordering start and finish with a fixed pattern of stock-holding, which is only varied if the pharmacist realizes that trend in demand is changing. With manual methods a significant amount of stock expires on the shelf, and reorder pack sizes are often inappropriate. The holding of very-slow-turnover drugs is usually too high.

A well tried manual method of reordering is the 'two card' system. In this system, each drug line possesses paired cards fixed into a slot on the front edge of the shelf in relation to the drug. Both cards bear the drug name, formulation, strength and pack size. The foremost card is coloured and the rear card white. As the stock line becomes depleted, the dispenser removes the front card to a box in readiness for reordering and, when appropriate, uses all cards waiting in the reorder box as the source of the order to the wholesaler. When supplies arrive, they are checked back on to the shelf with the coloured card. In its absence, the coloured card has left the white card in position as evidence of the depleted line, and of the fact that reordering is taking place. As a semiautomatic refinement of the two card system, the reorder cards bear identifying perforations and can be inspected sequentially from a carousel by a card-reading machine, which transmits electronic data through a modem and telephone line to the wholesaler (Siemmens).

Computer methods of stock reorder

The computer holds in memory an exact replica of shelf stock, which includes drug name, formulation and strength, pack size, quantity, maker's name, batch number, expiry date and source wholesaler for each item. Strict discipline must be maintained by pharmacy staff to ensure that drugs with shortest expiry dates are the first to be dispensed, and that restocks are placed behind existing stock held. All dispensing transactions result in simultaneous reductions in actual and memorized stock levels. The computer may even be programmed to prompt for the batch numbers and pack size that the dispenser should take from the shelf.

All consulting room prescriptions are written through the computer. Those written manually, for whatever reason, are copied into the main system at the next consultation session. Time and date should be noted for prescriptions dispensed out of hours, as these will attract a special fee.

The computer produces lists for drug turnover, taking each product's mean shelf life into account, and establishes those lines that are fast, intermediate and very slow moving. The computer will automate reordering of fast-moving lines, determining reorder quantity, pack size and basic holding levels. Holding policy for intermediate lines must be dictated by practice policy, and minimum levels are then set and input by practice staff, using a menu-driven software program. Smallest pack sizes are usually appropriate. The practice must also determine its policy for very-slow-moving lines, which will take local conditions and wholesaler response times into account.

Working from the above criteria, the computer compiles lists of reorder drugs automatically. To these the practice staff add new requirements taken from a 'picking list' on the computer. The order is then transmitted by computer through modem and telephone line to the wholesaler. Where more than one wholesaler is involved, the source wholesaler's code, included with the drug line data on computer, will be used to determine the source of each item, and separate lists will be prepared.

Checking in new stock

Stock replenishments from the wholesaler should first be checked against the computer's reorder list and the wholesaler's delivery list. Discrepancies will result in return and reorder. For all replenishments, not only the drug's identity but also the manufacturer's name, pack size, batch number, expiry date and price must be noted, and these data reconciled with, or added to, those in the computer reorder list as appropriate. Most systems allow sequential presentation of each reordered item on screen for checking in.

New stock should be placed behind existing stock on shelves to minimize the risk of expiry dates being overtaken. Total costs per delivery can be computed for comparison with the wholesaler's bill.

All dispensary systems have routines for dealing with incompletely redeemed prescriptions (sometimes termed 'owings'). These routines log deficits for items for which there is initially insufficient stock. After restocking, the computer then lists all deficits that can now be redeemed, and allows the dispenser to

Fig. 21.5 Dispensing screen: Global Clinical System's Dispensing Manager, incorporating stock control (Aremis Soft Healthcare)

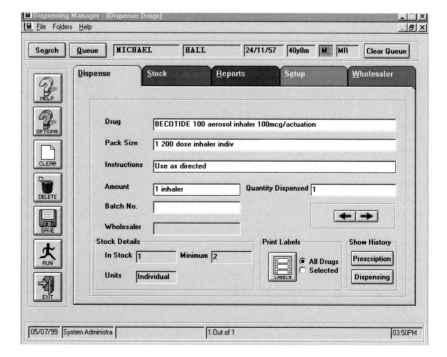

process each item in turn in the usual way, while resupplying label details retained from the initial print-run. The system must also list those items that are still outstanding because restocking has failed.

Shelf counts

In supermarkets computers control stock either by a tally of outgoing goods at the cash point or by periodic counts of goods left on the shelves. In each case the depletions from stock are the basis for reordering, but the two types of count give different answers. The difference is due to shrinkage (a euphemism for shoplifting), which depletes the shelves more rapidly than sales checkouts would suggest.

In a dispensing general practice, the tendency is for shelf stock to be inflated from several sources other than reordering – notably by drug company representatives, who often leave a liberal supply of samples on their visits to the practice. A discrepancy between stock issued and stock reordered still occurs, though in a reverse direction to that caused by shrinkage.

A periodic shelf count is therefore required, assisted by a computer printout of the electronic stock replica held on the system. Shelf holdings that do not correspond with the computer's replica are noted on the printout, and all amendments are entered into the system. Where deficits in shelf holding are revealed, their cause should be enquired into – some at least will be due to out-of-hours dispensing for which the prescription has not been issued on the system, and these costs can be recouped with the help of a computer prompt, which also issues a reminder that a night visit fee may be justified.

All dispensing stock control systems allow total stock valuation on demand, and it would require little extra effort to incorporate profit in a calculation of yield on capital.

21.21 DISPENSING PRACTICE INTERNAL COMMUNICATIONS

Communications between the consulting room and dispensary through the practice system offer advantages that are not available in non-dispensing practices.

- Prescribers can be warned of any stock that is due to expire after a further 6 weeks so that, where appropriate, these items may be preferentially prescribed.
- When prescribers attempt to prescribe an item which is out of stock, they can be warned by a program that also offers them possible alternatives.

- The drug batch number and maker's name should be transmitted from the dispensary database to the patient record to be stored there in accordance with EU directives on product liability.
- The dispenser can verify a patient's date of birth for the purpose of assessing prescription charge liability.
- The dispenser can verify from the patient record that a patient still holds dispensing status.

21.22 DISPENSING PRACTICE AND PRESCRIPTION PRICING AUTHORITY OPERATIONS

The powerful computer systems that the Prescription Pricing Authority (PPA) has installed to operate its Prescribing Analyses and Cost (PACT) and Indicative Prescribing Scheme (IPS) projects require keyboard input of data taken from handwritten or printed prescriptions. This wasteful transcription process will be terminated when all dispensing data are transmitted electronically to the authority. Payments to dispensing contractors are already made electronically by HAs.

It is important for the dispensing practice system to be able to provide reports that will support practice scrutiny of PPA operations.

- At the end of each month, total dispensing costs, numbers of prescriptions, numbers of items, and numbers of patient prescription charges should be provided.
- Each month, a cumulative tally of total prescribing costs should be compared with amounts that the PCG+T allocated indicative prescribing budget would permit per unit of time. The result should be expressed as a percentage, using 100 as the yardstick provided by the Indicative Prescribing Amount.
- PPA queries on disputed prescriptions should be resolved through electronic mail.

It would not appear to be useful at present to replicate PACT data by interrogating costs within therapeutic categories. Audit of cure and adverse response to drug treatment are dealt with in Chapter 11.

21.23 OTHER FORMS OF COMPUTER SUPPORT FOR DISPENSING PRACTICES

Just as it is helpful for the practice system to provide warnings of potential errors during the prescribing process, so the dispenser may be assisted by automated reminders. A notice 'to pay' printed on the bag label, a reminder to charge two prescription fees for combination packs, a reminder to instruct the patient to return for the balance of drugs on a partially redeemed prescription, and reminders to complete prescription endorsements should all be built into the system.

The system should print patient warnings automatically (e.g. 'Keep out of reach of children' or 'For external use only').

21.24   DRUG DATABASE REQUIREMENTS FOR DISPENSING PRACTICES

Dispensing practice computerization is heavily dependent on an adequate drug database. This must incorporate all those features needed for prescribing support (see Chapter 11) and dispensing stock control and reorder as used in pharmacy systems. The following components will therefore be necessary:

- Drug 'line' data – name, qualifying terms associated with the name, formulation, strength
- Normal dosage schedules
- Pack sizes
- Mandatory administrative instructions – the warnings as classified in the BNF for inclusion on labels (and preferably also on prescriptions)
- Prices
- An interactions matrix and relationally stored data to support automated checks on idiosyncrasies, dose for age, two prescribed drugs with the same action, contraindications and indications
- Drug status warning data – controlled drugs, ACBS drugs, prescription only medicines, withdrawn drugs, special reporting to CSM requirement, drugs not prescribable under the NHS, drugs cheaper than the prescription fee
- Textual display of the 20 drug attributes of importance to prescribers (similar to the information provided in the Data Sheet Compendium but in a synoptic and structured format)
- Electronically structured side-effect data
- Textual and electronically structured data on prescribing in pregnancy, lactation, liver and renal failure, the old and very young
- Other product-related dispensing data, such as multiple packs.

These data are available from, and are already provided to, most GP systems within the Multilex suite of drug databases. Martindale-on-line is a database providing for textual reference in dispensing.

SUMMARY

- The computer can search text for symbols, words or statements very rapidly and can replicate targeted data, or list or count those records in which targeted data occur. Multiple attributes may be searched for simultaneously. For later identification, data must have been entered in a form that makes them unique, and this is usually achieved by dictionary validation.
- UK general practices possess comprehensive health data about all patients in a defined population, and are therefore ideally placed to undertake research. Individual practice research is supported by the arithmetical functions and 'chart' graphics output of the practice computer. Some studies such as postmarketing surveillance and national epidemiology require collation of data on larger numbers of patients from multiple practices, and these call for the adoption of standardized terminology, minimum data sets, file structures, and recording techniques between practices. Data extraction software suitable for use in disparate GP systems must be used. Collation of data by PCG+T/HAs, by the chain of RCGP research practices and by the NCCA is required.
- Audit may be applied to practice structure, practice procedures, outcome of care, practice finances, prescribing, locality commissioning procedures, teaching, record-keeping and practice appointments. LANs and WANs enable professional performance to be monitored centrally by a system of clinical governance. Patient management procedures imposed by computer-based and other protocols must now be instituted by practices, and compliance with these policies will be monitored through PCG+T/HAs, who are accountable to the Commission for Health Improvement. Revalidation, performance-related bonuses, or castigation by the GMC are possible sequelae.
- Increasingly, point-of-care-testing and patient-held monitoring devices are interdependent with the practice computer – they may be scheduled by it, and may download time/date-stamped results to it for redisplay and analysis. Electrocardiographs, automated sphygmomanometers, spirometers, blood glucose meters, office-based biochemical autoanalysers, prothrombin time INR assay systems, and ultrasound scanning all now dovetail with PC-based software to provide enhanced functionality.
- Fewer than one in 10 practices dispenses, and dispensing practices (DPs) require a combination of

general practice and pharmacy computer systems that intercommunicate and share a drug database. Only in fully dispensing practices do prescribing and dispensing costs equate.

- Prescribing support requirements in a DP are the same as for other practices and include accurate, legible drug schedule specification, the automatic addition of patient and prescriber details with date, cross-checks on drug suitability and legal category, the use of a suitably formatted medication record, cost monitoring and adverse drug reaction reporting.

- Dispensing support can be provided for virtually all pharmacy activities – label print, script endorsement, stock control and reorder, new stock check-in and shelf counts, checks on PPA payments, payments to creditors, and accounts. The system can draw the dispenser's attention to such matters as the patient's fee payment status or multiple pack products.

- Communications between the prescribing and dispensing areas of a DP may be used to enable the prescriber to avoid drug expiry, to use stocked alternatives to an out-of-stock item, and to store batch numbers and maker's name on patient records.

- The need for a multifaceted and frequently updated drug database to support prescribing and dispensing is paramount, and only the Multilex group of databases currently approximates to GP requirements.

REFERENCES AND FURTHER READING

Research

Department of Health 1997 Research and development in primary care (National Working Group report). HMSO, London

Eimerl T S, Laidlow A T 1969 A handbook for research in general practice, 2nd edn. E & S Livingstone, Edinburgh

Fry J, Lindegard B 1980 Strategies for health service research. Update 15 October: 933

Greenhalgh T 1998 Meta-analysis and beyond: applying secondary research methods to primary care. British Journal of General Practice, August: 1540–1541

Hill A B 1966 Principles of medical statistics, 8th edn. The Lancet, London

Howie J G R 1980 Research in general practice. Croom Helm, London

Medical Research Council 1997 Primary healthcare (topic review). MRC, London

Swinscow T D V 1980 Statistics at square one, 8th edn. British Medical Association, London

Audit

Donabedian A 1966 Millbank MEM Fund Quarterly 44(3, part 2): 166

Fleming D M et al 1982 Workload review. Birmingham Research Unit, Royal College of General Practitioners. Journal of the Royal College of General Practitioners 32: 292

Fry J 1981 What can be done. Update 15 April: 1344

Gillings D B, Preece J F 1971 An analysis of the size and content of medical records used during an on-line record maintenance and retrieval system in general practice. International Journal of Biomedical Computing 2: 151

Hartropp P 1987 Audit of epilepsy management in a group practice. Update 1 February: 299

Lough M 1998 Audit program sets out to raise quality. Doctor 8 October: 56–58

Lawrence D 1998 Take first steps now. Medical Interface, November: 6

McColl A, Roderick P, Gabbay J et al 1998 Performance Indicators for Primary Care Groups: an evidence based approach. British Medical Journal 317: 1354–1360

Martin P B, Kerrigan P J C, Moulds A J, Millins 1982 Workload in practice. Update 1 July: 25

Royal College of General Practitioners 1985 What sort of doctor? Report from General Practice 23. RCGP Exeter

Secretary of State for Health 1998 A firstclass service: Quality in the new NHS. Stationery Office, London

Sheldon M G 1982 Medical audit in general practice. Occasional paper 20. Royal College of General Practitioners, London

Point of care testing and patient-held monitors

Bargery A 1995 How a GP's laptop reads ECGs. GP, July: 34

British Hypertension Society 1992 Caution urged over GP use of ambulatory BP monitors. Pulse 10 October: 20

Brueren M M, Schouten H J A, Leeuw P W D et al 1998 A series of self measurements by the patient is a reliable alternative to ambulatory blood pressure measurement. British Journal of General Practice 48: 1585–1589

Chambers J A, Marshall A J 1991 Cellphone ECG transmission. Cardiology in Practice, July/August: 19

Engel L, Delaney C, Cohen M 1998 Blood glucose meters: an independent head to head comparison. Practical Diabetes International 15(1): 15–18

Hilton S 1990 Near patient testing in general practice: a review. British Journal of General Practice 40: 32

Hobbs F D R, Broughton P M G, Kenkre J E et al 1992 Comparison of the use of four desktop analysers in six urban general practices. British Journal of General Practice, August: 317

Holwell D 1997 In-house ultrasound puts doctors at the helm. Doctor 10 April: 82–83

Lefever R 1984 Diagnostic facilities in general practice. The RCGP Members Reference Book. Sterling Publications, London

Murray E T, Fitzmaurice D A 1998 An evaluation of quality control activity for near patient testing in primary care. British Journal of General Practice 48: 1853–1854

Neville R G 1988 Introduction to new diagnostic aids in general practice. Update, May: 2311

Nickalls R W D, Ramasubram R 1996 Interfacing the IBM PC to medical equipment. The art of general communication. Cambridge University Press, Cambridge

Dispensing practice

Hammond V 1973 Pharmacy stock control. Pharmaceutical Journal 17 February: 140

Herd A 1990 Country matters. How does rural practice compute? Practice Computing, November: 7

Lewis J 1982 How to dispense from your surgery. General Practitioner 14 May: 53

Preece J F, Hunt N A, Skinner N J 1975 An integrated data system for the retail pharmaceutical service. International Journal of Biomedical Computing 6: 41

Preece J F, Ashford J R, Dunn L B, Pratt K A 1976 Stock control in retail pharmacy by bar code reader, tablet counter, and remote computer. Pharmaceutical Journal 21 September: 206

Preece J F 1992 A survey of dispensing practice software. Practice Computing, November: 13

22 Some specialized applications

22.1 PRACTICE BROCHURES

The 1990 contract has made it obligatory for practices to produce brochures (also known as practice leaflets) describing their services. Some health authorities have held local competitions to encourage good brochure design, with prizes being awarded to those considered to be straightforward, informative, easily readable and understandable, attractive, friendly and welcoming.

The classes of information usually included in practice brochures are:

- A list of staff, positions held and duties undertaken
- Surgery address, telephone numbers and opening hours
- A brief exposition of practice policy and ambit
- Surgery hours for each doctor, arrangements for appointments
- Emergency, out-of-hours and telephone consultations
- Home visiting arrangements
- Repeat prescriptions and special certificates
- Dispensing arrangements
- Dedicated clinics – antenatal and postnatal, family planning, child development, diabetes, asthma, stress, heart disease, health promotion, immunizations, cervical smears, over-74 checks
- Blood tests and other nursing services
- Minor surgery
- Private consultations
- Arrangements at the local A&E department
- Transport facilities
- Facilities for the disabled
- Patient participation groups, arrangements made for the practice to receive patient comment or complaint, and provisions made for the requirements of the Data Protection Act.

Production

Unless the GP system specifically provides for it, this is an application best undertaken on a freestanding PC using off-the-shelf software packages such as Microsoft Office or Lotus SmartSuite.

The four possible methods of producing practice brochures are summarized in Figure 22.1. The four types of output achieved are:

- text only
- text with simple monochrome line images
- text with colour images
- text with photographs.

Many practices have sought to make their brochures more interesting by incorporating images and, of these, the majority have opted for text with monochrome line images (as in Fig. 22.2).

It is clear from Figure 22.1 that greater degrees of sophistication in image production than this are more demanding of hardware and software. However, colour monitors must now be regarded as standard, colour printers lie well within most budgets, and the ability to import clip art, or create designs with the drawing and painting aids incorporated in bundled packages such Microsoft Office, all mean that considerable versatility in the production of images is now available to most home computer users. Digital camera images can also be downloaded for incorporation within art work (see below).

It is common for practices to create their own design but commission its replication from a local printhouse. Companies such as Neighbourhood Direct will of course produce a customized pattern, incorporate advertisements and provide brochures at a profit to the practice.

22.2 DIGITAL CAMERAS

Overview

Still digital cameras record an image as a digital electronic message, in place of the chemically reactive emulsion of a conventional film. A sequence of images is stored by the camera, which are later downloaded in a number of alternative ways to allow prompt

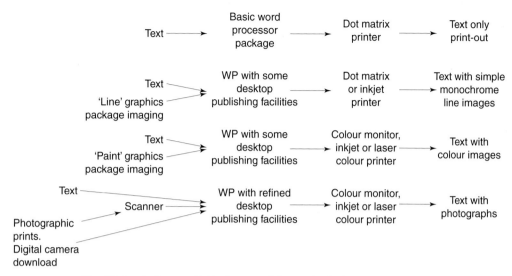

Fig. 22.1 Options available for assembling and printing practice brochures

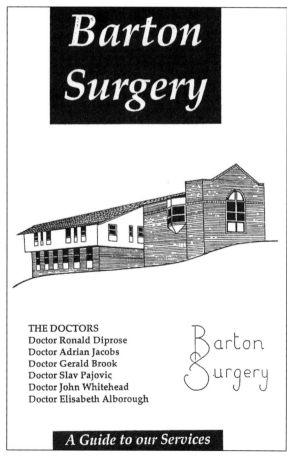

Fig. 22.2 An example of assembly of text and images for a practice brochure (courtesy Dr A Jacobs)

processing without the need for a photographic development agency. Digital photographs have a lower grade of picture quality than their film counterparts, but their method of processing and the way in which they can be presented are much more versatile. In general practice, images of morbidity recorded at consultation may be stored in relation to the patient's computer record, and may be transmitted in company with an e-mail letter to the consultant. Serial photographs allow progress to be monitored. At 10 cm distance the Olympus 840L camera takes a 12×8 cm image which corresponds to actual size.

Text may be superimposed on e-images for the purpose of creating practice brochures or practice websites. Images may also be displayed on television screens, or used in Powerpoint presentations.

Main features of digital cameras

Images may be downloaded directly from the camera to a digital printer, or to a computer that uses any type of colour printer. Although printing on photographic paper gives best results, this is expensive, and copier-grade A4 will suffice for most purposes. Downloading to a computer also allows the image to be modified by computer program (usually supplied with the camera) as regards subject matter, colour or contrast.

Features vary between brands of camera:

• Storage may be either resident in the camera, or else removable and provided either on floppy disks (which are extremely cheap), or on special memory cards, which are considerably more expensive. All forms of storage are reusable.

- The number of images that can be stored in a batch varies between cameras and with the type of image. High-resolution images are storage-hungry and may limit a batch run to six exposures. At the other end of the scale, up to 96 images may be accommodated in sequence before camera storage is full, at which point the memory card or floppy must be changed, or internally resident storage downloaded.
- Downloading to computer is by direct transfer from floppy disk, or by cable supplied with the camera for connection to the computer's serial port. Camera purchase usually includes the necessary software to drive computer downloads. Transfer takes several minutes, although the process can be accelerated by specially purchased readers and adapters, if these are marketed in relation to the camera model.
- Some cameras have a small LCD screen to show the user what is in focus, some can vary resolution, and some can compress the image to economize storage space by sacrificing some degree of resolution.
- Other variations between camera brands are similar to those that exist between brands of conventional still cameras, such as lens quality or built-in flash.

Computer requirements

The software packages used for making modifications to photographs on screen need at least 16 Mb hard-disk space. The production of a good quality image on a computer colour monitor will require 2 Mb of video RAM (V-RAM).

Digital cameras cannot be used to take VDU screen shots, as the scan rates of the two types of equipment are not synchronized.

Allied technology

Printed photographs can be scanned-in to computers for storage, transmission or modification. Storage may be on computer hard disk, floppy or CD. Photographic agencies now offer conversion of exposed conventional film to diskette or CD storage as an alternative to slides or photographic print production.

Video cameras are used for image transmission in telemedicine.

22.3 PATIENT INFORMATION LEAFLETS

Operational surveys have demonstrated that patients retain, on average, a mere 40% of the verbal data provided to them at consultation. Practices that have adopted the policy of issuing leaflets to patients on the nature and management of their condition not only obtain better compliance, but may avoid the unnecessary issue of a prescription.

Patient leaflets can now be downloaded from Internet sites such as Medical Legal Software (which follows Health on the Net Foundation guidelines), http://www.medical-legal.co.uk/patient-info, from the protocol packages SOPHIE, PRODIGY and ISIS, or from the MediDesk and Doctor's Desk modules (q.v.) and very many other sources.

PILs

In the early 1990s, GPs Tim and Beverley Kenny set up an electronic library of 200 patient leaflets coupled with a directory of 250 self-help groups under the title PILs (for patient information leaflets). The text-based version of this database was provided as a free upgrade to all EMIS users. PILs was tested successfully in 70 pilot practices, and is now offered as a GUI-based add-on package that can be used by any Windows-compliant GP system. GUI PILs incorporates anatomical diagrams.

PILs is accessible by the Read-coded term to which its data applies. It will interlink with the DERMIS and MENTOR packages, which also originated in association with the EMIS system and which, like PILs, are available to other Windows users. The PILs database provides the doctor with the necessary material to demonstrate on screen, and print out after consultation, advice to patients on the nature and management of their condition. The text of each leaflet is non-controversial, easily understood by the lay public, and has no bias with regard to prescribing. Most areas of general practice are covered, and each leaflet can be accommodated on one, two or, rarely, three sides of A4. The textual advice cannot be changed, but there is space at the top and bottom of the page to allow the doctor to print the patient and practice names and any extra comments. The titles within the database may be accessed from an alphabetical list, from sublists structured under each specialty, or through a keyword search using the first four letters of a subject name or synonym.

Installation is by diskette and a manual is provided (Patient Information Publications, 50 The Grove, Gosforth, Newcastle upon Tyne NE3 1NJ).

Fig. 22.3 Patient information leaflets – EMIS's PILs

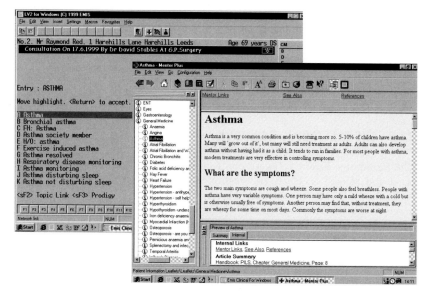

22.4 MINOR SURGERY

Two interesting programs have been launched that assist GPs in the management of minor operations, and Dr R L Kneebone has been closely associated with the development of both.

MINOPS

A description of the MINOPS program was published in 1994 by Kneebone and Tilson. The package provided full support for the management of minor surgery clinics.

- Paper forms and their equivalent electronic proformas were completed in parallel so that the patient's informed written consent could be obtained, paper-based histology report data could be keyed in, and system-based reports could be printed out. At the same time, all data were also retained on the computer database.
- A patient minor operations database and a computer dictionary of diagnoses linked to the terms used by the local histology department were maintained on the practice computer. Read coding was planned for use with the terms.
- Patient and procedural records were maintained using medicolegal standards.
- The system administered the patient's progress through the required steps of initial consultation, operation appointment, operation, histological report, complications (if any) and subsequent referral (if any).
- Waiting lists ordered by priority, and operating lists were created.

- Automatic monitoring of histology reports ensured that any necessary follow-up was not overlooked.
- Reports could be created to support claims to the HA for minor operations undertaken, and to check payments received.
- Audit was provided for workload, incidence of disease, procedures, malignancies, referrals, diagnoses, incidence of recurrence, postoperative complications, age bands, and waiting times for urgent and non-urgent procedures.
- The package could be used for training purposes.
- Minimum requirements were Windows 3.1, a 386 processor with 4 Mb of RAM and 10 Mb of available hard disk space. The program was written in Microsoft Access.

Minor surgery and skin lesions

This is a CD-ROM-based 'textbook' with data provided by Roger Kneebone and Julia Schofield. It is marketed by Primal Medical Information, and has received the formal approval and recommendation of the RCGP, through whom it may be ordered.

A colour atlas of 27 benign and seven malignant or premalignant skin lesions is provided, with reproduction of excellent quality. Management procedures related to each cover the management of the lesion and of the histology report that follows. Procedures are displayed in colour video with accompanying descriptive text.

The minor surgery section provides background information and details of suturing technique, instruments, minor surgery procedures, basic techniques, training sequences and local anaesthetics.

Patient education is well catered for, and help facilities are available. Navigation options are: file, search, 'go', bookmarks, patient education and help (RCGP, tel: (020) 7434 4300).

22.5 THE ELECTRONIC RED BOOK

The Computer Room software company has developed and refined an electronic version of the NHS Regulations (which include the Doctors' Terms of Service) and the Statements of Fees and Allowances (the 'Red Book') during the past decade. Arrangements have also been made to accommodate the variations in interpretation that occur between local health authorities. The Department of Health has granted the Computer Room distribution rights for the e-Red Book.

The e-Red Book module was originally based on:

- Department of Health data – the verbatim text in its original framework of the governmental edicts contained in the SFA and NHS Regulations
- individual health authorities' interpretative annotations of the Department of Health data as supplied, bundled and cross-referenced within the e-Red Book

- individual user notes and bookmarks – freestyle user notes and place markers for rapid retrieval of particular paragraphs as determined by the user.

The three types of data appear seamless, and are extensively cross-referenced by hypertext linkages. Searches can be initiated by the entry of any single or multiple words contained in the text, by entry of a word 'stem', by using a sophisticated thesaurus search routine which allows for synonyms, or by browsing an index.

Originally marketed by the developers, the e-Red Book has now been upgraded by the addition of a special program that calculates NHS fees due, and is bundled with the Radcliffe Press Text *Making Sense of the Red Book*. It is available on CD-ROM from Radcliffe Medical Press or *Doctor* magazine Book Service (tel: 01372 745815).

Other packages offering the Red Book's text in electronic format are now being launched. All will need to be updated regularly.

22.6 MEDICAL TRAVEL ADVICE

There are three main sources of electronic medical travel advice:

- MASTA, which primarily provides a telephone-mediated service

Fig. 22.4 The VP electronic Red Book as displayed on MediDesk

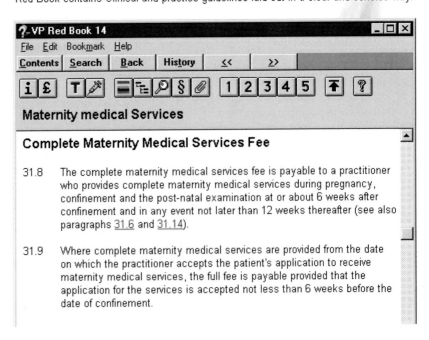

Red Book

Red Book contains Clinical and practice guidelines laid out in a clear and concise way.

- TRAVAX, a remote database accessible over the Internet, subject to subscription charges (except for doctors in Scotland)
- TRAVELLER, a diskette-based interactive enquiry program with monthly updates (also available through MediDesk).

MASTA (Medical Advisory Services for Travellers) maintains a central database that is regularly updated. Although this can be accessed on line, charges for doing so are quoted as £895 per annum. Alternative forms of access are:

- a telephone answering service with a prerecorded hierarchical structure, and calls charged at 60p per minute, which results in the preparation of a printed and posted individual schedule
- a telephone mediated answering service that not only provides a tailored schedule, but keeps a record of a subscriber's immunization history so that reminders can be issued. The annual subscription for the Regular Traveller's Service was £32 in 1999.

MASTA's data are validated by the London School of Hygiene and Tropical Medicine (Contact tel: 02392 553933).

TRAVAX, a remote database maintained by the Scottish Centre for Infection and Environmental Health, is accessible through the Internet on http://www.axl.co.uk/scieh. Applicants can sign up by accessing the website, and a subscription of £50 per annum is charged to practices situated outside Scotland. The database contains:

- general travel health information – general risks and countermeasures, and details of conditions such as jet lag and altitude sickness
- country-specific health risks and recommendations, with additional sections catering for children, expectant mothers, the elderly, and those suffering from specific conditions; alternative types of traveller are also provided for
- vaccine specifications
- vaccine schedules
- malaria prevention
- epidemiological updates.

TRAVELLER is provided on a monthly diskette that self-negates when out of date. It incorporates:

- immunization requirements
- malaria prophylaxis advice (an interactive anti-malarial calculator is incorporated)
- other medical travel risk prevention and counter-measure advice

- other tourist advice
- a description of the pathogenesis and principal features of each disease.

Searches can be made by resort or country. All types of travellers' risks are catered for, and the program can deal with complex multifactorial enquiries. Hotel-based, safari and backpacking travellers are dealt with separately. Preventive recommendations are tailored interactively to individual travel schedules, are displayed on screen, and are available on a plain paper printout for patients to take away.

Data are validated by the London Hospital of Tropical Diseases, and diskettes are virus-checked. Navigation is straightforward, and text and prompts are clear (Hadley Healthcare).

Other sources

- Shoreland Travel Health Information, at http://www.tripprep.com/index.html
- Stanford Travel Medicine Service, at http://www-leland.stanford.edu/-naked/stms.html

22.7 EDUCATION ON COMPUTER – INTRODUCTION

In most applications of the computer, the user depends to a very large extent upon the computer's memory. Education is an application in which doctors, their staff or their patients use the computer to enhance human memory. In years past, only the wealthiest of families could afford a personal tutor for their children, but computer-aided learning techniques, which can be used on home computers, make individual tuition available to everyone. So great an advantage is the one-to-one teacher–pupil ratio, that pessimists within the teaching profession fear the loss of teaching posts to classrooms in which each pupil has a computer terminal. Aside from considerations of school discipline, this is an overstatement that does not take into account the fact that talents involving self-expression, creativity and manual dexterity must be developed by methods other than the computer.

As regards the assimilation of knowledge, however, the computer offers techniques that are, for adults at least, demonstrably more effective in their results than other methods. The reasons for this are:

- Strictly personalized tuition that moves at the pupil's own pace.
- The system is impartial and emotionally neutral. The pupil recognizes that the program offers

Fig. 22.5 Medical advice for travel: Hadley Healthcare Solutions' Traveller package as displayed on MediDesk's Internet site

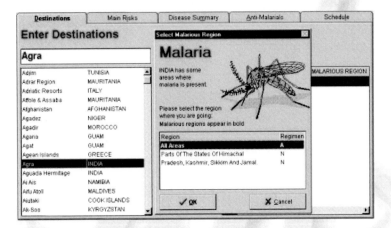

Using Traveller, it is quick and easy to look up vaccines for all parts of the world. Its simple interface allows you to select a holiday destination and then gives detailed advice on the vaccinations required. Also listed are risk factors for Malaria and Yellow Fever, with in depth guides to other diseases.

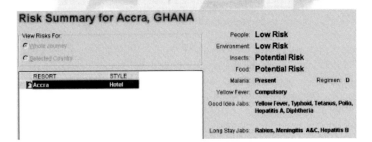

everyone the same rights of access, and that it possesses infinite patience.

- Interactive techniques are employed to stimulate the acquisition of knowledge and to show the pupil how well assimilation is progressing. Just as a teacher will ask pupils questions during a lesson, the computer can interrupt factual presentation with a question the answer to which can be selected from a menu list (multiple choice question).
- The computer can simulate problem situations in which a sequence of decisions must be taken by the pupil that will be audited by the system (patient management problems).
- Teaching programs sometimes adjust their presentation to suit the pupil's level of knowledge. If his answers show that the pupil is familiar with a section of material, that section can be discontinued; if material is not assimilated, it can be reiterated or reinforced.

- Visual aids are interspersed with text displays and are sometimes highly sophisticated. Diagrams, graphs and holograms, animation, colour and video may be used, and sound can be added (a package sometimes referred to as multimedia). A 'hold' facility allows the pupil to examine one frame in a film sequence, e.g. a barium meal or angiogram. Equipment must correspond with the medium employed.
- The computer keeps a performance score based on the validity of decisions made by the user, on the answers to multiple choice questions, and on the time taken to assimilate knowledge. These scores can be compared with peer averages and prove to enhance motivation. Scoring is immediate on completion of the programme.
- Material can be offered in a choice of formats – as, for instance, full text, synopsis, diagrams or a flowchart.

22.8 SIMULATION TECHNIQUES

Many a pilot has been helped to fly by a cockpit simulator that never left the ground. There is increasing use of simulation techniques in medicine as a means of training doctors in decision-making without risk to a live patient. As an example, the treatment of coma may be cited. In this programme the student enters results of a simulated clinical examination, and requests investigative and management procedures. The computer responds to each decision with new data. At the end of the programme the student obtains a score based on his clinical judgement in ordering appropriate tests for correct and rapid diagnosis, and accuracy in treatment.

Another application of this computer technique provides training in palliative care (the Macpac programme). Simulation training is also applied to procedures such as endoscopy. Movement of the endoscope in the surgeon's hands produces corresponding changes in a visceral image on the display screen. Correct technique and diagnostic skills are thereby cultivated.

Computer programs are available that model the physiological systems of the human body and their response to different pathological and pharmacological changes. Using these programs, doctors can test for themselves, for example, the effect of using various drugs in the treatment of heart failure, or the effect of administering thyroxine during pregnancy.

22.9 EDUCATIONAL DISKETTES AND CD-ROMS FOR PRACTICE USE

The first UK GP educational diskette to become widely available was the Phased Evaluation Program (PEP), produced by the South East Scotland RCGP Faculty with an ICI grant. As the fund of knowledge required for general practice is extensive, topics included in a trainee's 1-year curriculum must be highly selective, but the selection will be different for each trainee. The first PEP was a trainee assessment disk that was used to determine the pattern of strengths and weaknesses of individuals at the start of their training, so that areas of defective knowledge could subsequently be targeted.

The diskette contained 60 multiple choice questions spread over 11 areas of the medical syllabus to which answers of 'True', 'False', or 'Don't know' were invited. Patient management scenarios were then presented that simulated a general practice consultation, and required the trainee to call for elaborative and investigatory data, to interpret tests such as audiograms and ECGs, and to recommend treatment. Results were timed and scored, and the scores in each topic area were compared with estimates the candidate was asked to predict at the start of the program, and with the mean score of 200 peers. The program required an IBM-compatible PC, with an enhanced graphics adapter and an enhanced colour display. It lasted 90 minutes and could not be interrupted. The program could be rerun for comparison at the end of the training year. The success of the first PEP diskette led to the production of others in series, dealing with particular fields of GP activity.

Other educational diskettes have followed the same basic architecture of the PEP program and are proving very popular. Some diskettes provided by pharmaceutical companies offer a mixture of formal education, topical information, and practice resources such as programs for the construction of practice leaflets.

The PEP diskette established an important precedent in achieving accreditation for PGEA purposes. It is, as always with extraneous software, essential to insist on a 'virus-free' guarantee before loading all diskettes, and to check with the GP computer supplier that it is both safe and appropriate to proceed. Older computers using operating systems such as Xenix and BOS cannot run most of these diskettes, which are written in DOS or Windows, unless a special software interface is provided.

Because of its greatly superior capacity, CD-ROM is now the preferred medium for the local delivery of educational material. CD-ROM enables the use of colour video, sound, and the extensive dictionaries required by complex interactive procedures. Many operational software packages provided on CD-ROM now incorporate training modules using dummy data, and some encyclopaedic databases can ask questions as well as providing answers to them.

The recent dramatic reductions in the price of equipment needed to record CD-ROMs (from manufacturers such as Philips and Pioneer), and the ready availability of reasonably priced 'tools' software with a tuitional architecture, mean that CD-ROM-based educational packages can be crafted and distributed ever more readily and more cheaply (see also Chapter 19).

It would be very useful to have programs available to train staff in their duties as regards the completion of forms, the use of triage, their responsibilities for security, confidentiality and the DPA, and all activities set out in the practice brochure. Staff training in the use of the GP computer system and the use of the Red Book are already available as software modules.

Patient electronic medical education is now well catered for by commercial diskettes and CD-ROMs, the Internet, Kiosk technology, NHS Direct and the NELH.

22.10 REMOTE DATABASES FOR EDUCATION

In addition to permitting access to remote databases for interrogation, telecommunication is also used to transfer educational packages *en bloc* to local computers. In the USA, AMANET gives access to a collection of interactive medical courses prepared by the Massachusetts General Hospital, and these courses can be used to contribute to the postgraduate educational activities that are required for periodic reaccreditation.

In the UK in 1996, CIBA Vision pioneered and launched the first of its 'full cycle' GP educational packages on the Internet, entitled 'The Management of Dry Eye in General Practice'. This enabled doctors to download and print out tuitional text, to complete an assessment questionnaire which was returned to the company through e-mail, and to have the questionnaire autocorrected and sent back to the participant with model answers appended. On completion of the exercise, the doctor was sent a certificate that conferred 2 hours PGEA accreditation (http://www.cibavision.co.uk).

The Wisdom Project, pioneered in 1997 by the Department of General Practice at Sheffield University, provides Internet-based continuous learning packages for GPs. Relaunched as Wisdom 2000, it offers primary care teams free participation in educational programmes dealing with a range of issues that include evidence-based practice, clinical governance, PCG management, and change management. Background information, authoritative data resources, and discussion groups are available. PGEA accreditation is available locally, and it is intended that this should be extended nationally to support the process of professional revalidation (http://www.wisdom.org.uk). UKPractice.net Ltd provides on-line medical educational packages on behalf of the RCGP and these attract PGEA credits (http://www.ukpractice.net).

It seems inevitable that the requirements for revalidation in the UK will depend heavily upon the use of autovalidated distance learning packages, as reaccreditation has done in America. The joint RCGP–GMC schedule for revalidation combines self-assessment of needs for re-education or retraining with 5-yearly peer review by a team that includes the PCG+T clinical governance lead, an HA clinical adviser and representatives from the RCGP, the LMC and patient organizations. Reports are provided to the Joint Committee on Postgraduate Training. 20 quality indicators are used.

Educational programmes have also been transmitted by conventional and satellite television signal. Conventional broadcasts often transmit by night and require video storage by the recipient (British Medical-television).

22.11 PGEA ACCREDITATION SOFTWARE

The collation of attendance records in multiple categories for multiple doctors at multiple centres in multiple regions is an administrator's nightmare, yet each GP's PGEA accreditations depend upon the promptness and efficiency of this process.

A menu-driven database program developed by two GP tutors and a system consultant (Bowring et al 1991) promotes the entry of all relevant data, using electronic dictionaries. Up-to-date tallies of attendances may be viewed on screen and periodic printouts are obtainable (after the style of bank statements) that distinguish between full and incomplete accreditation.

The software package is housed on diskettes, and is first used by each local GP tutor or his/her secretary, who logs individual attendance details – doctor's identity, course categories and dates. The diskettes are then passed to the local postgraduate education centre staff for coordination with lists of doctors registered for local tuitional package deals ('season ticket schemes'). Finally, the diskette is sent to the HA, where all attendances for each doctor are collated from nationwide sources.

PGEA accreditation software is used to validate, but does not replace the need for, practice claims on FP/PEA forms, with their supporting documentation.

22.12 GENETIC COUNSELLING

GPs are under increasing pressure to provide their patients with advice on genetic risk, and secondary care does not possess the resources to deal with the increasing number of referrals that need to be made in this field.

The preparation of family trees, coupled with the assessment of genetic risk and the formulation of management strategies, requires decision support software that could be used in general practice to cope with patient demand, but such software packages as are currently available are too complex and abstruse for routine use in primary care.

Both the science of genetics and the design of counselling support software are areas of vigorous development with which most GPs are unfamiliar. A primary care genetic counselling package must first provide the GP with knowledge of the science and techniques used in diagnosis, then provide facilities for the construction of a pedigree chart that incorporates all the factors known to be relevant to the condition under investigation. Finally, the program must produce an assessment of risk in terms which both the doctor and patient can understand, together with appropriate case management guidance. Emery (1999) has reviewed available packages and found that none are currently suitable for use in general practice.

Further progress in software development can be expected to take place in response to demand. Secondary care packages presently deal with diagnosis, risk calculation and pedigree drawing, but none provides decision support based on the level of risk.

Emery considers the On-Line Mendelian Inheritance in Man (OMIM) database to be the most extensive electronic catalogue of human genes and genetic diseases currently available. It is accessible through the Internet, and has hypertext linkages with Medline.

REFERENCES AND FURTHER READING

Avery T 1999 Guide to the use of travel health databases. Prescriber 5 July: 85–87

Bowring D, Burton E, Rennison H 1991 GP Magazine, September: 7

Doctor Magazine 1996 Article on e-Red Book. Doctor 1 July: 66

Donald J, Thomson D 1992 Computer-aided assessment can PEP up training. Practice Computing, September: 8

Emery J 1999 Computer support for genetic advice in primary care. British Journal of General Practice, July: 572–575

Kneebone R L, Tilson P C 1994 Program cuts minor surgery red-tape. Practice Computing, Spring: 15–18

Muir Gray J A Preparing a leaflet for patient education. British Medical Journal 284: 1171

Practice Computing Magazine 1996 EMIS at the cutting edge of development. Practice Computing, Autumn: 19–22

Practice Computing Magazine 1997 The electronic red book. Practice Computing, Spring: 16–17

Practice Computing Magazine 1997 Article on traveller package. Practice Computing, Winter: 10

Rose P, Lucassen A 1999 Practical genetics for primary care. Oxford University Press, Oxford

Thomas J 1990 New episode for GP's TV channel. Doctor 22 March: 53

23 Clinical protocols and expert systems

23.1 INTRODUCTION

Each country has its own idiosyncratic behaviour patterns. World tourists who unwittingly yawn, stretch or blow their noses may, depending upon their location, be committing a grave social indiscretion.

In the medical field, idiosyncratic conduct on the part of doctors reflects differences of opinion that, unless it leads to alternative treatments of equal merit, will put some patients at a disadvantage. Protocols abolish this disadvantage. A protocol has been defined as a consensus strategy codified and used to determine future conduct. Protocols encapsulate expertise in a format that renders it universally applicable.

Medical protocols began as paper-based hierarchical flowcharts. Their transfer to computer resulted in increased sophistication and speed of access. The most highly developed protocols offer a considerable degree of decision support, sufficient to justify their designation as expert systems.

23.2 DISADVANTAGES OF PAPER-BASED PROTOCOLS

In contrast with their computerized counterparts, paper-based protocols have the following disadvantages.

- Use of the flowchart does not result in data entry.
- With computer systems, only the relevant decision node need be spotlighted. Access to paper-based protocols always involves viewing the entire flowchart – a slow and cumbersome process – and the flowchart may require more space than can conveniently be provided on a working document.
- Doctors are diffident about consulting paper documents in the presence of patients.
- Updating requires reprinting.

- Interactive dialogue between protocol and user is impossible.
- No interrogation of the patient record by the protocol is possible.
- The protocol cannot be tailored to the level of expertise of the user, nor modified to suit local needs.

Computer-based protocols overcome these problems and have the additional advantage that they can orientate themselves to be age/sex specific, situation-specific or target-specific. They can also be adapted as training modules.

Computerized medical protocols now play an important part in the management of modern UK general practice. They need to be given dedicated storage space on the practice server ('the protocol library'), to be accessible by all users on the practice LAN, to dovetail with patient clinical records and to be updated as upgrades become available. Protocols are now a key instrument in the imposition of clinical governance (see also Chapter 21) and are assuming increasing medicolegal importance.

There are three basic forms of clinical protocol – data entry routines, diagnostic protocols and patient management protocols. Patient management protocols, in turn, are of three main types – those used in preventive medicine, those used to help supervise the management of chronic disease or pregnancy (surveillance), and those used to suggest an appropriate path of management for a newly diagnosed case (Box 23.1).

23.3 PROTOCOLS THAT ACCELERATE AND VALIDATE DATA ENTRY

These protocols trap data in an efficient and rapid manner in situations where sets of multiple parameters constantly recur. Lengthy repetitive history taking

---

Box 23.1 Clinical protocols used on practice systems

Data entry protocols

Diagnostic protocols

Patient management protocols

- preventive medicine
- surveillance of chronic disease
- decision support

- First generation

    EMIS Templates
    Wolfson Computer Laboratory
    Multilex prescribing monitor

- Second generation

    SOPHIE
    MENTOR
    ISIS

- Third generation

    PRODIGY
    MENTOR UPGRADES
    MediDesk

- Fourth generation

    Expert systems

---

that follows a fixed pattern is well catered for, such as occurs at the first antenatal consultation, at the assessment of a comprehensive medical case, or during an occupational medical check. Involved physical examinations such as are employed for neurology, or for examination of the cardiovascular or skeletal system, are also suitable for protocol data entry. Data entry protocols act as *aides-memoire*, helping to ensure that nothing is omitted, and they promote consistency in recording so that comparisons can be made between cases and with previous consultations (sometimes a patient's previous entries are displayed in parallel at the time of data capture). Increased speed in data entry is achieved by prompting for appropriate answers and requiring only minimum data, or default entry, in return. Accuracy is obtained by validation with reference to internal dictionaries of values for each parameter within each field. Morbidity and intervention (procedure) codes are allocated at the time of entry that provide conformity for subsequent search procedures. Some suppliers have constructed specialized data entry protocols that provide for the summarization of records at take-on to computer, or for the entry of multiple pathology test reports. Data entry protocols may also be user-defined to accommodate practice research or other special interests.

Examples of two sophisticated data entry tools, Clinergy and Visual Read, have already been described in Chapter 6.

23.4 DIAGNOSTIC PROTOCOLS

The diagnostic process is sometimes straightforward, when it may be represented by simple flowcharts (Fig. 23.1).

By contrast, it may be highly complex, involving three elements – a single flowchart or several overlapping flowcharts, a probability listing, and pattern recognition. Computer programs that combine these three elements fall into the category of 'expert' systems (see below).

In addition to trapping data, some less expert protocols can analyse the results obtained, and compute possible diagnoses, listed and weighted in order of probability. Most of the research and ongoing applications of computer diagnosis have taken place in hospital, where the computer's probability listing facility has proved superior to human judgement in dealing with such matters as acute abdominal pain, jaundice, non-toxic goitre, some endocrine diseases, dyspepsia and congenital heart disease.

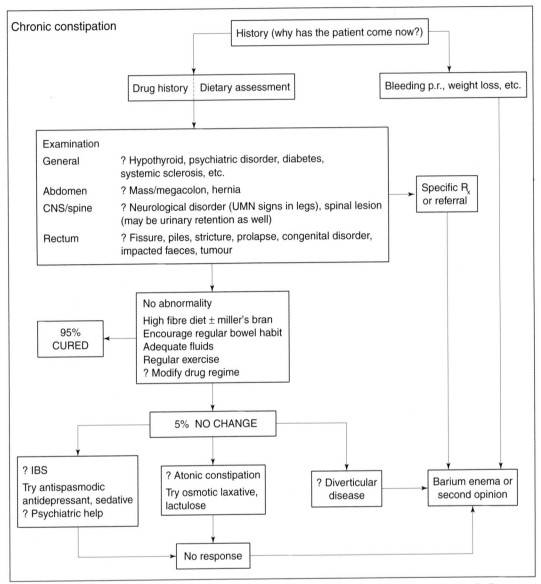

Fig. 23.1 A simple diagnostic protocol (Courtesy of Dr David Preston, Louth County Hospital)

In order to arrive at a probability listing, symptoms and signs must not only be recorded but allocated a weighting factor by the examiner, a process that inevitably introduces an element of subjective judgement.

In general practice most clinically complex cases need to undergo hospital-based investigation before a diagnosis can be made. As a result, computer diagnosis has a much less significant role to play in general practice affairs than it does in hospital. The diagnostic art of the primary care physician is for the most part a clinical rather than an investigatory one, involving the elicitation of symptoms and signs before pattern matching begins. Some treatments can be instituted on a provisional basis without a firm diagnosis. Fears that computers will replace general practitioners would seem to be unfounded.

23.5 PREVENTIVE MEDICINE PROTOCOLS

Commonly used preventive medicine protocols prompt for, and validate the data entry for, all procedures needed when screening well men, well women, over-74-year-olds, new patients, children and cervical cytology. They are also employed in immunization programmes.

23.6 SURVEILLANCE PROTOCOLS

Surveillance protocols support the supervision of chronic conditions such as diabetes, asthma, hypertension or hyperlipidaemia, and are used in antenatal care or contraception programmes (see also Chapter 9).

Unlike preventive medicine protocols, which simply furnish straightforward check lists and validate data entries, surveillance protocols must interleave with a number of other applications on the system, allow for care to be shared with other health professionals, and follow strictly defined guidelines laid down by authorities such as NICE, the British Hypertension Society or the British Thoracic Society. In addition to the need to prompt for and validate the entry of data relating to the procedures required to monitor chronic disease, surveillance protocols must provide for:

- decision support at the point of care
- a shared surveillance record which displays the results of serial readings of the same parameters over time, and which enables data entries by both doctor and nurse, using a subprotocol that defines their respective responsibilities; surveillance is usually organized by running dedicated 'cohort' clinics
- care and records to be shared with other health professionals, such as diabetologists, chiropodists, ophthalmologists and physiotherapists
- the incorporation of the results of all investigations, including those obtained from point-of-care and patient-held monitoring devices; PHM devices may need to be scheduled from the practice system
- close linkage with the repeat medication routine, the reappointment routine, the consultation log and summary records
- patient education facilities to include patient education screens and patient instruction leaflets, and subprotocols to monitor patient self-treatment and to ensure compliance
- process of care to be audited both as an aid to improving performance, to provide data for annual reports to the PCG+T/HA, and to support claims for management allowance.

The organization of surveillance of chronic disease in the UK has become considerably more complex during the past 10 years. This is largely the result of initiatives launched by authoritative special interest and patient pressure groups, together with government intervention through the Department of Health. Payment of a special management allowance for diabetes and asthma is now dependent upon the demonstrable use of official guidelines, a policy that is likely to be extended to cover the treatment of other chronic conditions. The following measures must therefore be taken:

- *Authoritative guidelines* for surveillance of chronic diseases must now be incorporated into a formal and declared practice policy with the approval of the health authority and local provider. Objectives, targets and criteria must be defined. This policy document should be stored on the practice computer so that it can be used within a decision support system for patient care at consultation, can be amended when necessary, and can be replicated for HA scrutiny in support of the management allowance.
- *A list of patients suffering from the condition under review* must be capable of being compiled by computer, so the exact criteria that will need to be identified by the search process must be included in each patient's medical record. For some chronic conditions this list must be available to the HA.
- *An individual management plan* must be formulated and stored on the computer for each surveillance patient. The plan will take into account the measurement of all parameters needed to fulfil the requirements of the minimum data set and the authorized management protocol for the condition. Dedicated data collection routines must then prompt for, validate and record these values.

23.7 DECISION SUPPORT PROTOCOLS – AN OVERVIEW

Attempts to codify, and commit to computer, the intricate sets of rules by which doctors reach decisions have absorbed very considerable amounts of time, effort and money, particularly in the USA. Limited success has been achieved in some areas, and further development continues apace.

In UK general practice, given the magnitude of the task, development of decision support has necessarily been piecemeal and has taken place in a series of phases. If we use Figure 23.2 to represent the sequence of events involved in the doctor's management of the patient, then it should theoretically be possible to offer decision support at any point in the chain, although most individual software developers have understandably limited themselves to particular areas.

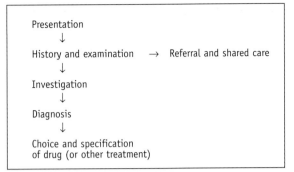

```
Presentation
      ↓
History and examination    →    Referral and shared care
      ↓
Investigation
      ↓
Diagnosis
      ↓
Choice and specification
of drug (or other treatment)
```

Fig. 23.2 The sequence of events involved in patient management

Thus the Multilex designed prescribing monitor seeks to eradicate all predictable prescribing errors (see Chapter 11), the Wolfson Computer Laboratory designs assist in the choice of appropriate laboratory tests and define the boundaries and individual responsibilities of shared care, simple data entry protocols assist in recording history and examination, and PRODIGY and MediDesk give support to the linkage between diagnosis and treatment. Currently, only the upgraded version of MENTOR can, in many instances, start with presentation and proceed through the chain to diagnosis and treatment.

The progressive development of GP decision support is described in Box 23.1 as taking place, historically, in a series of 'generations'. Early development began at the Wolfson Laboratory in the 1970s, Multilex's designs and EMIS Templates were launched in the 1980s, and second- and third-generation packages became operational in the 1990s.

23.8 THE WOLFSON COMPUTER LABORATORY PROTOCOLS

A number of the foremost suppliers' systems can now dovetail with the Wolfson Computer Laboratory (WCL) suite of protocols. WCL programs are protocols with inbuilt expert system technology that support, but do not impose, decisions on the patient management process. The doctor is able to 'toggle' between a patient record screen and the expertise support program so smoothly that use of the protocols imposes no increase in consultation duration. The programs justify the use of the term 'expert protocols'.

WCL protocols have been constructed to deal with diabetes, hypertension, hyperlipidaemia, anaemia,

asthma, paediatric surveillance, and pathology laboratory sampling and investigation (see Chapter 12). Protocols dealing with numerous other areas are under development. The programs have been developed in cooperation with specialists in primary and secondary care, and with reference to nationally agreed guidelines, but are capable of a certain degree of modification in the light of local needs.

Each program first interrogates the patient record, identifies and prompts for missing and new data, and then offers advice on examination and investigation. Finally, warnings, then therapy and other management recommendations including referral are issued, together with a suggestion for a review interval.

The program is arranged in the computer as a protocol, together with a lattice-work of background expert information that is called into use in context by keywords selected by the user. A hypertext framework is used to display this text in layers of progressively increasing detail, should the user so wish, and this will be accompanied by appropriate illustrations in the form of line diagrams, 'chart' or artwork graphics.

The WCL programs accurately define the boundary between primary and secondary care, thus helping to eliminate unnecessary referrals. The pathology services support module makes similar economies in pathological investigations by suggesting those most appropriate to a given clinical situation.

23.9 EMIS TEMPLATES AND PROTOCOLS

The lead in EMIS Template development was taken by members of the EMIS National User Group (NUG) who cooperated with each other in order to simplify data entry routines, and to devise ways of refining the Read 4-byte set of codes. The result of their deliberations was a set of data entry frames incorporating Read-coded terms, and written in a computer file format that could be keyed in to their system – the so-called EMIS Templates. Enthusiasts swapped their own Templates through the User Group, and later used the Internet to do so (http://www.emisnug.prg.uk/) through an appointed company Web-master.

In a further development, some EMIS Templates were upgraded so as to incorporate authoritative guidelines. These became known as EMIS Protocols. The introduction of Read 5-byte codes removed the need for the EMIS modifications that had been applied to the 4-byte set.

By 1990, there were 70 5-byte EMIS Templates and 17 5-byte Protocols.

Fig. 23.3 An EMIS data entry template

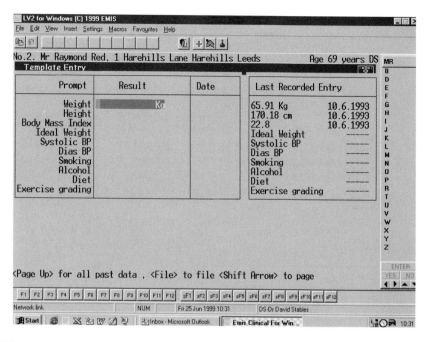

23.10 AAH MEDITEL'S SOPHIE

AAH Meditel responded to the entrepreneurial activities of the EMIS NUG by developing a more sophisticated data entry and clinical guideline-based protocol engine linked to Read codes and the patient record. The acronym SOPHIE stood for 'Screening Of Patient Health in an Interactive Environment', and the software was developed by the company itself.

- Each of SOPHIE's introductory screens offers advice on the use of the protocol being accessed, and provides basic information taken from the patient record, such as identifying details and the date of the last check. The user is also offered the option to view or amend registration details (Figs 23.4, 23.5).
- History and examination screens follow, in which information missing in the record is prompted for and, when entered, validated and Read-coded. Free text can be added to the clinical screens.
- The option to prescribe is then offered, for which Multilex-based cross-checking routines are used. This is followed by prompts to carry out additional related procedures, if appropriate, such as influenza immunization, antismoking counselling, NHS claim submission, or reappointment.
- Patient advice leaflets may then be printed out on the basis of the information obtained, and the protocol's findings are added to the patient's notes.
- The questions SOPHIE displays are context-sensitive to the individual patient record, and the soft-

ware runs automatic checks on the patient's record to produce opportunistic reminders where these are appropriate (termed 'watchdogs').

SOPHIE can be customized to incorporate local guidelines or to form the basis for the individualized delegation of responsibilities.

When the second version of SOPHIE was released in 1992, it incorporated the following 'off-the-peg' protocols:

- Well man screening
- Well woman screening
- Geriatric surveillance (75 and over)
- New patient questionnaire
- Quick version of the new patient review
- Diabetic interim review
- Heart attack risk score
- Oral contraception (with FP1001 issue)
- Hypertension.

Since 1992 the SOPHIE protocol library has been steadily increased. As well as providing fast input of clinical details, it streamlines the entry of laboratory results and claim submission.

23.11 ISIS

Medical Care Systems (MCS) also developed their own protocol generator for use in client practices. This was designed along broadly similar lines to SOPHIE, and offered Read-coded data entry routines

Fig. 23.4 A SOPHIE II data entry screen (Torex Meditel)

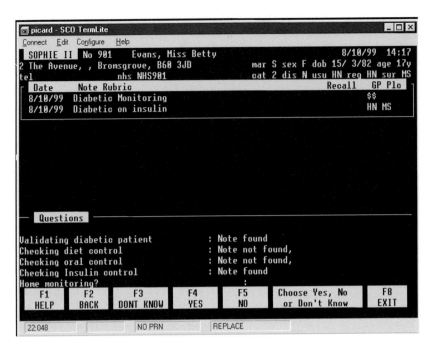

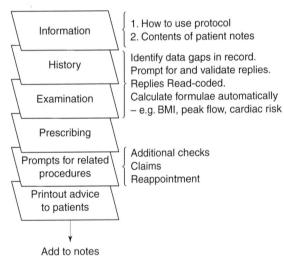

Fig. 23.5 The architecture of a patient management protocol (based on SOPHIE)

for frequently encountered clinical or administrative situations.

- Guidelines were incorporated to enable decision support, and opportunistic reminders were integral.
- Patient advice leaflets based on responses to questions could be printed out.
- The system was able to compile claims, and provision was made to allow billing for fees due from private practice, solicitors and insurance companies.
- All forms of certification were catered for.
- Software for the protocol generator was supplied to practices and was bundled with a suite of ready-made protocols.

Practices creating new ISIS protocols are able to exchange them with each other by post, or through the MCS website (http://www.torex.co.uk/medical) under Torex 2000. MCS is now part of the Torex Health Group.

23.12 PRODIGY

Overview

In 1994 the Department of Health took note of the second-generation protocol software being developed by GP system suppliers, and tasked the NHSE with constructing and testing its own prototype, with a view to promoting the twin aims of clinical governance and the more efficient use of NHS resources. To avoid the criticism that this would impose the practice of medicine by diktat, the use of PRODIGY at the point of care was to be made discretionary, but the project was widely regarded as yet another means of producing downward pressure on prescribing costs. PRODIGY, which by a stretch of the imagination can be derived from the full title of 'Prescribing RatiOnally with Decision support In General practice studY', was selected as the acronym for the fledgling software. Its design was originally based on the Prescriptor system, which had already been piloted in 50 Dutch practices. In principle, PRODIGY is bolted on to any GP clinical system, and cuts in at the point at which the GP enters a diagnosis, so as to interpose tree-branching logic that will lead to an optimal intervention.

Implementation

- GP system suppliers were invited to cooperate, and AAH Meditel, EMIS, Genisyst, MCS and VAMP were the original responders to make the necessary modifications that integrated the software.
- Expenses were met from Department of Health Research and Development funds, and the software was provided free of charge to GPs, apart from maintenance costs.
- The project was based at the Sowerby Centre for Health Informatics at the University of Newcastle.
- Data were originally derived from the Liverpool Medical Adviser Support Centre in the form of clinical guidelines, and drug information was based on the British National Formulary. In the longer term, PRODIGY will take its data from the National Institute for Clinical Excellence.
- Audit of the use of PRODIGY will continue to investigate its effect on outcome, costs, and the process of consultation from both the doctor's and patient's point of view. 'Before and after installation' video recordings of the consultation have been used.
- The ability to incorporate PRODIGY is now a requirement for system accreditation.
- PRODIGY's advice can be followed, over-ridden or customized by the GP.
- When GPs enter a Read-coded diagnosis, they are presented with data subdivided into 'aims of treatment', 'management of condition', and the option to view references. 70% of primary care presentations are catered for.
- Advice is provided on further investigation, referral, alternative regimens of suitable medication, and other appropriate treatments.
- Prescribing regimens are checked against the patient record for allergies, drug interactions and contraindications.
- Drug costs are shown if alternatives have the same efficacy or the original choice offers only marginal advantages. Where products are equivalent, PRODIGY will recommend the generic alternative.

- Advice is context-sensitive and tailored to the requirements of the individual patient.
- Screens are provided for joint access by doctor and patient, in order to assist in the decision process.
- An advice leaflet can be printed out for the patient on the blank side of form FP10 comp. which details the nature and treatment of the condition.
- PRODIGY can be used as an educational tool.
- PRODIGY's website (http://www.schin.ncl.ac.uk/prodigy) in March 1999 listed 150 protocols that were either completed or scheduled for completion by 2002.

Figure 23.6 is taken from PRODIGY's website demonstrator screen, and illustrates both the strengths and weaknesses of trying to codify the practice of medicine.

The frame's content implies that the first line of treatment for otitis media should be a tailored prescription for pain relief together with a patient leaflet, and that antibiotics should only be used in selected cases.

Let us view this advice in perspective. Some 40 years ago ENT wards admitted a constant stream of children for emergency tympanotomy to prevent otitis media developing the sequelae of chronic suppurative otitis media, mastoiditis, and death from intracerebral infection. The introduction of antibiotics removed the need for tympanotomy, the occasional penalty thereafter being fibrosis of the ossicular joints if the case had not been properly monitored.

In the example, the PRODIGY screen needs to spell out, at the stage of its first-line advice, how cases should be selected for antibiotics, in order to avoid creating the impression that the use of these drugs is regarded as exceptional.

- PRODIGY phase 1 pilot testing involved 137 GPs, ran for 3 months in the spring of 1996, and was limited to advice on the three most cost-effective drugs for a given diagnosis. 94% of GPs who used the module thought it was worth developing.
- PRODIGY phase 2 ran from 1997 to 1998, involved 900 GPs and 63 HAs, and exhibited drugs by class rather than as individual selections. Half the GPs who used the phase 2 module considered that further improvements were needed, but most were prepared to continue using it.
- In November 1998, the Health Minister announced the full roll-out of PRODIGY to all GPs in England who wished to use it. Initially, phase 3 of PRODIGY will concentrate on chronic disease management. PRODIGY is obtainable free of initial cost through GP system suppliers.

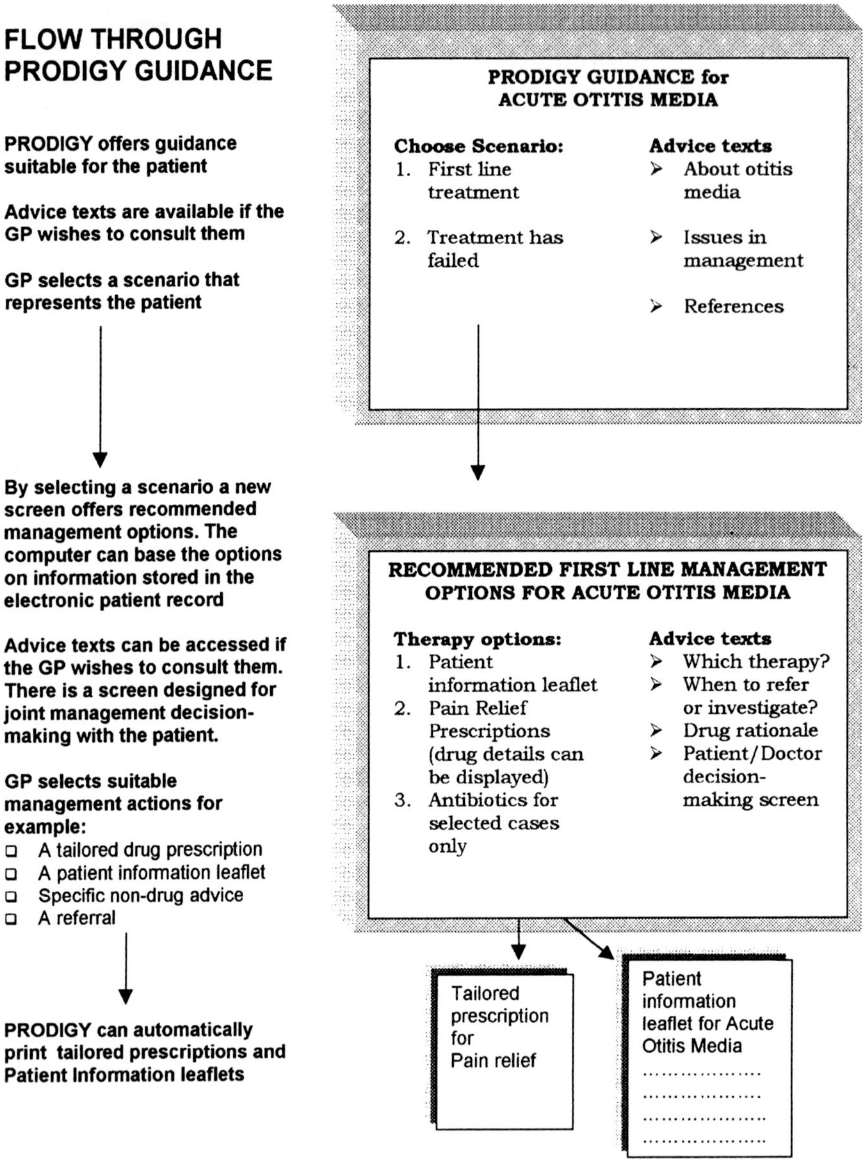

FLOW THROUGH PRODIGY GUIDANCE

PRODIGY offers guidance suitable for the patient

Advice texts are available if the GP wishes to consult them

GP selects a scenario that represents the patient

By selecting a scenario a new screen offers recommended management options. The computer can base the options on information stored in the electronic patient record

Advice texts can be accessed if the GP wishes to consult them. There is a screen designed for joint management decision-making with the patient.

GP selects suitable management actions for example:
❑ A tailored drug prescription
❑ A patient information leaflet
❑ Specific non-drug advice
❑ A referral

PRODIGY can automatically print tailored prescriptions and Patient Information leaflets

PRODIGY GUIDANCE for ACUTE OTITIS MEDIA

Choose Scenario:
1. First line treatment
2. Treatment has failed

Advice texts
➢ About otitis media
➢ Issues in management
➢ References

RECOMMENDED FIRST LINE MANAGEMENT OPTIONS FOR ACUTE OTITIS MEDIA

Therapy options:
1. Patient information leaflet
2. Pain Relief Prescriptions (drug details can be displayed)
3. Antibiotics for selected cases only

Advice texts
➢ Which therapy?
➢ When to refer or investigate?
➢ Drug rationale
➢ Patient/Doctor decision-making screen

Tailored prescription for Pain relief

Patient information leaflet for Acute Otitis Media
....
....
....
....

- PRODIGY takes the GP through current recommendations for the treatment of a condition.
- PRODIGY aims to use high quality reference sources including the Cochrane Library, Effective Health Care Bulletins, Effectiveness Matters, evidence-based journals and medicine reviews, key peer-reviewed journals including the Drugs and Therapeutics Bulletin and databases including Medline and Embase.
- A national validation panel with representatives from the Royal College of General Practitioners, Royal Society of Physicians, Royal Pharmaceutical Society of Great Britain and General Medical Services Committee endorse the clinical content.
- PRODIGY is able to support guidelines developed by the National Institute for Clinical Excellence (NICE) and has been included in the recent NHS documents ' A First Class Service' and 'Information for Health'.

Fig. 23.6 PRODIGY's demonstrator screen on the Internet

Fig. 23.7 PRODIGY data incorporated within patient information dictionary: In-Practice Systems' Vision system, using PILs text

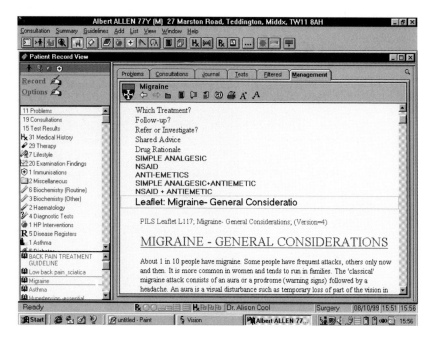

When fully operational, it is likely that PRODIGY will be used as a vehicle for urgent Department of Health or CMO messages to general practices. PRODIGY guideline upgrades will also link with secondary care assistance – assistance in distinguishing between a high and low risk of cancer will be matched by fast-tracking of referred cancer cases.

23.13 MEDIDESK

Against the background of PRODIGY, which was regarded by many as an attempt by government to intervene in the prescribing process, a rival software package, named MediDesk, was launched in October 1998.

Aware that the government would be likely to oppose any GP computer system that carried advertising, the 20-pharmaceutical-company consortium that contributed to the original funding of MediDesk formed a non-profit-bearing trust and gave the project's management autonomy. They also invited and obtained the cooperation of software and communications companies, the most prominent of which were Microsoft, Mitsubishi Electronic, BT Syntegra and BT Health. Unsurprisingly, MediDesk was one of the first organizations to be granted full NHSnet code of connection.

Ready made medical applications were contributed by:

- Health One (GP medical record)

- Pro-choice Applications (travel health advice)
- Visual Productions (Visual Read)
- Healthworks (electronic health and medical information).

Some 3 months prior to launch, MediDesk merged with the health care connectivity and desktop applications company Trident Health. This company already had a 5-year track record in the medical field, which included the design and management of the notably successful Sandwell Network Strategy Pilot, a project linking hospital, pathology laboratory, GPs, community health services, the health authority, the social services, and mental health clinics.

Like PRODIGY, MediDesk assembles a library of guidelines. These are selected by an independent advisory board under the chairmanship of Sir William Asscher. User feedback is furnished by a panel of GPs. Guidelines are provided for use across the whole therapeutic spectrum and include forms of treatment other than prescribing, with data drawn from multiple authoritative sources, which in future will include NICE. Regional and local guideline variations will be taken into account. MediDesk did not initially incorporate its guidelines within patient management protocols.

MediDesk software is configured to run in tandem with existing GP clinical modules and is supported remotely. Although it will take time for MediDesk to achieve the degree of integration enjoyed by PRODIGY, Trident Health's expertise in the health field, and the influence exerted by BT, Microsoft and

Fig. 23.8 MediDesk's exemplar desktop screen

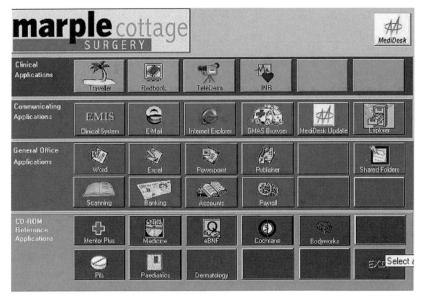

Mitsubishi are likely to accelerate development. System design is deliberately directed towards implementing both a common electronic health record and the Department of Health strategy embodied in *Information for Health*. MediDesk claims that it will provide a single platform upon which all practices can mount diverse applications of their choice. It will certainly facilitate communications between health professionals.

MediDesk deals with clinical, administrative and financial aspects of practice management, and Trident Health's operations at Sandwell are probably a microcosm of what is ultimately to be expected from further MediDesk development. The Sandwell pilot implemented 14 different clinical and administrative messages:

- Pathology requests (200 possible tests)
- Pathology results
- Radiology results
- A&E attendance notification
- Pathology supplies ordering
- Contract Minimum Data Sets from providers
- Day case referrals
- Breast clinic reports
- OP clinic referrals
- Early diagnosis referrals (endoscopy, anorectal and haematuria clinics)
- Clinic correspondence
- Cancer registry entry
- Admission and discharge notification
- A library facility.

The Sandwell pilot also offered electronic waiting list and practice pay scales information, and preconfigured healthcare leaflets. 'Bedside e-data' was already provided within the Trust hospital. ISDN dial-up was used with e-mail to submit Microsoft Word and Microsoft Excel transfers. Standalone Sandwell intranet workstations accessed diverse GP system software packages by terminal emulation. Unfortunately, the Sandwell system used the OS2 operating system, which gave rise to difficulties in accessing NHSnet. As a result, MediDesk has diversified into other, less insular, intranet configurations.

23.14 OXFORD CLINICAL MENTOR

Overview

The most adroit and attractive of the decision support packages currently available to GPs is the Oxford Clinical Mentor (OCM), published by the system supplier EMIS in conjunction with Oxford University Press. OCM's architecture delivers precisely what GPs need in the format in which they want it. Unlike PRODIGY, whose operation is dependent upon the entry of a Read-coded diagnosis, OCM lists differential diagnoses in response to the user's entry of one or more symptoms or signs, whether or not these are supported by test results. This differential list of possible diagnoses also serves as a picking list, selection from which enables the user to 'jump' to an elaborative text relating to the term chosen. Having browsed one or more such elaborative texts, users decide which diagnosis they consider to be appropriate, 'click' on to it, and thereby proceed

Fig. 23.9a and b Examples of MediDesk's clinical guidelines screens

Fig. 23.9a

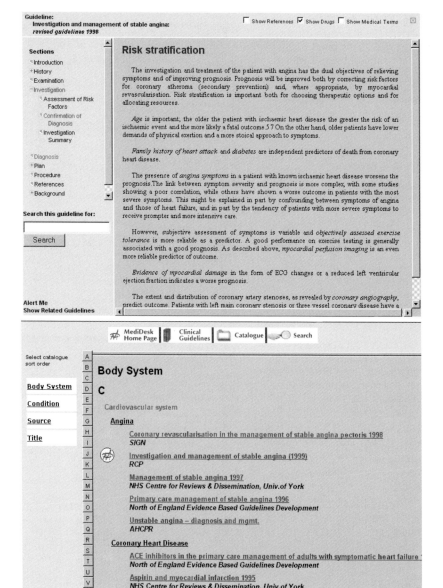

Fig. 23.9b

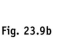

to a screen that details management. Elaborative texts are backed with references which can be summoned by embedded hypertext links, and a direct hypertext linkage with Medline is also available.

Further details

- Entry of symptoms can be made:
  - by typing in the full term
  - by typing in part of the term and thereby calling up a short picking list
  - by searching full-length picking lists, which may be assembled alphabetically, counter-alphabetically, by frequency of occurrence, or in the reverse order to that in which updates have been made to the data.
- Symptoms can be weighted by using answers to the questions 'How long?' or 'How much?'
- Searches may be made on all keywords within the database, or by browsing chapters, titles, syndromes, or drugs.
- The differential diagnosis screen is subdivided into four discrete lists. The first three of these nominate

Fig. 23.10 MENTOR's differential diagnoses listings, displayed as the result of the user's entry of two presenting symptoms. Differential diagnoses are subclassified according to whether they occur commonly, uncommonly or rarely

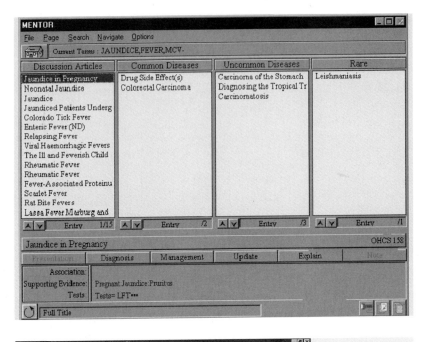

Fig 23.11 An example of a MENTOR elaborative text displayed as a result of 'clicking' on a term in the differential diagnostic list

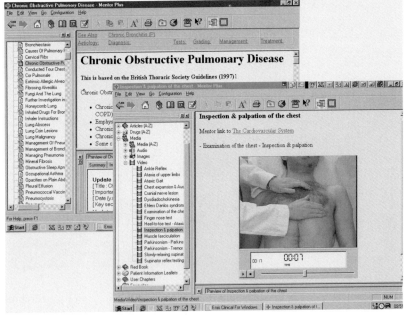

the common diseases, uncommon diseases, and rare diseases that may apply to the presentation whose details have been entered. The fourth list offers access to related discussion articles.
- The management screen suggests suitable investigations, as well as proposing medication or other forms of intervention. If alternative treatments are suitable, these are quoted, with references.

- Over 200 high-resolution colour images are provided.
- Users can add their own notes to the data displayed.
- The data shown are suitable for use in general practice, and for use as first-line treatment in hospital. They are also designed so as to anticipate the questions most frequently asked by patients.

- Texts have been written by GPs together with clinical specialists. They draw extensively on material from the *Oxford Handbook of Clinical Specialties*, the *Oxford Handbook of Clinical Medicine* and the *Oxford Handbook of Clinical Rarities* to provide for the requirements of evidence-based medicine and best practice. Details of over 2000 diseases and 25 000 medical terms are incorporated. National guidelines for common disorders have been included. Provision has also been made to allow locally used guidelines to be added to the database.
- The OCM is provided on CD-ROM but updated monthly on-line. Updates are searchable both by date and importance, as well as being accessible in their proper context.
- The package runs on Microsoft Windows and is suitable for all computers using this operating system. It requires a minimum of a 486D 66 MHz processor with 8 Mb of RAM, 35 Mb of available hard disk space, a VGA 256 colour 640 × 480 monitor, a CD-ROM drive, mouse, sound card and speakers.
- Single-user prices were quoted in 1999 as £119.83 for single users, with annual update charges of £58.75. Those additionally purchasing the PILs and Dermis packages are able to link between the three modules.
- A further development of OCM termed MENTOR Plus enables the decision support module to interact with the EMIS clinical software and its Read code directory.

23.15 PRECONSULTATIVE HISTORY-TAKING

In studies conducted to determine the relative importance of all procedures used in reaching a medical diagnosis, the taking of an adequate history proves to be by far the most significant. Unhappily, the deficiencies of conventional history taking are such as to undermine this importance. Because it requires more time to take a good history than can usually be allowed, manual histories tend to be disorganized, incomplete and sometimes illegible. These deficiencies are not confined to general practice. Hospital experience has shown that risk factors which would have been detectable in the patient history, and which should have modified management, are overlooked in a high proportion of outpatients. Failure to act on such risk factors is a major reason for litigation in the USA.

Two solutions to the problem have been tested, the use of paper questionnaires and computer-based interrogation. In each method, either the patient enters his/her responses (using a simple keypad with 'Yes', 'No', 'Don't know' options for the computer), or a nurse or midwife records responses on the patient's behalf. Both methods act as an *aide-memoire* and are capable of recording a comprehensive family, social and past medical history.

The advantages of computer-based histories over paper questionnaires are:

- They are fully legible.
- They avoid irrelevant questions, given a knowledge of the patient's age, sex and main complaint.
- Because computers appear to be impersonal, patient responses to them are less inhibited.
- Because they use ramifying logic, positive responses lead to enquiry in greater depth and detail on relevant matters.
- The computer can identify, and bring to notice, risk factors in the history, offering suggestions on actions which should be taken.
- Given an adequate history for some symptoms (such as dyspepsia), the computer can list possible diagnoses in order of probability and quote an index of probability for each.

Paper questionnaires and computer-based histories cannot fully replace the clinician's interview with the patient. The slant given to symptoms by the patient's own misinterpretation, and innuendos inherent in tone of voice and facial expression, cannot be represented. It is a fundamental principle of good history-taking that patients must be allowed to describe their problem in their own words before being cross-questioned – only in this way can questions be avoided to which the patient feels a particular answer is implied. The real strength of questionnaires and computer histories lies in their comprehensive coverage of details for which there is scant time at consultation. They are adjuncts to the doctor–patient interview that save time for the doctor, and afford both time and opportunity to patients to make their contribution towards diagnosis.

Despite the advantages of computer interrogation over the patient questionnaire, it is the latter that is now extensively used to preface patient attendance at hospital outpatient departments. The time taken by the patient to respond to a list of questions extensive enough to cover his family, social and past medical history may be as long as 90 minutes, and questionnaires are therefore sent by post to be completed at home.

If this exercise was to be carried out on a computer at hospital, it would necessitate patients arriving 90 minutes earlier for their appointments, and would require the provision of a bank of outpatient terminals. Outpatient computer histories, as opposed to paper questionnaires, have been reserved for a few specialties, such as initial antenatal attendance when the history is taken by the midwife.

In general practice, preconsultative history taking, either on paper or on computer, has been employed in the following circumstances:

- When a patient first joins a practice (full medical, social and family history) – this provides practitioners with a background knowledge of medical history, and alerts them to ongoing problems, risk factors and the need for preventive procedures
- Prior to a routine consultation appointment, in order to assess the need for, and therefore provide the chance to offer, opportunistic preventive procedures (preventive procedure history only)
- Prior to a consultation for psychiatric problems (standardized psychiatric symptom and history questionnaire)
- Lifestyle assay – interrogation of risk factors present in a patient's lifestyle, with the corollary that the computer calculates reduction in life expectancy and suggests desirable changes; the doctor may augment these suggestions
- Nutritional assay – representative data on a weekly dietary intake are asked for by the computer, and entered by the patient. The computer then recommends changes in line with the needs of subjects of either normal or excess weight.

23.16 EXPERT SYSTEMS – AN INTRODUCTION

If the English guarded their linguistic heritage as jealously as the French, and rejected out of hand the bastardization of words that occurs when jargon is coined, then computer experts would be left speechless. A sally into the study of artificial intelligence leaves the uninitiated head buzzing with 'buzz' words, most of which have been borrowed from a different context, and whose meaning has been distorted in the process. These words are not necessary to a basic understanding of the subject and of its potential – a subject which is of considerable importance to future medical practice.

Calculating machines apply arithmetical rules to data that are supplied to them. Computer record systems contain patient records and add further data, using rules for record construction. Computerized prescribing uses a complex set of rules for writing and validating prescriptions, and interrogates a large structured drug database and the patient record in the process. *Artificial intelligence* (AI) programs achieve a still greater level of complexity and, when they interrogate a very large structured database that is authoritative and comprehensive in its field, an *expert system* is created.

Apart from the complexity of data and rules, the main differences between the ordinary computer program and artificial intelligence programs are as follows:

- Ordinary programs follow rules based on certainty – decisions are either right or wrong. With artificial intelligence programs, many rules are based on probability.
- With artificial intelligence programs, subdecisions are often interdependent, and alternative routes must be compared before a final path is selected.
- Advanced programming allows progression of the computing process in the absence of some items of data – the jigsaw picture can be completed even though one piece is missing.
- In artificial intelligence, phrases and link-words to build up a text commentary are mapped on to the paths taken by the rules. This text commentary may be displayed, and may be supported by references to the evidence on which the choice of path was based.
- An artificial intelligence program can be checked by a validating program, which tests the performance of its rules against a set of cases of known presenting features and outcome. The validating program will identify decision points in the original program at which changes might be made to improve performance – almost a self-learning function.
- Like the human brain, powerful computers can be configured not only to react to stimuli but to have dedicated storage subunits in which a bank of experience is built up as a result of exposure to a succession of stimuli. Cumulative changes progressively modify the computer's response to further stimuli (Neural Networks).

23.17 APPLICATIONS OF EXPERT SYSTEMS

Most developments of artificial intelligence in medicine have taken place in the USA.

Expert systems have been used to assist:

- systematic case investigation
- differential diagnosis and definitive diagnosis
- case management after diagnosis – therapy and monitoring
- teaching.

The clinical areas of application have included infectious disease, interpretation of pulmonary function, ventilator management, oncology, ophthalmology, coagulation disorders, rheumatology, serum electrophoresis, digitalis administration, and ventricular arrhythmias in coronary care. Using artificial intelligence techniques, electronic models of physiological systems have been created that allow the putative testing of therapeutic regimes to take place 'in vitro'. Conversely, AI methods applied to diagnosis often use models of abnormality rather than normality.

Differential diagnosis and patient management are procedures for which simpler computer protocols have been used. Expert systems offer a much more sophisticated approach which attempts to employ all the medical knowledge and decision pathways of a practising physician. The expert system either adopts a policy of making direct and positive recommendations, or may invite the doctor to enter clinical data and diagnostic and management decisions of his/her own, so as to be able to respond with constructive criticism (*critiquing system*).

Critiquing systems only provide comment if the decisions they offer are as good as, or better than, the physician's. As with other advanced expert systems, they back up their comment with references to source data. With critiquing systems, the risk–benefit ratio of each decision is weighed against alternatives. Critiquing helps doctors to identify areas of knowledge and judgement in which they are out of step with current medical practice, as mirrored in the system.

SUMMARY

- Idiosyncratic policies in practice put some patients at a disadvantage, and this can be avoided by the use of protocols. Protocols are more convenient and more efficient if they are lodged on computer rather than on paper. Computerized protocols capture, standardize, validate and encode data. Protocols that additionally analyse the captured data can produce probability listings for diagnoses which are often superior to those compiled by doctors.
- Computerized medical protocols now play an important part in the management of modern UK general practice. They need to be given dedicated storage space on the practice server ('the protocol library'), to be accessible by all users on the practice LAN, to dovetail with patient clinical records, and to be updated as upgrades become available.

Protocols are now a key instrument used in the imposition of clinical governance, and are assuming medicolegal importance.

- The three basic forms of medical computer protocol are those designed for data entry, those that assist in diagnosis, and those for patient management. Patient management protocols may be applied to preventive medicine, surveillance of chronic disease, or to the total control of a new case from the point of presentation onwards, taking into account symptoms and signs, investigations, treatment and referral.
- The development of decision support software for use in general practice has been piecemeal and has taken place in phases. Multilex's prescribing monitor, the Wolfson Computer Laboratory's designs for assisting the commissioning of pathology tests and improving shared care, and the EMIS User Group's data entry Templates were early developments in this field. AAH Meditel's SOPHIE, EMIS's MENTOR, and MCS's ISIS all produced more elaborate models bridging the gap between diagnosis and treatment.
- In 1994 the government tasked the NHSE with producing PRODIGY, with a view to controlling the efficiency with which NHS resources are used, and the pharmaceutical industry responded, enabling the development of MediDesk. Both these packages produced further refinement in the assistance given to doctors in reaching decisions on treatment, once a diagnosis had been made. PRODIGY has now been rolled out to all English NHS practices who wish to use it.
- The MENTOR package underwent further intensive development, and now offers support for decisions throughout the chain of processes required for patient management from the point of presentation onwards. It is now marketed jointly by EMIS and Oxford University Press as the Oxford Clinical Mentor.
- Preconsultative history-taking provides greater detail in family, social and past medical matters, but paper questionnaires are usually employed because of the slowness of the task. The method is used for hospital outpatients, and occasionally in general practice.
- Expert systems using artificial intelligence make decisions based on probability as well as certainty, can deal with incomplete data, accompany decisions with textual commentary, and use validation programs to test their own performance. Expert systems have been applied to case investigation, diagnosis, patient management, and teaching in a variety of clinical fields. Recommendations may

be made directly, or provided obliquely as constructive criticisms of the clinician's recorded decisions.

REFERENCES AND FURTHER READING

Adams I D, Chan M, Clifford P C 1986 Computer-aided diagnosis of acute abdominal pain: a multicentre study. British Medical Journal 293: 800

Asthma Working Party of the RCGP 1986 Protocol for the care of patients suffering from asthma. Royal College of General Practitioners, London

Board of Patient Care Magazine (ed) 1982 Patient care flow chart manual. Wadsworth International Group

Davenport P M, Morgan A G, Darnborough A 1985 Can preliminary screening of dyspeptic patients allow more effective use of investigative techniques? British Medical Journal 290: 217

De Dombal T 1981 Who needs a computer? World Medicine 30 May: 36

Dove G 1982 The computer doctor. Computer Update 1(4): 96

Engle R L, Davis B J 1963 Medical diagnosis: past, present and future. Archives of Internal Medicine 112: 512

Evans C R 1972 Psychological assessment of history taking. In: Abrams M A (ed) Spectrum 71. Butterworths, Sevenoaks: p. 9

Hampton J R, Harrison M R G, Mitchell J R A et al 1975 Relative contributions of history-taking, physical examination and laboratory investigation to diagnosis and management of medical outpatients. British Medical Journal 2: 486

Johnson P 1991 Flexible protocols at a touch of the keyboard. Practice Computing, November: 30

Levy M, Hilton S 1992 Asthma in practice. RCGP Enterprises, London

McDonald C J 1976 Protocol-based computer reminders, the quality of care and the non perfect ability of man. New England Journal of Medicine 295: 1351

Miller P L 1986 Expert critiquing systems. Springer Verlag, New York

Peters M 1992 To refer or not: the use of clinical decision support. Practice Computing, July: 19

Royal College of General Practitioners 1995 The development and implementation of clinical guidelines. Report from General Practice 26. RCGP, London

Scadding J G 1972 The semantics of medical diagnosis. Biomedical Computing 3: 83

Sheldon M 1982 The use of patient questionnaires in practice. Medicine in Practice: 320

Somerville S, Evans C R, Pobgee P J et al 1979 Mickie – experiences in taking histories from patients using a microcomputer. Proceedings of Medical Information. Springer-Verlag, Berlin: p. 713

Somerville S 1983 The electronic notebook. Practice Computing, August: 18

Waine C (ed) 1992 Diabetes in general practice. RCGP Enterprises, London

24 Portable computers – cooperative systems – rota compilation

24.1 PORTABLE COMPUTERS – INTRODUCTION

Unenviably, the USA hosts the world's highest litigation rate against the medical profession. It has been estimated that at any given point in time the American doctor will be facing an average of three pending law suits for negligence. Approximately half these cases will turn on the allegation that an important factor in the medical history was overlooked.

The trend towards the formation of larger practice units and larger out-of-hours service combines that has occurred in the UK in the last two decades makes it increasingly likely that a doctor will see a patient with whom s/he is unfamiliar, and whose medical record is not readily available. In this situation, any important details in the medical history that the patient forgets to mention may be overlooked by default. There need be no such hiatus. New computer technology can allow replicated patient records to be downloaded on to a portable machine at the surgery for use during routine home visits, and the need to provide records in an emergency can be met by downloading them over the telephone or radio-telephone to a remote unit.

The term portable or mobile computer should be taken to mean any form of computer that is designed to be carried around by the user as a personal accessory. Portable computers are of two principal types: A4-sized, briefcase-styled 'notebook' or 'laptop' computers with carrying handles, and pocket-book-sized 'palmtop' computers designed to fit the pocket or handbag. Input to both types may be by keyboard, screen sensing, or a mixture of both methods. In contrast with portable word processors, portable computers are not provided with integral printers.

Portable computers differ widely in cost, size, functionality and efficiency. They communicate with the practice's main computer in a variety of ways –

floppy disk, cable, infrared signal, direct radio signal, modem and PSTN, ISDN and terminal adapter, and radio telephone.

Portable computers now provide for the same broad range of global communications as desktops and, in addition to data telephony, include fax, short messaging services (SMS), e-mail, access to the Internet and bulletin boards, conferencing and the use of on-line services.

Computer access using radio telephony demands that all linkages and hardware in the chain of data transfer shall be fully compatible. As remote computers will be accessing the practice server and patient files stored upon it, it is essential that the GP system supplier should be closely, if not directly, involved in setting up a system's remote extension. The following additional components will be required to configure access:

- A server modem or terminal adapter and telephone line
- Communications software, including provision for file conversion and file transfer (most communication software packages now cope with all intermediary functions)
- A digital radiotelephone (analogue kits will be limited to voice traffic)
- A cellular data card or network adapter
- A portable computer with cabling or cradling connection to the radiotelephone kit
- The services of a cellular network provider.

A GSM compatible phone (Global System for Mobile Communications, which sets Europe-wide standards) uses encrypted digital data and includes provision for short messaging (SMS) of the characters which can be stored until retrieved.

Rapid enhancement is taking place in the field of portable computer development, which leaves in its wake a wide variety of functionality and price. A prospective purchaser should identify carefully the features required and budget available before 'shopping around'.

Assistance in funding portable computers has sometimes been obtainable from local out-of-hours development funds.

24.2 NOTEBOOK COMPUTERS – OVERVIEW

Designed and priced as a business accessory, the notebook computer was formerly known as the 'laptop'. Most models are built in the style of a small, thin briefcase, whose lid opens to rather more than a right angle and contains a liquid crystal display. The base of the case is occupied by the computer's main components, over the top of which is mounted a keyboard of sufficient size for touch typing.

As the notebook computer approximates to its desktop equivalent in terms of functionality, it may be used for a wide range of tasks in general practice, in addition to that of porting patient electronic records.

Most 'notebooks' weigh 2.5–3.5 kg and have displays of a diagonal dimension around 13 inches. They are more expensive, more prone to damage, and more likely to develop faults than their equivalent desktops. Although improvement continues to take place in battery design, batteries usually have to be recharged after 1½–4 hours use.

The portability of 'notebooks' makes them a prime target for thieves.

24.3 NOTEBOOK COMPUTERS – MAIN FEATURES

Before purchase, the specification of a notebook computer should be compared very carefully with a user's requirements.

Processors

Earlier 486 processors cannot cope with modern Windows applications, so a Pentium CPU is the only realistic choice of notebook for general practice. Until recently, 133 MHz units were the slowest CPUs fitted to new notebook models, but even these are now being phased out. It is wise to choose a processor such as an Intel mobile CPU, which has been designed specifically for portables, as this will confer greater power economy. Another useful option is to select a notebook with an upgradable CPU, cache, chipset and memory.

Memory

The minimum realistic requirement is 16 Mb, and memory should be upgradable.

Hard disk

Hard disk requirements will be determined by the number and size of the applications involved. A hard disk holding less than a gigabyte may well prove restrictive. The relative cost of a greater volume of storage is small nowadays, making it a good investment.

Preference should be given to an easily removable hard drive (some need unbolting), as this offers the advantages of potentially unlimited storage, and options for off-site data security and backup replication.

Display

Colour displays are markedly superior to monochrome for Windows applications.

Dual scan displays (also known as passive matrix or DSTN) have less vibrant colours and a smaller angle of view – i.e. they can only be seen 'square-on' – but are less power hungry and less expensive than their TFT counterparts. TFT (thin film transfer displays, also known as active matrix displays) have noticeably better colour reproduction and can be viewed over a wide angle.

A display's *resolution* is measured in terms of the number of light points per unit area (pixels) that it provides. Colour 'variability' is quoted in terms of the number of bits used to define each pixel's colour. The 'refresh rate' is the frequency with which light points have their charge renewed in order to maintain light emission.

Video RAM (VRAM) is the memory that supports the display. 1 Mb of VRAM supports 24-bit colour at 640×480 pixels; 2 Mb of VRAM support 24-bit colour at 800×600 pixels; 4 Mb of VRAM support 24-bit colour at all resolutions. A refresh rate of at least 72 Hz should be attained at any resolution to ensure viewing without optical fatigue.

Keyboard

The spacing and ease of use of a keyboard's keys should be checked. Function keys vary between models as regards their design and convenience. A *tracker ball* or *joystick* will be provided in relation to the keys, and the ease of use of these and of the cursor movement keys should be checked. Some notebooks have a clip-on external mouse, and some have a wrist rest at the front of the keyboard.

NCR makes a notebook computer without a formal keyboard whose data entry takes place via an electronic pen and sensitive screen (the NCR 3125 Notepad). A simulated keyboard, icons and menus are visible on the display when required, and upper and lower case handwriting are recognized, as are a range of penwritten signals ('gestures'). Output is viewed on the same screen.

Expansion

All notebooks can accept floppy disks and, in some, the floppy drive can be replaced by a CD-ROM drive when required.

The number of drive bays and card slots provided as standard varies between models. These allow access to networks, telephony, printers, graphics, encryption and CD-ROM drives. *Port replicators* and *docking stations* are pieces of equipment that can be purchased separately and bolted on. The former doubles the number of serial and parallel ports, and the latter allows access to a range of additional facilities, such as multimedia presentations on a larger monitor, additional disk drives, or the use of a full-sized keyboard.

The more facilities that the notebook uses, the shorter the battery life between charges, and software is available that shuts down those facilities that are not immediately required for a particular application.

Sound

Some notebooks are equipped with speakers and a microphone adjacent to the keyboard, Soundblaster software, and a 16-bit sound chip, so as to achieve Microsoft Sound System compatibility. Sound facilities provide for dictation and conference recording, with playback. An external microphone and speakers can also be supported.

Software

The sale of notebook computers is usually bundled with software such as Windows 98 or above, plus Microsoft Office or Lotus SmartSuite, which include word processing, spreadsheet, database management and fax. Other commercial packages may be added.

Power

Notebooks can take their power either from batteries (which require the use of a recharger) or AC transformers. All three of these items are relatively heavy.

It is important that the notebook should register its batteries' residual charge, and that the charger should be able to prevent an overcharge. If batteries are not drained before recharging they lose capacity, and if they are overcharged they deteriorate.

Lithium ion (Li-ion) batteries are now used in place of the less effective nickel metal hydride (NiMH) and the inefficient nickel cadmium (NiCad) alternatives. Some notebooks provide for two battery packs to be used alternately. Battery life between charges varies with the task in hand, and between models, from 1½–4 hours, although manufacturers usually claim longer effectiveness.

Other considerations

A carrying case, which is relatively cheap, helps to give added protection. Warranties should preferably offer 3 years of cover with a free replacement service during repairs. On-site repair warranties are expensive. Some suppliers offer a year's free insurance with purchase, and one supplier (Daewoo) offers a free upgrade service.

Subnotebooks

Subnotebooks are scaled down versions of notebooks. The diagonal dimension of their displays is usually 8.5–9.5 inches and their keyboards are proportionally smaller, which may make touch-typing difficult. So far, subnotebooks have proved neither significantly lighter nor cheaper than notebooks.

New or second-hand?

Designs tend to be upgraded even more frequently for notebooks than for PCs, so that second-hand models are easily available. As with used cars, knowledge of the provenance of a second-hand computer is all important, as is the availability of a guarantee and repair facilities.

24.4 PERSONAL DIGITAL ASSISTANTS – AN OVERVIEW

The paper-leafed, ring-bound pocket book, which was formatted to accommodate addresses, telephone numbers and personal schedules, and which became fashionable in the 1980s as the 'personal organizer', was displaced by its electronic counterpart during the 1990s. As ever-greater functionality was added to the latter's design, the resulting product came to resemble earlier versions of the notebook computer in all but size, and the name 'electronic personal organizer' was changed to 'personal digital assistant' or PDA.

Nowadays, PDAs have all the communication potential of notebook computers, and use specially modified versions of some of the principal software packages employed by larger computers. Despite all this, the PDA still fits into a coat pocket, though the scaled down computer has its disadvantages. Because the screen and keyboard are miniaturized, only a few lines of normal sized text can be read at a time, and touch typing is impossible. The PDA weighs and costs about one-fifth as much as a notebook computer, and runs on conventional batteries that last upwards of 10 hours. To date, PDAs have not been equipped with hard disks, and do not have to 'boot up'. The terms 'palmtop' and 'handheld' have sometimes been applied to pocket-sized computers that possessed more advanced functionality than the original electronic personal organizer, but all pocket-sized computers now come under the banner of PDAs.

24.5 PERSONAL DIGITAL ASSISTANTS – MAIN FEATURES

Input

As with notebooks, input to PDAs may be from a button keyboard, from a sensitive screen display, or from a mixture of both. PDAs that use a button-operated keyboard have cursor control keys and function keys. PDAs do not have tracker balls, joysticks or mice.

Screen-sensitive displays usually occupy most of the upper surface of a flat box which contains the computer, and such screens may be sensitive to finger touch, an inert stylus, or an electronic pen, depending upon the model. On sensitive screens, icons and menus allow selection, a simulated keyboard allows text input, and handwriting and drawn symbols ('gestures') may be recognized digitally. Drawings can be stored.

Standard functions

The standard functions of a PDA are: address book, diary, 'to-do' lists, clock with alarm, calculator and freestyle notepad.

Additional software

Newer PDAs use either Epoc 32, or Windows CE 1.0 or 2.0 operating systems, the latter being a specially adapted version of Windows 95. Application programs offer word processing, database management and spreadsheet facilities. Spellchecks, thesaurus, graphs, route planning, presentation software, mathematical and financial packages, drawing programs and games are also available, depending upon the model.

Screens

Screens are liquid crystal, may be monochrome or colour, and although all are small, still vary considerably in size and shape. The Casio BN 20 manages to accommodate 20 lines, each of 53 characters, but inevitably, character size has to be reduced to achieve this. PDA resolution is inferior to that found on quality notebooks.

Processor and memory

PDA processors are less powerful and slower than those of larger computers, and are designed specifically for power economy, so that applications such as multimedia cannot be supported. Operating systems and application programs are resident in ROM and so are instantly available when the equipment is switched on. Data interaction and temporary storage of user data takes place in RAM, of which most PDAs possess 256 Kb–2 Mb, usually expandable to 4 Mb by the use of extra cards. Standby mode, which is dependent upon a minimal, but continuous, supply of electricity, retains user data in RAM when other functions are in abeyance. The PDA is supported with a permanently resident lithium battery, which cuts in while the conventional batteries are being changed.

Communication

PDAs may communicate with PCs or Macintosh computers and networks, typically through cable, infrared port or telephony, in order to download subsets of files, or upload data. Medical records may thus be accessed from the patient's home, and PDA data may be backed up, printed and permanently stored in this way. PDAs also port directly to printers.

E-mail, the sending and receiving of faxes, and Internet access are available, and a Web browser may be provided. Voice and data telephony may be triggered from a list of contacts held on the PDA, and Short Messaging Services are available through GSM-compliant network providers.

Other considerations

PDAs can be run from mains transformers, but PDA battery life is considerably longer than that of notebook computers. The quality of sound produced by the microphone, speaker and recording facility attachments of PDAs has so far been poor.

Companies that are prominent in the marketing of PDAs are Apple, Casio, the GO Corporation, Hewlett Packard, Psion, Sharp, Toshiba and VPi.

24.6 COMBINED PORTABLE COMPUTERS AND CELLPHONES

The need for portable computers to link with mobile phone technology led to the development of combined equipment in the mid 1990s. Two of the earliest models were the MS-DOS-5.0–based Hewlett Packard Omnigo, in which the telephone and computer could be used separately or docked together, and the Nokia Communicator 9000, in which the two elements were incorporated into a single handheld device weighing 397 g. Both these models combined the facilities of a sophisticated PDA with the ability to communicate with a PC, send digital voice, data, and fax traffic, and access the Internet. A range of later models is now available.

Further miniaturization of PDAs and mobile phone technology has produced BT's wrist top communications tool, worn like an oversized wristwatch by a strap on the forearm. This equipment combines telephone, video phone, fax, computer, watch and paging device. The 'wrist top office' weighs around 120 g, and may be powered thermoelectrically by body contact.

24.7 PAGERS AND MOBILE PHONES – INTRODUCTION

Pagers and mobile phones enable doctors and nurses on home visiting rounds, or at leisure, to stay in contact with their operating base. Compact lightweight equipment can be carried on or near the person that will alert the recipient to the presence of an incoming call. The amount of data and type of response available to the recipient vary extensively with the level of service provided.

Pagers are restricted to incoming signals. Tone pagers provide only 'alert' signals, to which the recipient must respond by finding a telephone and calling base. Other types of pager and mobile phones have small LCD screens. Alphanumeric pagers display a message of limited length that has been relayed by an intermediary operator. Numeric pagers display a pre-agreed numeric code which the sender has keyed-in through a touch-tone telephone.

Mobile phones provide interactive voice contact through radio transmission, either between two mobile users or between a mobile user and the conventional telephone network.

Mobile phones can make use of the short messaging service. Some screen-based pagers, and most mobile phones, can accept messages relayed from the phone network company website that have been sent from computers with modems. Digital mobile phones are able to transmit data from computers, and thus access other computers, send faxes and e-mail, and link with the Internet (see portable computers, above).

24.8 PAGERS – SPECIAL FEATURES

- The main pager network companies are BT, PageOne and Vodazap, and coverage of the country is more complete than it is with mobile phones. Compared with the mobile phone's bundled first annual charge, a pager is much less expensive to own, but more expensive to call (up to £1.50 per minute from a phone box). The least expensive pagers come with an added monthly charge. Others are bought outright.
- Most pagers weigh less than 70 g and have clips to attach to clothing. Optionally, audio alert signals may be exchanged for vibration. Screen pager messages are stored, are limited in length and number, and are time-, or time/date-stamped. Brand-specific extras are appointment alerts, news flashes, football and lottery results, scrolling of messages, and time settings for on–off switching.
- Some screen pagers accept messages originating from computers with modems, sent through the network company website. In these cases, virus-checked motive software for the computer can be downloaded free of charge from the company website.
- In a 1998 survey, the Consumer Association found that a fifth of all pager calls sent were not received. No provision was made for notifying the sender of contact success or failure – a distinct disadvantage in a one-way communication system.

24.9 MOBILE PHONES – SPECIAL FEATURES

- The phone network companies are Cellnet and Vodaphone (which offer GSM services), Orange and One 2 One (which operate on PCN protocols), and TIW. Although coverage is extensive and serves well populated areas effectively, it has not yet spread to all remote country districts. In some areas that are covered, the signal may be defective, and some suppliers offer a 2-week free trial period in order to allow users to validate their services. While some handsets can be purchased from warehouse outlets such as Comet on a 'cash down' basis to which are added monthly fixed fees (or alternative types of 'top-up' voucher, some of which may be issued subject to a minimum level of use), most business is done by service providers (SPs). The latter are specialist retail outlets who subcontract with the network companies. SPs offer a range of tariffs in which the monthly fee and call rates are reciprocally related, and the handset is provided at a discount, with a binding annual contract. All told, mobile calls cost more than calls made from home, whether sending or receiving, and charges for Internet access may also be higher. The most prominent SPs are Cellcom, Martin Dawes, Motorola, Telco, Singlepoint V4 and Uniqueair.

- Having ensured that the area in which they wish to operate is covered by a network, and selected the tariff that most nearly favours their projected use of calls (frequency, distance, time and duration), prospective users must take into account any additional services on offer and purchase a handset appropriate to the chosen network company. Analogue networks are being phased out, and all four network companies offer digital networks that will allow faxes and data traffic. GMS companies also offer short messaging services (charged for sending but not for receiving).

- The mobile phone user is automatically informed if contact with the recipient has not been established. If the phone is switched off, incoming calls can be transferred to a voice mailbox. Some sound-alert signals can be adjusted for volume, some are unalterable and too quiet for use in noisy surroundings, and some can be transformed to provide a silent vibration.

- The handset has electronic memory, mostly in the form of an SIM card that contains details of the user's contract and phone number. The memory also stores a 'memory dials' facility from which autodial can be triggered by keying-in (or occasionally by speaking-in) a name code. Details of the last few calls made are stored, and may be retrieved, and the incoming number is displayed. Call duration may be displayed and may be pre-limited by the sender. The time and number of a missed incoming call may be displayed.

- Mobile phones are powered by NiMH or Li-ion batteries and should incorporate a battery life indicator. Battery life is optimally about 100 hours talk time and 350 hours on standby. Batteries are recharged through desktop, in-car, or trickle chargers. As batteries deteriorate if they are overcharged, a charge monitor and cut-off should be used.

- An interface card allows a digital mobile phone to transfer fax, e-mail, data and Internet access to a computer.

- The short messaging service (SMS) provides for up to 160-character text messages to pass to and from mobile phones. In addition to the numeric signals they transmit, the buttons on the phone pad can each be used to represent several alphabetical letters, and sequential key depressions will allow the user to cycle through the options, so that a particular letter can be reached and registered. SMS messages compiled in this way are charged for sending but received free. Messages from computers with modems can be sent free through network company websites to mobiles but, in order to do this, motive software from these websites must first be downloaded. SMS can also be sent through Internet 'gateways' to be found on the Web under the terms 'SMS' or 'text messaging'.

- Both GSM- and PCN-based network companies offer NHS GPs discounts under the NHS Mobile Phone Agreement, a 24-hour helpline service, and special insurance arrangements. All discounts are handled by Astec Communications. For further details contact one of the companies or phone the NHS-Wide Networking Infoline on tel: 0121 625 3838.

24.10 COOPERATIVE SYSTEMS – AN OVERVIEW

Rationalization and delegation of out-of-hours (OOH) services in the form of cooperatives and deputizing agencies have enhanced the lifestyle of general practitioners to a greater extent than any other factor since the inception of the National Health Service. These reforms have also improved response times and achieved high levels of customer satisfaction.

The compression of call handling, which is required to allow more intense but less frequent stints of duty at unsociable hours, would not have been possible without the use of call handling software and the computer-aided logistical control of a field force that is enabled by radio contact. Similar computerized management systems are already well established and in general use throughout other emergency services.

Since the Bolton GP Dr Krishna Korlipara initiated the GP cooperative movement in 1996, the development of cooperative computer systems has progressed so rapidly that they now constitute one of the most advanced applications of IT in the medical field. The majority of UK GPs now work in cooperatives. Adastra Software Ltd supplies around 70% of co-op sites, with smaller companies such as Knight Owl bringing up the rear.

24.11 COOPERATIVE SYSTEMS – THE LOGISTICS

The four primary steps in information handling for out-of-hours (OOH) service provision are:

- Call receipt
- Triage, prioritization, and message transmission to the field force
- Action recording
- 'End of duty' collation reporting to the patient's own GP the following morning (the so-called 'dawn report').

In addition, cooperative logistics require the provision of IT support for financial adjustments within the consortium, which take the form of colleague billing and fee payments, in order to redress any inequities in the share of duties undertaken by individual members. It is also usual to levy a membership fee.

Variations in working methods between cooperatives relate to the following:

- *Triage.* 25% of practices now employ nurses for this purpose, whereas others rely on trained receptionists. Increasingly, computerized protocols are used. In some co-ops triage is carried out by a GP.
- Many co-ops now use dedicated fleets of *cars* with chauffeurs.
- *Radio communication terminals* may be:
  - voice cell phones
  - electronic two-way messagers (such as Cognito) with small screens and printers using a fixed-cost radio-packet network (such as Paknet)
  - cell phones linked to small computers possessing keyboards, which use screens mounted on the car's dashboard or sun visor to display their data.
- *Action reports* may be handwritten on a triplicating notepad whose leaves are a suitable size for inclusion in a 'Lloyd George' wallet. One copy is given to the patient, one copy is faxed to the patient's GP, and one is retained at co-op headquarters. Electronic action reports countersigned by the doctor may be used. In future, electronic action reports will be relayed to the patients' own prac-

tices and autofiled in the patients' computer records after perusal by the GP.

24.12 ADVANCED COOPERATIVE SYSTEMS

A fully featured cooperative system is capable of providing the following facilities.

- Call handling software logs the details of patients and their requests, allows allocation and prioritization, logs times of all transactions to

Table 24.1 Call volume planning for cooperatives (Courtesy of Adastra Software). GP cooperative – incoming call volume reckoner (daily averages over one year – all co-op calls including advice and base referrals); calls assessed per 25 GPs in membership

Hour of receipt	Mon–Fri	Sat	Sun
From Midnight	0.78	0.85	1.03
1.00 am	0.60	0.57	0.69
2.00 am	0.48	0.54	0.59
3.00 am	0.45	0.45	0.46
4.00 am	0.39	0.49	0.43
5.00 am	0.44	0.39	0.57
6.00 am	0.31	0.36	0.86
7.00 am			1.82
8.00 am			5.14
9.00 am			6.71
10.00 am			5.00
11.00 am			4.43
12.00 pm			4.14
1.00 pm		3.50	2.75
2.00 pm		2.76	2.84
3.00 pm		2.76	2.92
4.00 pm		3.00	3.06
5.00 pm		2.97	3.39
6.00 pm		3.03	3.45
7.00 pm	2.79	2.75	3.36
8.00 pm	2.47	2.54	3.19
9.00 pm	2.14	2.43	2.44
10.00 pm	1.67	1.75	2.12
11.00 pm	1.00	1.18	1.18
Day total	13.51	32.32	62.56

For Bank Holidays reckon as follows:
1st day of Christmas = Sunday less 30%
2nd day of Christmas = Sunday plus 20%
3rd day of Christmas = Sunday plus 50%
4th day of Christmas (when it happens) = Sunday plus 90%
New Year's Day, Good Friday, Easter Monday = Sunday plus 25%
May and August holidays = Sunday plus 10%

create an audit trail, and dovetails with call despatch programs. A permanently displayed status bar shows the number of calls (with their respective priorities) waiting to be passed on, those pending action, and those completed. Computerized call handling and despatch are four times faster than methods that depend upon paper and cellphone.

- The system automatically identifies the incoming caller's telephone number and logs it.
- A bank of prerecorded comments from cooperative practices relating to patients likely to call is automatically interrogated by the system. Any such comments that can be matched with a new incoming call are appended to the new call data.
- A cumulative database of all past call details is compounded. All previous records relating to a patient making a new call are automatically appended to the new call data.
- A separate database of all voice conversations, date/time-stamped and with cross reference to serial log numbers, is compiled automatically.
- Once basic details have been logged by the telephonist, a trained nurse speaks to each caller to determine whether either a home visit or patient attendance at the primary care centre (PCC) should be recommended. If a visit is needed, the nurse allocates and logs a priority for it, which s/he also quotes to the patient. If attendance at the PCC is required, the nurse makes an appointment. If telephone advice will suffice, then s/he gives it and keeps a record of it. Guidelines for triage should be set for the co-op. Nurse triage software such as the TAS package has proved very successful (see Chapter 25).

- Tracking systems allow intermittent radio signals emitted from visiting doctors' vehicles to report their geographical position to the co-op's headquarters. With reference to postcodes, the most appropriate vehicle can thus be detailed to respond to the call.
- The call details and priority are beamed to the selected car, from which automatic acknowledgement of receipt is triggered.
- Route planning programs are available for use on the car's IT display that demonstrate direction, and comment on road conditions.
- The visiting doctor records the case's clinical, medication and disposal details, which are then relayed back to base and subsequently Read-coded.
- Collated contact details for each work shift for each practice are bundled electronically, and used to compile 'dawn reports'. Each practice receives its own dawn report across the locality intranet or NHSnet, peruses all contact details and autofiles them.
- Colleague billing and fee payments are computed each month and submitted to practices with lists of contacts, disposals and response times.
- All staff log on and off electronically, and payroll is computed.
- Night visit claims are prepared monthly for each practice by computer from logged data. Electronic transmission allows these to be checked by the practice and forwarded to the PPSA.
- Statistical analysis is used for search and report on: call incidence, calls by age groups, disposals, morbidity in relation to demographics, response times by priority, peaks and troughs, night visits, and lists of frequent callers by practice.

Fig. 24.1 Triage outcome screen: Adastra cooperative system

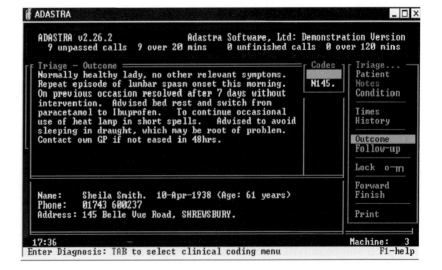

```
ADASTRA                                                        _□X
ADASTRA v2.26.2              Adastra Software, Ltd: Demonstration Version
  9 unpassed calls   9 over 20 mins    0 unfinished calls   0 over 120 mins

Triage - Outcome                              Codes    Triage...
Normally healthy lady, no other relevant symptoms.     Patient
Repeat episode of lumbar spasm onset this morning.   N145.    Notes
On previous occasion resolved after 7 days without           Condition
intervention.  Advised bed rest and switch from
paracetamol to Ibuprofen.   To continue occasional          Times
use of heat lamp in short spells.   Advised to avoid        History
sleeping in draught, which may be root of problem.
Contact own GP if not eased in 48hrs.                       Outcome
                                                            Follow-up

                                                            Lock  o─┐

Name:    Sheila Smith.  10-Apr-1938 (Age: 61 years)        Forward
Phone:   01743 600237                                       Finish
Address: 145 Belle Vue Road, SHREWSBURY.
                                                            Print

17:36              _                             Machine:   3
Enter Diagnosis: TAB to select clinical coding menu        F1-help
```

Fig. 24.2 Outstanding call screen: Adastra cooperative system

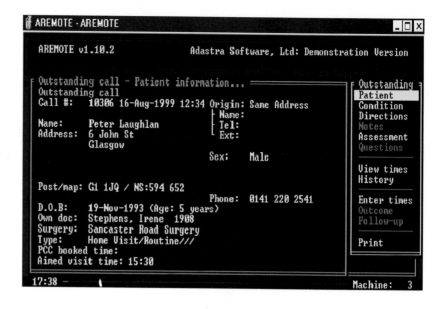

Audit of a co-op's activities should be used as an aid to improving standards, and should take into account government and health authority guidelines. Expenditure should also be audited, with particular regard to the use of manpower, which absorbs 80% of a co-op's costs.

- Monthly and annual accounts are prepared by computer.
- Rota duty schedules are best compiled by computer, for which several efficient software packages are available (see below).
- Adequate security should be provided in the form of power-failsafe telephones, UPS, backup, security printout, antivirus software, and encryption of transmitted data.
- Support should comprise the provision of adequate manuals, contracts that include maintenance and upgrade provision, a helpline, training seminars and training packs, and user groups.
- Methods of maximizing co-op income should be explored, such as renting out the primary care centre during the daytime, using the call centre for community nursing or social services, and collecting all income on time. Economies are derived from bulk purchase of drugs and expendables. The National Association of GP Co-operatives has organized a series of exclusive discounts for GPs setting up cooperatives, which include costs of hardware, software and medicolegal insurance for non-medical staff.
- A computer file of patient complaints, and the cooperative management's responses to them should be maintained.

Government quality guidelines for cooperatives

- A doctor on duty should be at least a trainee GP.
- Co-op doctors should send medical reports to the patients' own GP as soon as possible following service delivery.
- Co-op members should be told if staff employed by the organization are insured, and if they use protocols.
- Co-ops must set out and use guidelines on dealing with patient requests and home visits.
- Requests for care should be recorded separately from clinical records for the purpose of response analysis.
- Complaints about the service should be logged, and action taken in conjunction with the patient's own GP.

In addition, health authorities will have the right to investigate co-op (or deputizing agency) standards and, subject to LMC concurrence, will have the right to stop GPs using an unsatisfactory service.

24.13   ROTA COMPILATION

Before computerization, the compilation of the out-of-hours duty roster was a thankless task. Suspicions of inequity often followed its preparation, and a succession of revisions was demanded by the discovery of factors that had previously been overlooked.

The degree of difficulty experienced in computing a roster is proportional to the number of its

Fig. 24.3a Rota compilation. Allocation of shifts for duty on the practice reception desk; allocations can be performed automatically provided availabilities and templates are available (Easy Rota Staff Scheduler, courtesy of PCTI Solutions)

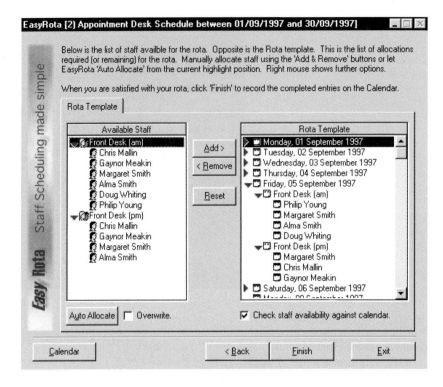

Fig. 24.3b Rota compilation. Retrieval of prepared schedules (Easy Rota Staff Scheduler, courtesy of PCTI Solutions)

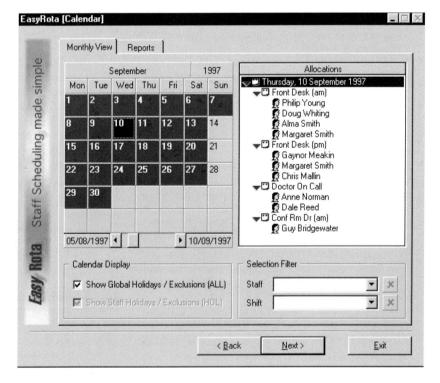

participants. Consequently, the needs of a large cooperative can only be met realistically by a computer program. IQ Software's Rota Master can cope with an unlimited number of doctors in a cooperative and is highly sophisticated. Smaller packages such as EMS's Rotashift are of more limited scope, cost a great deal less, and are suitable for smaller cooperatives or use within practices.

Rotashift from EMS, 59 Bolingbroke Road, Cleethorpes DN35 0HF (tel: 01472 694954) runs on MS-DOS, Windows 3.1 or Windows 95, minimally requires a 386 PC with 4 Mb of RAM, and costs about £200 plus VAT.

The program can cope with up to 99 rota members, and up to four shifts a day whose timing is determined by the user. Shifts are allocated per full-time doctor, with half shares for half-timers. The roster is constructed as a single computation, with amendments being made mutually at participant level by individual members.

Schedules can be printed out for the integrated roster or for individual participants, and provisions can be built in to accommodate shifts from which individuals must be excepted. There is a helpline.

Rota Master from IQ Software (UK Ltd), Spring Wood House, 12 Stocksmoor Road, Midgley, Wakefield, West Yorkshire WF4 4JQ (tel: 01924 217693) runs on Windows 95 or NT (a Windows 3.1 version is also available), requires a 75 MHz PC with 16 Mb of RAM and 30 Mb of available hard disk space, and is priced on a sliding scale around £1500–2000 plus VAT that is determined by the number of participating doctors. There is also an annual maintenance fee.

The package can handle any number of participants, whether as an aggregate or split between several cooperatives and constituent practices. Shifts may be of any duration and number. Equitability can be calculated per participant or per practice, and can be based on the doctor's whole-time or part-time commitment to practice, on list size or on the number of partners per practice.

Rota Master splits the compilation of the roster into two phases. Initially, a block of shifts is allocated to each practice as a whole. Beside each practice's shift block there is a series of empty slots, each of which represents an individual shift. Partners within the practice must then agree and enter individual names within all slots so as to satisfy the total practice commitment. Subsequently, each individual whose name has been entered has the option to offer to depute the shift if someone else wishes to take it on.

In the second phase, those participants wishing to take over shifts from those seeking to depute them register their choice, and the final version of the roster is produced.

A sophisticated program is employed to maintain a balanced distribution of frequency and type of shift between participants. This program can be varied by weightings introduced by the user. Macros are available that enable the inclusion of positive or negative preferences, and the exception of shifts that the individual is unable to fulfil. Time limits may be applied to all modifications.

Schedules can be printed out for the whole rota, for constituent co-ops, for each practice, or for each participant, together with a statistical breakdown of shares and any weightings introduced. Reminders for individual doctors can be produced. All reports can be posted, faxed or e-mailed.

Rota Master integrates with both Adastra and Knight Owl cooperative software. A helpline is provided.

Other packages

- DR Duty (Analytical Databases Ltd, tel: 07771 960074)
- Easy Rota (PCTI Solutions, tel: 01977 690977)

SUMMARY

- Litigation for negligence frequently hinges on the allegation that an important fact of a patient's medical history has been overlooked. The trend towards the formation of larger GP combines increases the chance that a patient's full history will be unknown to the newly attending doctor. Computer records need to be accessible, and can be provided on portable computers, either by a cabled download from the practice server prior to the day's home visits, or through radiotelephony on an *ad hoc* basis out of hours.

- Portable computers are of two basic designs: notebook computers are the size of a small briefcase, have most of the functionality of a desktop PC, are more expensive than their PC counterparts, can run from mains transformers or batteries, but have a relatively short battery life between charges. Personal digital assistants (PDAs) are small enough to fit the coat pocket or handbag, and have reduced functionality as compared with a PC, partly because they have no hard disk. The miniaturization required of the PDA screen and keyboard also limits their functionality. The only way to secure a permanent record of user data on a PDA is to download them.

- Portable computers can communicate with a server through floppy disk, cable, infrared signal, and radio or conventional telephony. External communications can include fax, short messaging services, e-mail, Internet access, conferencing and bulletin boards. All remote access by terrestrial telephony requires modems and communication cards (or their counterparts), communications software including file handling, and a telecommunication services provider. Radiotelephony additionally requires the use of a digital cellular telephone in conjunction with the remote computer. As all links in the chain must be fully compatible, and users need to access the practice server and practice records, the GP system supplier must be closely involved in installing and maintaining remote access.

- Pagers and mobile phones are conveniently small and portable pieces of radio equipment that enable their users to keep in touch with their operational base. Cover is almost nationwide. Pagers are restricted to incoming signals, and tone pagers provide only 'alert' signals, to which the recipient must respond by finding a telephone and calling base. Alphanumeric pagers have a small screen, which displays a short message that has been relayed by an intermediary operator. Numeric pagers display a preagreed numeric code that the sender has keyed in through a touch telephone.

- Mobile phones provide interactive voice contact through radio transmission, either between two mobile users or between a mobile user and the conventional telephone network. There are a few rural areas where mobile phones cannot operate. Only digital radio telephones can transmit computer data. Having purchased a mobile telephone, services are paid for in various ways, which include regular subscriptions, air time tariffs or 'top up' vouchers. It is more expensive to transmit calls by radio than by the conventional telephone network. There are five cellular phone network companies: Cellnet, Vodaphone, Orange, One 2 One and TIW.

- Sophisticated computer systems are required by GP cooperatives, and these must provide for call receipt; triage, prioritization and message transmission to the field force; action recording; 'end of duty' collation reporting to the patient's own GP; and billing of, and fee payment to, participants.

Cooperatives often employ nurses for triage, and chauffeur-driven cars for out-of-hours visiting. Triage classifies incoming calls according to whether a home visit, an attendance at the primary care centre or advice only is required, and in the last case the nurse provides advice and records it. Advanced co-ops now equip their cars with cell phones linked to small computers possessing keyboards, which use screens mounted on the car's dashboard or sun visor. Co-ops must be aware of, and comply with, government and HA guidelines.

- Rota compilation is a thankless task if performed manually, and is much more simply undertaken on a computer. Rota compilation packages vary considerably in price and functionality, but a large cooperative will need to choose one powerful enough to cater for all its participants and permutations.

FURTHER READING

Anaoka M 1996 The masters of electronic arts. Doctor 15 August: 34

Bean S 1997 Best buy notebook computers. Medeconomics, August: 45

Bromley P 1998 Think twice before you purchase a notebook PC. GP 10 April: 103

Cembrowicz S 1996 Is palmtop computer out-of-hours answer? Pulse 7 September: 66

Consumers Association 1998 Palm reading and writing. Which? April: 30–33

Consumers Association 1998 Pagers vs mobiles. Which? May: 16–23

Kennedy S 1996 Best buy palmtop. Medeconomics, February: 70–71

Mimnagh C 1997 How to choose between a laptop and a palmtop. GP 26 September: 79

Newsome C 1994 Portables join the age of the Pentium. PC User, November: 50–52

PC Magazine 1995 PC Magazine Guide to Mobile Computing

PC Magazine 1998 Mobile Pentium II notebooks

PC User Magazine 1994 Lab test: high-end portables. PC User, October/November: 134–171

Practice Computing Magazine 1996 The Nokia Communicator. Practice Computing, Autumn: 8

Practice Computing Magazine 1996 The peripatetics of GP computing. Practice Computing, Winter: 18

Ramster C 1997 Choose the best mobile phone. Medeconomics, April: 69–71

Practice computer facilities for nurses and patients

25.1 PRACTICE NURSES NOW NEED TO BE COMPUTER LITERATE

The past two decades have witnessed the steadily increasing contribution, importance and responsibility of the practice nurse. To the 'handmaiden's' tasks of dressing application, venepuncture, ear syringing and urine testing have been added those more highly specialized skills of sharing care in chronic disease management, running prevention clinics on an autonomous basis, and being the first point of contact for acute disease management. Progressively, nurses are becoming the gatekeepers of the NHS, manning NHS Direct call centres, and using triage to determine how cooperative out-of-hours calls should be managed and whether requests for same-day practice consultations or visits should be conceded. With special training and protocols, nurses can even run their own primary care consultation sessions. When the overall management of a new general practice in Chellaston, Derbyshire, was vested in the practice nurse, with the salaried doctor playing second fiddle, shock waves were felt throughout the establishment, but the development was merely an extrapolation of an underlying trend.

The expansion of the nurse's role has called for additional training in the fields of prescribing, triage, family planning, travel medicine and minor illness. It also requires that the boundaries of medicolegal responsibility are redefined. There is now ample evidence that delegation to nurses saves doctors' time, makes the nurse's task more fulfilling and is well received by patients. In particular, triage has halved the home visiting rate and the same-day consultation rate, given that satisfactory alternative forms of help were made available. From the government's point of view it has proved to be an economy to have more general practice work delegated to nurses, given the higher pay scales that doctors command.

The creation of Nurse Practitioner and Nurse Consultant grades serves to emphasize the increasing importance of the nurse's role in general practice. The practice nurse now requires to access the practice computer system as extensively as does the doctor (Table 25.1) and it is important that the expertise needed in order to do so should be acquired during a nurse's formal training.

25.2 COMPUTER FUNCTIONS USED BY PRACTICE NURSES

Although the extent to which computers are used by nurses varies considerably from practice to practice, the practice nurse and nurse practitioner will probably need to be familiar with the following:

- Supplier software which accesses the consultation appointment list and the clinical record for patients on that list, and which provides the facility for 'toggling' between the two
- Condition orientated records, the data entry and patient management protocols related to the chronic condition being supervised, and the repeat medication routine that dovetails with these
- The structure of preventive medicine records, the use of opportunistic prompts for preventive procedures, and the mechanism of recall using search and mailmerge
- Data entry routines for registration checks, preventive procedures, and family planning, with the construction of electronic claims relating to these services and the ability to check target achievement levels
- Travel medicine software (such as *Traveller*)
- Computerized protocols for minor illness management

Table 25.1 A practice nurse's roles and the related use made of the practice computer system

	Service provided	Associated computer use required
Dressing Room	Apply dressings, syringe ears, venepuncture, test urine	Patient clinical record
Shared care of chronic disease	Diabetes, asthma, hypertension, obesity, epilepsy, psychiatry, warfarin monitoring, family planning and HRT	Condition orientated patient records, shared care protocols, repeat medication
Autonomous clinics	Immunization, cervical cytology	Data entry screens for Imm & CC Target achievement checks & claims
	Well man (WM), well woman (WW)	Opportunistic prevention, recall Data entry screens for WM & WW clinics
	Registration checks	Registration programs Claims
	Travel medicine	Travel package, e.g. 'Traveller', claims
	Other screening procedures	Appropriate data entry screens
Acute illness consultation	Minor illness management Referral of cases if outside remit	Protocols Clinical records Prescribing software Nurse prescribing subset in practice formulary
Triage	For cooperatives For requests for same-working-day visits and consultations For NHS Direct	Triage software, e.g. TAS, call handling software Practice protocol DoH-licensed US triage software

- Practice system prescribing software, and the use of the nurse prescribing subset of the practice formulary
- Practice protocols, the more complex of which will need to be computerized, for the triage of 'same-working-day' visits and consultations
- For use in the management procedures of GP cooperatives:
  - Call triage software such as the Telephone Advice System (TAS), a sophisticated computer application dealing with over 130 disease presentations. TAS runs on a 100 MHz Pentium PC with 16 Mb of RAM, using Microsoft FoxPro for Windows. At the end of a phase of questions, a summary, conclusions and treatment are suggested, and a report is produced (for enquiries, tel: 01923 829743).
  - Call scheduling software such as that provided by Adastra or Knight Owl
- For the purposes of NHS Direct, the Department of Health has licensed an extensively tested US software package based on best evidence and using a framework of algorithms. The line of enquiry starts with a symptom, which prompts a series of

questions directed initially towards eliminating the most serious possibilities. If this can be done, further questions are posed whose answers will lead to a conclusion.
- Portable computers can be taken on home visits by nurses in order to use data entry protocols for registration checks for patients over 74 years of age, for monitoring elderly patients who are mentally or physically infirm, or for domiciliary midwifery. Patient records are downloaded from the practice server for use in the field, and the amended portable version is subsequently uploaded when the nurse returns to the medical centre. Community nurses have used a similar configuration with portables downloading the day's schedule of work for each nurse from the central Community Health Services server, together with the appropriate patient records. Amended records are subsequently uploaded to the server. The 'Minimum Data Set' assessment system using button/touchscreen portables to record medical, behavioural, dietary, physical and social factors in elderly patients in residential homes was developed in the USA to quantify

dependency and determine care charges. 18 recommended care protocols backed by research evidence are automatically triggered if appropriate. MDS is now being used in the UK.

25.3 TRIAGE AND MEDICAL HELP LINES

Experience with medical help lines in the USA and Scandinavia prompted trials of their use in the UK. Specifically trained nurses take calls from patients and, working to strict protocols, give treatment advice if they deem this to be appropriate. If verbal advice would not suffice, they recommend referral to an alternative agency, which may be a GP's routine surgery, an out-of-hours primary care centre, an A&E department, an emergency dentist or pharmacist, or the social services or community mental health team. By siphoning off calls that do not require a higher professional level of expertise, nurse triage seeks to bring about a more appropriate and economical use of all health services, but particularly those provided by GPs and A&E departments.

25.4 THE AVAILABILITY OF PAST MEDICAL HISTORY DURING THE TRIAGE PROCESS

Nurses advising from a practice will have the relevant patient's computer record to guide them when assessing the case. Nurses working from cooperative or deputizing agency control rooms have cumulative databases of past calls to which they can refer. Other agencies do not, as a rule, have the benefit of past records, and this may be a serious disadvantage.

A range of agencies that are unrelated to the patient's general practice now offer *ad hoc* medical advice over the telephone. These include:

- Health Call, which offers advice on 200 health topics, with telephone calls charged at 50p per minute on 09001 600600
- Commercial answering service agencies, which contract with cooperatives and group practices to filter incoming calls from their respective patients – such calls are usually charged at local call rates: Cambridge Answering Service (on fax: 01223 214899); Border Medical Answering Service (on tel: 01244 355005)
- NHS Direct, the government sponsored national scheme which offers free medical advice over the telephone, and has call centres located at sites such

as ambulance trusts and GP cooperatives. Typically, cooperative doctors on call are used as medical referees and accessed through mobile phones. The NHS Direct national telephone number is 0845 1888, later to transform to the '888' system. NHS Direct advice is also obtainable over the Internet.

25.5 REQUIREMENTS OF THE COMPUTERIZED TRIAGE PROTOCOL

In 1997, following the death of an infant whose parents had been given prior advice by a cooperative nurse, recommendations were made that triage protocols should include a special paediatric section, that nurses should employ questionnaires that use and record both positive and negative questions, and that detailed notes or, preferably, voice recordings should be kept for further reference. Patients should always be given the option to phone back later, and should be given clear instructions as to the circumstances that should prompt them to do so.

A helpful resource pack for professionals on conducting telephone advice has been prepared by the Guy's–King's–St Thomas' Medical School. It can be obtained from Marilyn Peters, OOH Project, Department of General Practice and Primary Care, GKT Medical School, Weston Education Centre, Cutcombe Road, London SE5 9PJ.

25.6 NURSE PRESCRIBING

The Medical Defence Union advises nurse members to use written protocols for the administration of medicines, if nurses are expected to administer prescription-only medicines without the doctor first seeing the patient. The venue for nurse prescribing should be limited to a hospital or a health centre and not extend to a private practice.

A prescribing protocol needs to conform with the legal requirements of the Medicines Act 1968, as well as the requirements of the UK Central Council as set out in its Standards for Administration of Medicines 1992.

In 1997 the Department of Health commissioned a review of the prescribing, supply, and administration of medicine by health professionals, in association with which it required an interim report on the supply and administration of medicines by nurses under group protocols. The review team defined such a group protocol as 'a specific written instruction for

Table 25.2 Nurse prescribing protocol (from Interim Report to Ministers from a DoH-commissioned review on the supply and administration of medicines by nurses and other health professionals under Group Protocols, 1998 – source: *Journal of the Medical Defence Union*)

Clinical condition to which the protocol applies	Characteristics of authorized staff	Description of treatment	Management and monitoring of group protocols
Clear definition of the clinical condition, including criteria for confirming it	Details of necessary professional qualification	Name, dose and route of medicine to be supplied under the protocol	Names of professionals drafting protocols
Description of the additional clinical criteria which mean a patient can be treated using the protocol	Specialist qualification, training and experience necessary and relevant to condition to be treated	Follow-up treatment required	Names of professional advisory groups which have approved the protocol
Description of the criteria which exclude a patient from being treated using the protocol	Requirements for continued training of staff treating patients under protocol	Advice, including any written advice to be given to the patient	Name of the manager/employer who has authorized the use of the protocol
Action to be taken for patients who are excluded		Instructions for identification and management of possible adverse outcomes	Identification of the health professional providing the treatment, the patient and the medicine being administered
Action to be followed for patients who do not wish to be treated under the protocol		Arrangements for referral to medical advice	The protocol should be dated
		Facilities and supplies to be available	A review date should be set after which the protocol will no longer be valid
		Details of treatment records required, including a clear audit trail	
		Special consideration for patients receiving any other medication	

the supply or administration of named medicines in an identified clinical situation'. The findings of the Review's interim report were summarized by the MDU and are shown in Table 25.2.

It would be appropriate to use the criteria listed by the MDU as a template upon which to construct a nurse prescribing protocol for each clinical situation for which responsibility is delegated. The template and all protocols should be stored on the practice and PCG+T computers.

A dedicated subset of the practice or group formulary must be allocated for nurse prescriber use and this subset must clearly distinguish those drugs which the nurse can authorise on her/his own initiative in case management (as 'independent prescriber') from those specifically deputed from a management plan already authorised by a doctor.

25.7 INFORMATION TECHNOLOGY FOR PATIENTS

The necessary brevity of the average GP consultation restricts the amount of verbal health information that can be imparted by the doctor, and such instructions as they do receive are only partially retained by most patients. The health educational deficit needs to be made good by opening up other channels of communication. A number of different methods are available. Where appropriate, some representative examples are given.

Rack-mounted, generic, preprinted leaflets
Generic health information leaflets, usually provided free by health agencies or pharmaceutical companies, are frequently offered in the reception area of doctors'

surgeries. A Mori survey, carried out to assess their usefulness, found that the number of topics covered by these leaflets varied, but was limited to a maximum of 60, and that the option to take a leaflet was exercised by a mere 15% of patients.

Advice leaflets on conditions specific to the consultation

At the completion of consultation, the doctor uses the practice computer to print patient instructions linked to the diagnosis made, and sometimes also to the treatment given (see also Chapter 22).

Audio tapes, video tapes and telephone helplines specific to the condition

A wide range of these facilities is offered by patient self-help groups, pharmaceutical companies and medical Royal Colleges in relation to specific conditions (see also the section on helplines above).

A particularly interesting form of telephone-based behavioural therapy has been developed at the Bethlam and Maudsley Trust, in which the patient is given a PIN number by the doctor to access a remote computer. Using the touch-tone telephone keypad and a 24-hour freephone line, the patient inputs codes for clinical information in response to voice-mediated instructions. The computer then sets a task, on completion or failure of which the patient calls again for further instructions. The doctor receives a printout of data that maps out the patient's state of mind, and these include warnings of any suicidal tendencies.

The approach is suitable for treating mild or moderate obsessive–compulsive disorder and depression, and can be extended over many weeks. Relapse rates are lower than with drugs and the method has no side effects. (For further information, contact Behaviour Therapy Steps, tel: (020) 7919 3366.)

Diskettes and CD-ROM disks (see also Chapter 19)

Patient self-help groups and pharmaceutical companies produce numerous diskettes on specified conditions related to their field of interest.

Doctor in the House (Dr Hilary Jones) is an interactive medical encyclopaedia on CD-ROM to be used by patients at home. It offers a symptom analysis questionnaire, with provision of advice about the condition identified as likely to be the cause, healthy lifestyle advice, a child development section, and emergency medical care, together with other useful material (Windows; Global Software Publishing Ltd, tel: 01480 496575, and high street outlets).

Ticket Window is basically a hotel, travel ticket and car hire booking program loaded from diskette, which also provides access to travel health data (PC/Mac and modem; Minerva On-Line Access, tel: (020) 8402 3350).

Anxiety Self Help and *Computer Assisted Relapse Management for Alcoholics* are diskette- and PC-based programs for use by patients. Each uses a database of coping strategies and a question and answer format. They have been developed by Dr Fred Yates of the Northern Regional Health Authority's Alcohol and Drug Addiction Unit.

The *Patient Wise* diskette contains clear explanations of over 300 conditions and enables doctors to display and print out elaborative information for patients (DOS/Windows; John Wiley & Sons).

The *Oxford PILs* directory contains over 200 patient information leaflets and a list of 500 self-help groups from which the doctor can print out selections for patients (see also Chapter 22).

The Internet (see also Appendix A)

The following websites are of general health interest to patients:

- Canadian Health Network, http://www.hwc.ca/ (in French and English)
- Duke Community and Family Medicine Home Page, http://dmi-www.mc.duke.edu/cfm/cfmhome.html
- Guide to Women's Health Issues, http://asa.ugl.lib.umich.edu/chdocs/womenhealth/womens_health.html
- Healthwise, http://www.columbia.edu/cu/healthwise
- Worldguide: Health and Fitness Forum Welcome Page, http://www.worldguide.com/Fitness/hf.html

An increasing number of general practices and Health Trusts are now launching websites, which are targeted at patients as well as other healthcare professionals.

25.8 KIOSK TECHNOLOGY

Computer terminals employing touchscreens or keyboards for public use have been set up in the waiting areas of doctors' surgeries, and in pharmacies. These mirror the use of computer kiosk technology for sales promotion at sites within hotels, shopping malls and railway stations.

At the outset of its development, the cost of kiosk technology was greater than could be justified for its use as an adjunct in general practice. However, prices are falling for some kiosk packages and, being screen-based, these information systems offer the prospect of offsetting costs by selling associated advertising space.

The following kiosk systems have been operational in general practice or pharmacy settings:

- In-Touch With Health: touchscreen provision of patient information on medical conditions, surgical operations, prevention, travel health, NHS services and patient support groups (Brann Ltd, Phoenix Way, Cirencester GL7 1RY, tel: 01285 644744)
- the CALM Computer Assisted Lifestyle Package: a keyboard-based patient questionnaire on lifestyle, health, stress, nutrition and fitness, with printout of interpretation (CALM Corporation (UK) Ltd, tel: 0161 428 5529)
- the Hollings and Conatry Health Information System: keyboard-based display and printout of data on medical and surgical topics, local health services and self-help groups (East Surrey HA and South Thames region)
- the ELFIN Health Information System: based on the use of a simplified keyboard, a broad range of health topics is covered, and opportunistic prevention is promoted. The interactive software monitors the collective use made of the system to allow audit of health concerns in the practice population (Professor Ian Stanley, Department of General Practice, University of Liverpool)

- the INFOTRAC Computerized Health Library: an American CD-ROM and keyboard-based system that offers patients an on-screen questionnaire, covers a wide range of health issues and provides patient advice leaflets; the system was trialled by Southampton University in a local practice and local hospitals in 1994
- A Question of Health: an on-screen, keyboard-and-PC-based lifestyle questionnaire with print-out of scores (Dr Ian Thomson, Beechtree Surgery, Selby, North Yorkshire, tel: 01757 703933, with Glaxo sponsorship)
- Born Santé: an interactive and informative touch-screen computer system from which pharmacy customers can obtain healthcare information (a Unichem Development)
- PharmAssist: a touchscreen-based system sited adjacent to a hospital pharmacy that instructs patients in why, how, when and how long to take their specified medication. The pharmacist keys in the appropriate medication code and the patient selects a national flag to determine which language will be used. A game-style program appraises the patient's assimilation and an instruction leaflet is printed (Lewisham Hospital Pharmacy, London SE13 6LH, tel: (020) 8333 3205).

26 Security

26.1 OVERVIEW

When the Gulf War against Iraq was imminent, the entire Allied campaign was jeopardized by the theft of a loaded computer that had been left in the unattended car of a senior British Air Force officer. The cost of the loss of the portable computer could have been measured in four figures, but the value of the data in money and lives was incalculable. Paper records are only destroyed *en masse* by fire – a mercifully rare event – and can be read in ones or twos by the unauthorized if carelessness permits. With computer records, all the eggs are in one vulnerable basket. Fire, theft, wholesale corruption or destruction due to system malfunction, viruses, hacking, and global unauthorized disclosure are the compounded risks of which the computer record user must be acutely aware.

The need for practices to take system security seriously is further reinforced by the system suppliers, who unanimously and specifically disclaim all responsibility for backup, insurance, Data Protection Act (DPA) notification for registration, clean electricity supplies, virus prevention and the protection of electromagnetic media. On pain of being prosecuted under the DPA, and being sued for damages by patients, practices are made legally responsible for the accuracy and protection of personal record data.

It has been rightly claimed that computer records are more secure than their manual counterparts, but this can only hold true if punctilious training, staff discipline, and security procedures have been implemented.

In 1994, the National Computing Centre (NCC) published the results of a survey of IT security breaches that it had undertaken in conjunction with the DTI and ICL. The report disclosed that during the 2 years prior to the survey, 850 of Britain's major companies had together shared an estimated £1.2 billion loss as the result of electronic fraud or failure. Fraudulent transactions proved to be the largest single headache in the business computing world, a risk unlikely to be experienced in medicine, save in the context of e-banking or commissioning, but all the other risks listed by the survey can and do apply (Table 26.1).

During the period surveyed, half the respondents had experienced system failure, one-third network failure, and one-third reported virus intrusion. In 2 years, the rate of theft had doubled, and the victimized were revisited by thieves (who knew the equipment would have been newly replaced) an average of three times. GP surgeries are at risk of burglary, not only by reason of their computer equipment, but because they are a source of drugs and prescription pads.

26.2 FIRE, WATER, AND LIGHTNING DAMAGE

Although these risks should be covered by a specific computer insurance policy, precautionary measures to be taken by the practice must include:

- Implementing fire regulations and the recommendations of the local Fire Prevention Officer. Power cables should be checked by a qualified electrician. A fireproof safe should be installed to house backup tapes and copies of all working programs. If a sprinkler system has been installed, waterproof dust covers should be applied to equipment overnight.
- Where a possibility of flooding exists, equipment should, wherever possible, be sited above levels of threat
- An exterior lightning conductor should be fitted, power circuitry should be adequately earthed, and

Table 26.1 Summary of computing security risks and countermeasures

	Counter-measures	Insurance	Maintenance contract
Physical risks			
Fire	Implement fire prevention officer's recommendations. Check cables	+	–
Water damage	If possible site equipment above level of threat of flooding. Waterproof dust covers at night	+	–
Lightning	External lightning conductor, check earthing of power cables, surge proof uninterruptible power supply (UPS)	+	–
Other accidental damage			
Theft or malicious damage	Implement crime prevention officer's recommendations for premises and equipment	+	–
Power failure or interference	UPS, consider emergency generator for large installations, separate ring main for system	–	–
Network failure	Network management/security software	–	+
Hardware failure	Adequate maintenance contract	–	+
Degradation of magnetic media	Diskette, hard disk and tape discipline	+	–
Logical risks			
Hacking; tapping telephone lines, branch surgery landlines or cellular telephone networks	Firewall, router, encryption, modem hygiene	–	–
Unauthorized access to system	Password and log off protocol, engineer's access protocol with backup, audit trail, planned siting of terminals	–	–
Operator or user error	Adequate staff training	–	–
Software failure	Backup, with fireproof safe storage of programs and daily practice data. Adequate maintenance contract with on-line patching	–	+
Consequential data loss due to system malfunction	Backup	–	–
Viruses	Router; firewall; floppy disk, bulletin board, e-mail and Internet hygiene, antivirus software	–	–
Fraud	e-banking and commissioning fund transaction access limited to specified individuals by password. Audit trail	–	–
DPA related liability	Adequate staff training	–	–

Where available, adequate insurance cover should be obtained for all risks for which maintenance contracts do not fully provide

The DPA, Health Authority system supplier and medical defence organizations are all legitimately involved in the process of GP computer security

Increasingly, security features are specified as a component of the DoH's requirements for system accreditation (RFA)

a surge-proof uninterruptible power supply (UPS) should be installed (see below). The latter will protect the main processor, but during lightning storms all other equipment should be disconnected.

26.3 THEFT

Preventive measures must be applied both to the premises and to the computer equipment:

- The advice of the Crime Prevention Officer (or, if building anew, the Police Architectural Liaison Officer) should be obtained. An alarm system (British Standard BS 4737) linked to the police station may be fitted. External door five-lever locks (BS 3621/80) and adequate window locks are required. Steel shutters may need to be added to windows. Audio or visual intruder alarms may also be needed (the National Approved Council for Security Systems will supply a list of approved installers). Attention must be paid to skylights, flat roofs, fire exits and security lights. Medical centres should be designed so as to provide an easily visible single point of access to the building and a clear surrounding area. The NHS Security Manual issued by the National Association of HAs and Trusts, and the NHS Guidelines on minimum security standards (BS 8220) both detail practice security obligations, and the GMSC and Department of Health have set up a national database of computer crime against GPs, so that problems and their solutions can be identified.
- Computer processors, laser printers and backup drives should be armoured and anchored. Where practicable, six-sided armoured enclosure cabinets should be used, failing which, four sided designs that incorporate overlapping flanges may be acceptable, provided that the exposed surfaces of the enclosed equipment are tamper-proof. All armoured cabinets should conform with specifications issued by the Loss Prevention Council. The design of the cabinet must allow adequate machine ventilation, and obviate static build-up. Armoured cabinets should be bolted to immovable desks, floors or walls. Preferably, computer terminals should not be visible from the outside of the building. Alarms are available that activate if any items of equipment are moved or tampered with, and these either emit a 'screech' signal when activated or else trigger a pager link with an appointed member of staff.

26.4 PRACTICE COMPUTER SECURITY PROCEDURE

1. One member of staff must be appointed to take overall responsibility for maintaining all security procedures, and for ensuring that all members of staff not only have a list of these procedures but are adequately trained in their use. A deputy security officer should be appointed to cover holidays.
2. The Crime Prevention Officer should visit and advise the practice.
3. The Fire Prevention Officer should visit and advise the practice.
4. The system supplier's maintenance contract should be checked to verify which of the risks listed in Table 26.1 are covered by it and which are not.
5. Computer insurance should be taken out to cover as many as possible of the eventualities left uncovered by the maintenance contract. Makes, models and serial numbers of all equipment should be recorded, and notified to the company.
6. The procedures called for by the Data Protection Act should be reviewed.
7. The member of staff charged with overall security responsibility should carry out a review of existing arrangements on a regular basis and list them, showing which should be upgraded. NHS Guidelines on Minimum Security Standards (BS 8220), and the Department of Health 1995 *Handbook of Information Security: Information Security Within General Practice*, refer.
8. A copy of the security review should be sent to the HA with an application for funding approval for those upgrades that are required.

26.5 COMPUTER INSURANCE

Maintenance agreements with suppliers are essential, and it is not sensible to separate maintenance arrangements for hardware and software, because of demarcation problems (see Chapter 27). Also, the day when practices could afford to ship their equipment back to the workshop to await repairs without replacement has long since passed. But maintenance agreements do not cover all hazards, and simple surgery contents insurance policies do not cope with the specialized needs of system users. A tailor-made computer policy is required to compensate for the following risks:

- Fire, water damage, other forms of accidental insult to equipment, and theft (including loss of portables)
- Hardware breakdown due to other causes not included in the maintenance contract – misuse,

malicious damage, lightning, power supply failure, or negligence

- Reconstitution of data after system breakdown. Although the use of assiduous backup and program safekeeping policies will limit the cost of reconstructing data, there may still be some extra wage bills to pay, towards which HAs seem unduly reluctant to contribute. Serious data corruption problems may need the intervention of a data restoration specialist – an expensive option. It is important to note that consequential liability following data loss or corruption remains the practice's responsibility.
- Incidental expenses incurred in taking action to pre-empt damage (due, for instance to flooding) or to adjust hardware or software to an updated system specification following breakdown. Satisfactory policies to cover most of these risks are marketed by companies such as the Medical Insurance Agency.

26.6 CLEAN ELECTRICITY

The power supplied to computers should be invariable. If voltage is insufficient, data in RAM may be lost, or the system may 'go down', but excessive power can corrupt data or damage equipment. Computers are designed to operate within the narrow band of voltage that the electricity companies are tasked to provide, but whose constancy cannot always be guaranteed at the ultimate point of delivery. There are several possible reasons for this:

- Electrical equipment in the same building may cause voltage interference. This is usually avoided by using a separate ring main for the local network. Electrical sockets for all computer equipment should be carefully located so as to minimize the chance of their being switched off inadvertently.
- Storms with cable damage, lightning strikes, and sudden changes in the demand for industrial or domestic power may temporarily destabilize local supply. Failure may be total ('black-out'), partial ('brown-out'), or rapidly intermittent ('line noise'). Excessive peaks are known as *spikes* or *surges*. Partial interruption (sometimes referred to as 'pollution') may not be severe enough to 'hang' the system, but its existence may be inferred following the occurrence of an otherwise inexplicable corruption of data or loss of files.

Suppliers' contracts and the provisions of the DPA make it abundantly clear that regularization of the power supply to the practice computer is the prac-

tice's own responsibility. Dereliction of this responsibility that resulted in data loss or other damage would find insurance companies, defence organizations and the HA unsympathetic.

The definitive answer to the threat of power corruption is the uninterruptible power supply (UPS) unit. This consists of a battery pack, coupled with power security software, which is installed on the practice system. Power failure triggers audiovisual alarm signals. The battery pack provides sufficient auxiliary power to allow an orderly shut down of the system, and the batteries recharge automatically when the mains power supply resumes.

There are two forms of UPS: off-line and on-line. The off-line unit triggers battery operations as and when the mains power fails, and does so with delays that are so small that computer operations are unaffected. Off-line units only restore failed power supplies and do not usually provide surge or spike protection.

The on-line unit uses the battery pack as a filter, which supplies the computer with power at all times, and which is continuously recharged from the mains. On-line units protect against surges, spikes and all 'line-noise' pollution. While the on-line unit is clearly the preferred option, it may prove twice as expensive as the off-line equivalent.

Three types of UPS alarm alert the user to power failure: a continuous or interrupted sound emission, a visual signal on the UPS unit itself – which may be either the extinction of a small light bulb or the activation of an LCD display – and the appearance of a text message on all users' VDU screens.

Emergency battery operation will provide sufficient auxiliary power in the event of mains failure to allow the continued operation of the computer system for a further 7–15 minutes, during which time users have the opportunity to shut down their system in a disciplined manner, and avoid data loss or corruption. Small UPS units are designed to be compact enough to fit beneath one side of an office desk, but large practices are likely to need a battery pack of greater height and footprint.

The capacity of a UPS unit is measured in volt-amperes, and must accurately match the power rating of the equipment for whose support it is installed. The power rating of a practice's equipment is the sum of the ratings of each of its components – fileserver, terminals, printers and other peripherals. The power rating of all equipment should be marked on its casing by the maker.

Power security software must be included with the purchase of a UPS unit and must be installed on the practice server. An appropriate interface that dovetails with the practice's operating or networking system must also be specified.

Batteries in UPS units are of the sealed lead-acid type and should require no maintenance. Newer UPS designs meet approved standards for factors such as safety, and the absence of radio frequency interference or input harmonics.

A UPS is one of those critical pieces of equipment, as are the fileserver and backup unit, that should always be covered by a supplier's maintenance contract.

26.7 HACKING

Hacking is electronic eavesdropping, which takes place through the telephone network. The eavesdropper may also have the ability to corrupt or alter data. Branch surgery landlines and cellular telephone networks are the configurations most vulnerable to hacking, although it has to be said that the risk in either case is small.

In the absence of physical damage to the telephone network, and in the absence of demonstrable criminal intent, there is currently little legal redress against those obtaining unauthorized access to other people's electronic messages.

In all developed countries, some form of legislation exists to punish those hackers who, in addition to eavesdropping, attempt to commit a crime such as fraud, blackmail, data corruption or system damage, but it is often exceptionally difficult to obtain the necessary proof to bring prosecution. Prevention is therefore all-important.

- Network security software packages, which are suitable for use on both a regional or a world-wide basis, offer a combination of protective features:
  - *End-to-end security* (one type of 'firewall') is a process in which the computer at each end of the transmission, challenges the authenticity of the other (one example of this procedure is the CHAPS Challenge Handshake Authentication Protocol, widely used by banks when transferring money)
  - *Message content integrity* can be monitored during transmission and the message can be proved electronically to have originated from the authenticated sender and received by the authenticated recipient.
- Most incidents of hacking are directed towards the penetration of remote computer databases. As a barrier against interlopers, a remote database must restrict external access to a read-only area of storage, within which each subdivision is earmarked for, and limited to use by, an identifiable interrogator or interrogators. This is the 'mailbox' principle.
- Data compaction, and more particularly encryption, impede the hacker. Encryption disguises plain text by converting it into a coded equivalent, and the degree of sophistication of the most advanced forms of encryption has delivered virtual impenetrability.

Encryption has now become so powerful a tool of concealment that governments have recognized the potential threat it represents if misused by the international criminal fraternity in order to coordinate their activities. In response, Israel, France, Russia and China have banned encryption. The US government placed an embargo on the export (other than to health agencies) of encryption software that incorporated more than 40 bits in its technology, but this merely served to defer the inevitable as several European developers have now achieved virtual impenetrability. The concept of 'key ESCROW' has been proposed as a compromise, whereby a copy of relevant de-encrypting software is lodged with law enforcement agencies to enable them to continue to 'bug' communications, as they do with conventional telephones.

In the UK, the political status of refined encryption is still under review, but the BMA's insistence that patient data on NHSnet should be encrypted will have to be accommodated. The implementation of encryption will, of course, increase costs.

26.8 UNAUTHORIZED ACCESS

- Terminals should be carefully sited so that they are only legible to those with authorized access.
- A terminal should only be operated by the user who has logged on to it. Terminals should not be left logged-on and unattended. Logging off must always conclude terminal use by each individual.
- In some instances it may be useful to restrict access by the use of a terminal lock and key. All staff contracts should include clauses that ensure the respect of patient confidentiality and observance of the provisions of the DPA. Signed guarantees to maintain confidentiality should also be furnished by system engineers, data collection representatives, and casual visitors to the practice. Software correction via modem should be similarly protected.
- Logging on to the system must involve the use of a personal password known only to the individual, and to the computer manager who is responsible for password allocation. The password will serve

to determine the level of access gained by each user of the system to the patient files (no access, read only, or read-and-write). The password will also equate with the flag of authorship attached to each data entry for audit trail purposes. Passwords are usually changed periodically to maintain secrecy.

- Responsibility must be allocated for the deployment and storage of diskettes and tapes used for backup and other purposes. Old diskettes and tapes must be wiped of all data or else destroyed. A shredder will be required to allow disposal of old printout.

- A doctor must assume responsibility for monitoring the validity and anonymity of data passed to a data-collection agency. Any research project using personally identifiable data must have the informed consent of the patient, and local ethical committee approval.

26.9 BACKUP

If system or electricity supply failure occurs, then data in RAM will be lost. The extent to which software resists corruption is one test of its quality, but nevertheless system or supply malfunction can lead to partial, or occasionally total, destruction of data stored on the hard disk. The effects of this potential disaster can only be averted if the contents of the hard disk have been copied to an independent storage device from which the hard disk can be reconstituted.

- The computer manager must be responsible for backup, and this should be built into the contract of employment.

- Backup should be undertaken daily, and will need to take place outside working hours. Many practices now use a different copy for each working day of the week, overwriting the oldest on each run. Following system disruption, data will be reconstituted as at the point of the latest backup.

- Diskettes were originally used to back up GP systems, but the number of diskettes and the total time required for this method are excessive and impracticable. Magnetic tapes ('tape streamers') are now almost universally employed, and recording is frequently on to digital audio tape (DAT). Alternatives are an independent second hard disk drive, or a rewritable optical disk – the latter will run at speeds of up to 800 Mb per 12 minutes. Storage technology is undergoing rapid innovative development, and is set to provide ever faster access and greater capacity.

- More sophisticated backup procedures are configured to reduplicate all changes to data as and when they occur – a tandem system that incorporates full audit trails. These systems allow total data reconstitution when taken in conjunction with the full daily copy of the hard disk contents.

- Backup procedures should be undertaken automatically by the system, and the computer protocol should incorporate a prior check on the integrity of data on the hard disk (file check program), a subsequent check on the validity of the copy (copy verification program), and a facility to allow the user to inspect one of the transferred files on a system VDU for confirmation, if required.

- Backup copies should be kept in a separate premises in a fireproof safe in company with the original copies of diskettes or CD-ROM disks bearing the supplier's programs and the latest versions of the morbidity, drug and protocol dictionaries.

- Full backup should be undertaken before all system upgrades, engineer visits and remote software patching.

26.10 PRESERVATION OF HARD DISK INTEGRITY

Hard disk drives can be damaged by rough handling. Jolts may cause the reading head to deface the platter, a problem that can be avoided in some drives by the use of a housekeeping program that immobilizes the head in a neutral position while the computer is moved. Maintenance contracts may disclaim responsibility for damage due to system relocation unless this has been carried out by the supplier.

Careful planning of the disposition of electricity sockets will make it less likely that terminals are switched off accidentally – the latter event may corrupt data stored on hard disks. For a similar reason, applications should be closed down in the reverse order to that in which they were opened, prior to switching off the system. The high speeds maintained for long periods by hard disks limit their working life, and replacement should be considered if otherwise unexplained access failure occurs after 3–4 years of use (see also the section on the Scan Disk program, Chapter 2).

26.11 DISKETTE, TAPE, BULLETIN BOARD, INTERNET AND E-MAIL DISCIPLINE

No data from diskettes, bulletin boards or Internet files should ever be loaded on to the practice computer without the system supplier's express approval.

Blank diskettes should always be obtained new and unused from reputable sources 'shrink-wrapped'. The platter surface should not be handled or otherwise insulted, and the diskette should not be subjected to heat, nor to the magnetic fields of electrical equipment other than the terminals (even a ringing telephone is capable of causing magnetic damage). Once a diskette's contents have been installed on the practice system and the diskette has stopped rotating, it should be removed from the diskette port until needed again. Working copies of diskette-based suppliers' programs should always be used in preference to the originals, in order to preserve the latter. The same physical care should be applied to magnetic tape as to diskettes.

The practice computer should only use NHSnet for e-mail, and only access the Internet through NHSnet's secure outbound gateway. Other forms of Internet and e-mail access have proved vulnerable to virus infection.

26.12 VIRUSES

Overview

In 1989 a criminal gang giving a Panamanian address flooded the world's computer user base with mailed diskettes containing a virus that rapidly rendered systems inoperable. In Britain alone, 20 000 diskettes were distributed in this way. With calculated irony, the diskette's wrapper claimed to advise users on their risk of infection with the AIDS virus. A screen message then demanded a ransom payment of $378 for the provision of the virus antidote.

Viruses originated as esoteric pranks but later became vehicles for extortion. Perpetrators of virus crime put themselves at risk of prosecution under the Criminal Damage Act of 1971. Viruses are fragments of computer program, as distinct from user record data, which have the ability to infect and replicate, as do their biological counterparts. Viruses can insinuate themselves into any area of processor memory, hard disk or diskette that is not restricted to read-only access, and can be transmitted through cable or telecommunication in company with other data. Each virus is restricted to the operating system for which it was written. Originally, the majority of viruses were DOS-based, because DOS was the most widely used operating system for off-the-shelf utilities, but other environments, particularly Windows and Macintosh, are now being colonized.

Virus infection nearly always results from contamination via extraneous diskettes, freeware and shareware, bulletin boards, e-mail and the Internet. Rarely,

it has been known to be imported with third-party software distributed by GP system suppliers, or to be resident on newly purchased hard disks.

Viruses disorganize the host programs to which they are attached and thereby destroy both program and document data. .exe and .com files are those most commonly infected. Virus designers often contrive to present bizarre screen effects or banal messages as the destruction proceeds. The appearance of the Chernobyl virus, which could irreparably damage the BIOS circuitry, and of the SATAN and other viruses on the Internet, sent shock waves throughout the IT community. By 1999, there were approximately 20 000 known computer viruses, since when the total number has increased inexorably, but a handful of these together account for over 90% of reported infections. Some viruses now have the power to damage hardware beyond repair.

Viruses are commonly categorized by extravagant terms that describe their manner of operation. 'Worms' act insidiously, slowly corrupting data as the system is used. 'Logic bombs' ('time-bombs') lie in wait until triggered unwittingly by the host system, such as by a date change, so that backup data copies are likely to have been corrupted before the infection is discovered. 'Trojans' ('Trojan horses') conceal their malignancy within an apparently desirable utility such as free software. 'Stealth' viruses are formulated so as to defy detection by antivirus software. Although some writers treat viruses, trojans and worms as different entities, such distinctions serve no useful purpose. All are self-perpetuating destructive rogue program material, and will be referred to here collectively as viruses.

The ingenuity of virus creators knows no bounds and computer users must be constantly on their guard against new developments.

Countermeasures

● The most important countermeasure is prevention. No diskette from an unauthenticated source should ever be introduced into the practice computer. Some practices make it an offence for staff to bring any diskettes on to the practice premises other than those specifically provided by the system supplier. Particularly suspect sources are computer games and free software passed between computer enthusiasts. Freeware and shareware should never be used on the practice system, nor should bulletin boards be accessed from it. E-mail for, and Internet access from, the practice system should be confined to the NHSnet.

- It is possible in some systems to house programs in 'read only' areas of the hard disk so that they cannot be contaminated.
- Antivirus software (AVS) packages are marketed that enable users to detect and to eradicate viruses. These may be used to act preventively in memory on all incoming data, or else to determine whether infection has already occurred on disk. AVS acts in two principal ways:

  - *Scanning.* A dictionary is provided showing the unique section of program code that can be detected in each virus. This allows AVS to search the host system's files for all known viruses. The package may also remove the virus. Virus scanning can be performed periodically, or on every occasion when a file or program is accessed (real time scanning). New viruses and self encrypting viruses cannot be detected by this method.
  - *'Fingerprinting'.* The AVS inspects each host program file and generates a unique check number as a result of its calculations. Each time the host program file is used, the check number is recalculated. An alteration in check number demonstrates intrusion by a virus, and the method detects known, new and self-encrypting viruses.

The most popular AVS packages have been those provided by McAfee, Dr Solomon, Norton, Central Point and Sophos. McAfee and Dr Solomon's packages are now jointly owned by Network Associates, and the Norton packages are marketed by Symantec. Sophos is the most commonly used European-based package. It is important to choose an AVS package with an NCSA certificate (Table 26.2).

AVS purchase and update costs are related to the number of users on site. Updates may be provided monthly or quarterly, and are a vital feature of the AVS contract, since more than 200 new viruses appear each month. Updates should be provided on diskette, so that even viruses resident in the 'boot up' procedure will be covered.

Table 26.2 A number of packages that are certified by the NCSA (Courtesy of *Health Service Computing*)

Manufacturer	Program name	Operating systems covered
Alwil	AVAST32	DOS, Windows 3.1, Windows 95, NT Workstation, NT server
Computer Associates	Inoculan Anti-Virus VET anti-virus	Windows 95, Windows NT, Netware DOS Windows 95, NT workstation, Windows 3.1
Command Software	Command Anti-Virus	Windows 95
Data Fellows	F-Secure Antivirus	Windows 95
Aladdin	eSafe Protect	Windows 95
GriSoft	AVG	Windows 95, NT workstation
Ikarus	Virus Utilities	Windows 95
iRiS	Antivirus	Windows 95
Kaspersky Lab	Antiviral Toolkit Pro	DOS, Windows 95
Network Associates International (NAI)	VirusScan, NetShield	Windows 95, Windows NT Server
Norman Data Defense Systems	Norman Virus Control	Windows 95
Panda	Panda Antivirus	DOS, Windows 3.1, Windows 95, 98, NT Workstation, NT server OS/2
Sophos	Sweep	Windows, NT Workstation, NT server, Netware
Trend Micro Inc.	OfficeScan ServerProtect	Windows 95, Windows 98, NT Workstation, NT Server, Netware
Symantec	Norton Anti-Virus	DOS, Windows 95, Windows 98, NT Workstation, NT Server, Netware
	Norton AntiVirus Corporate Edition	Windows 95, NT Workstation, NT Server

Unless expressly authorized, two different AVS packages should not be used simultaneously. Combination packages offering AVS combined with network monitoring and a firewall (and in one case also encryption) are marketed under the general heading of 'security software'.

AVS providers should offer hotline facilities and news letters, but the quality of both varies between packages.

It is wise to run AVS checks after system engineers or software patching teams have accessed the practice system, and before the backup tapes taken before external intervention have been rerecorded.

In 1995, the Department of Health issued the *Handbook of Information Security: Information Security within General Practice* (ref. E5209) as its recommended policy document.

26.13 DATA OWNERSHIP

Since the introduction of the NHS, the Department of Health has been the provider and the undisputed owner of the pages on which the general practice record is written. Each page carries a printed reminder that this is so. Because it was inseparable from the page, data ownership by the Department was assumed by default.

The data collection schemes, and splits in partnership in which both estranged partners laid claim to a copy of the practice records, have raised the question of ownership of electronic clinical data. In 1989 a spokesman for the Department sought to establish government ownership of GP data in a Parliamentary reply. The GMSC and RCGP take the view that the doctor who creates the data owns them, whereas the DPA in effect puts the case for the patient. Some system suppliers have asserted that electronic data are ephemeral and that nobody owns them. In the final analysis it is once again clear that, as with paper records, the owner of the record storage medium controls the data and that in the case of the GP computer this will be the doctor. Contracts with Data Collection Agencies, and partnership agreements, should recognize and define this right of control.

26.14 THE DATA PROTECTION ACTS

Doctors have always protected the confidentiality of their patient records, but the enforcement of a code of practice in relation to electronic personal records became law with the Data Protection Act of 1984. Some minor amendments were made to the Act in 1998 to bring it into line with a new EU directive, but the underlying principles remained substantially unchanged. All general practices using patient record systems, whether held manually, on computers, or on word processors, must submit notification in order to register with: the Data Protection Commissioner (formerly the DP Registrar), Office of the Data Protection Commissioner, Wycliffe House, Water Lane, Wilmslow, Cheshire SK9 5AF, by requesting, completing and submitting the relevant set of forms and enclosing the appropriate fee. Submission of notification for registration will have to be renewed every year, and all amendments required to the form's contents must be declared as they occur. There is no charge for amendments. The register of users is publicly available, and failure to register renders a user liable to prosecution.

Notification for registration involves describing those persons controlling and those processing the data, the persons to whom the data apply, the data classes, sources, purposes of use, those to whom the data will be disclosed, and where subjects may gain access to their records. As omissions may be penalized and supernumerary entries cost nothing, it is important to allow for all present and future eventualities when completing the form. Practices should register as a partnership, quoting all partners but not the names of other practice staff, and nominating one spokesperson as contact for DPA affairs. Staff employed by the Health Authority and by the system supplier must be included as processors. Although, for the most part, practices will be acting as data controllers, they should also apply to be recognized as data processors (a subsidiary role), in order to cover any use they may make of personalized data that have originated electronically from their HA, the community health services or social services, or their accountant. The purpose of data use will be primarily for general medical services, but may include staff or trainee administration (payroll application is exempt), social service administration, research or teaching. Disclosures must include those made to the HA, provider Trusts, pathology laboratories and, where applicable (and with strict anonymity), the data collection agencies. Acceptance of notification for registration confers obligations on controllers and processors, and rights on the subjects to whom the data refer.

26.15 THE EIGHT PRINCIPLES OF THE DATA PROTECTION ACTS

Documentation on the Data Protection Acts now extends to a considerable amount of fine detail, which it would be inappropriate to reproduce here. This documentation is, in any case, available to every practice applying to notify registration. It is also available on the Internet, to which those seeking further information are referred.

It is, however, important that readers should understand the overall significance of the Acts, which is embodied in their eight principles and which may be summarized in six paragraphs:

- Personal data must be obtained and processed fairly and lawfully, in accordance with the declaration made in the notification of registration, and in accordance with the rights of data subjects. The data shall be adequate, relevant, not excessive for their purpose, accurate and up to date.
- Personal data must not be kept for longer than is necessary to fulfil the purpose for which they are processed (but the subject can require access to personal records extending retrospectively over unlimited periods of time – see next section).
- Appropriate technical and organizational (i.e. security) measures shall be taken against unauthorized or unlawful processing of personal data and against accidental loss or destruction of, or damage to, personal data.
- Subjects have the right to see data relating to them by applying in writing to a nominated member of the practice, unless those data are 'likely to cause serious harm to the physical or mental health of the data subject or other person'. Response must be by printout if requested, must be made within 40 days, and a fee may be charged.
- Data subjects have the right to require correction or erasure of inaccurate data, and can sue for any breach of the Act – not merely if they suffer damage as the result of the use of inaccurate or improperly protected data (including unauthorized disclosure), or if they suffer damage as a result of the loss of data.
- Under special circumstances, data may be divulged to proper authority in accordance with statute, court order, the need to prevent serious crime, or with the written consent of the subject.

26.16 CHANGES TO THE DATA PROTECTION ACT INTRODUCED BY THE 1998 AMENDMENTS

These may be summarized as follows:

- There are some minor semantic alterations, which do not affect the overall import of the 1984 Act. The DP Registrar becomes the DP Commissioner, data 'users' become data 'controllers' (a data con-

troller determines the purposes for which, and manner in which, personal data shall be processed), data 'bureaux' become data 'processors' (a data processor means any person, other than an employee of the data controller, who processes data on behalf of the data controller), and Registration under the Act now becomes Notification.

- Data covered by the 1998 Act are now defined as specific information relating to an individual which is held in a structured, readily accessible filing system. The processing of data is now very comprehensively defined and includes obtaining, organizing, disseminating, combining and retrieving information. Data processing in breach of an obligation of confidence is unlawful.
- The data subject's right of access is extended to include manual medical records as well as electronic records.
- Data controllers are required to ensure that where a data processor processes data on a controller's behalf there is a written contract between the parties, whereby the processor agrees only to act on the instructions of the controller, and to abide by the provisions of the security principle.
- In addition to the right of data subjects to obtain personal data about themselves, subjects now have the right to obtain a description of those data, the purposes for which they are being processed, a description of any potential recipients of those data, and information as to the sources of the data.
- The processing of 'sensitive personal data', such as medical data, now requires the explicit, informed, and by inference written, consent of the data subject. (Presumably this will be incorporated in the process of patient registration with a practice.)
- The data subject now has the right to require access to records extending retrospectively over unlimited periods of time. (The 1984 Act limited the retention of data to that duration which was necessary for the purposes for which the data were used.)
- A single charge must be made to cover all abstractions taken from the record (in place of charges made for each abstraction).

26.17 JOINT GMSC AND RCGP GUIDELINES FOR THE EXTRACTION AND USE OF DATA FROM GP COMPUTER SYSTEMS BY ORGANIZATIONS EXTERNAL TO THE PRACTICE – A SUMMARY

- The external organization must appoint a medical officer to be responsible for, and guarantee, confidentiality and maintenance of data validity.

- The operation must be monitored by the Committee on Standards of Data Extraction in General Practice (COSODE).
- Data ownership remains with the GP.
- No patient must be identifiable, other than to the GP, without that patient's informed consent.
- No practice must be identifiable within the data, without the practice's consent.
- The external organization must supply the practice with a statement that stipulates the categories and purpose of data extraction. The GP must give informed consent.
- Data extraction must be copied to, and verified by, the practice. It may be performed either:
  - by a technician visiting the practice and using a diskette, under the supervision of the GP or an authorized staff member
  - by the general practitioner who has personally been trained to extract data, before verifying them and transmitting them through e-mail or storing them on diskette.
- External organizations must, prior to a maintenance visit by their staff, confirm the purpose of the visit, guarantee that data access will be restricted to the engineer on pain of dismissal, and assume legal liability for the destruction of any confidential replicated data following the operation.
- The external organization must be registered with the DPA in respect of its actions.

26.18 ESCROW

Supplier bankruptcy could result in serious maintenance continuity problems for users, unless a copy of the system's source code is placed in trust with a neutral legal guardian. This procedure is termed ESCROW.

26.19 DONGLES AND DISABLING SYSTEMS

A *dongle* is a removable ROM chip, which is attached exteriorly to the processor but is needed to complete the system's housekeeping circuitry. Although software manufacturers sometimes use dongles to protect the copyright of their software, these devices may also be used as keys to control user access to systems. At the end of a working day, a dongle attached to a practice system may be removed to a safe, so that theft of computer equipment overnight would not result in breaches of patient confidentiality.

Some practice systems have the power to disable the system if a succession of invalid attempts is made to log on by password. The number of attempts may be specified by the user. Once the system has been disabled, it will require the intervention of the supplier to restore it. As systems may be left running overnight for e-mail transmission, disabling systems offer a better means of secure access than dongles.

FURTHER INFORMATION

Data Protection Act

The Data Protection Commission provides a series of free booklets as guidelines to the DPA, and the GMSC has published three elaborative handbooks describing the implementation of the DPA in general practice. The GMSC handbooks, which may be obtained from the British Medical Association, BMA House, Tavistock Square, London WC1H 9JP, are:
Guidance to General Medical Practitioners on the Subject Access Provisions of the Data Protection Act
Guidance to General Medical Practitioners on Data Protection Registration
The Data Protection Act. A code of practice for general medical practitioners
Website information: Data Protection Act 1998, http://www.hmso.gov.uk/acts/acts1998/19980029.htm; Data Protection Act 1984, http://www.open.gov.uk/dpr/dprhome.htm.

Other security topics

Department of Health and Primary Health Care Specialist Group 1990 Guidance on security standards for primary health care practitioners. HMSO, London
Department of Health 1995 The handbook of information security: Information security within general practice (ref E5209). HMSO, London
Herd J 1990 Outbreak. Health Service Computing, May/June: 34–36
Mayo J L 1989 Computer viruses; what they are, how they work, and how to avoid them. Windcrest Books, Blue Ridge Summit, PA
NHS Guidelines on Minimum Security Standards (BS8220). HMSO, London
NHS Security Manual NAHAT Birmingham Research Park Vincent Drive, Birmingham B15 2SQ tel: 0121 471 4444
NHSE Information Management Group booklet: Play it safe – a practical guide to IT security for everyone working in general practice. NHSE (obtainable through health authorities)
NHSE Information Management Group 1995 Training video on information security. NHSE (obtainable through health authorities)

27 Agencies concerned with practice computers

27.1 GP SYSTEM SUPPLIERS

Support

It has taken GP system suppliers a long time to develop an efficient level of support for their users. During the 1980s, when hardware and software were in any case less reliable, harrowing stories of delay in fault correction abounded. Happily, 'down time' of several weeks is now a thing of the past, although support standards still do not match those found in computing for banks, air travel or the Stock Exchange. The greater the range of practice applications transferred to the computer, the more patients are put at risk by system malfunction or non-function. We should not forget that motoring organizations vie with each other to provide on-site assistance within the hour.

Ideally, system suppliers' support should comprise:

1. Hardware repair or, failing this, replacement. Engineer availability should be not less than 9 am–5 pm from Monday to Friday, and response should be provided within 8 working hours.
2. Software fault correction via modem and telephone line. Faults should be investigated within 4 hours, leading to prompt 'patching' or circumvention advice.
3. Routine software enhancements involving 'debugging' and streamlining of existing software modules
4. A help-line, manned between 8 am and 6 pm from Monday to Friday. Queries should lead to action being initiated within half an hour. Outside working hours, an efficient mechanism for logging calls, with subsequent return of call, should be available.
5. A reference manual dealing with all features of the system
6. A maintenance contract guaranteeing minimum support levels and defining the rights and obligations of both parties

7. System training on-site
8. Hardware upgrades
9. Major software upgrades and new software modules.

Although these standards can hardly be considered unreasonable by comparison with those obtaining elsewhere in mission-critical computing, they are not achieved by all suppliers, nor, in the past, have they been comprehensively specified in the requirements for system accreditation.

Support costs vary between suppliers but are usually between 10% and 15% of the capital outlay per annum, and should at least cover items 1–6. Training may also be included, or may be billed separately. New software modules and hardware upgrades will usually be billed as separate items.

Maintenance contracts

Maintenance contracts stipulate the levels of service, terms of trading, and rights and obligations of the parties. To be equitable, contracts should not be slanted, and to be binding they should be specific. Some contracts are heavily weighted in favour of the supplier, even to the extent that they attempt to waive responsibility for eventualities for which common law inevitably holds them responsible. (In common law, the Unfair Contract Terms Act may be invoked to redress the balance of a seriously slanted contract clause.) Other contracts are extensively compromised by the overuse of terms such as 'reasonable endeavours' or 'best efforts' in relation to the suppliers' obligations. Most of the maintenance contracts investigated by *Practice Computing* in 1992 were considered to be fair and workmanlike, but if small print is held to be a measure of concealment, then these documents should be read with great care before contracts are signed.

In line with principles laid down in the Requirements for Accreditation, contracts should be binding for 1 year in the first instance and subsequently be terminable by either side after giving 90 days notice.

There is considerable variation between the contracts of different suppliers, but for the most part they deal with the following issues:

- *The level of support provided* – hardware repair or replacement; software fault correction, enhancement and upgrade; helpline; call-out; documentation; staff training
- *Fees* – frequency and method of payment, the mechanism for their increase, the penalties for non-payment and arrangements for renting systems
- *Security* – transfer to the customer of total responsibility for backup, insurance, DPA notification for registration, the provision of clean electricity, virus prevention and the protection of magnetic media
- *Logistical cooperation on the part of the practice* – telephone points must be provided near terminals so that problems may be described, suitable access to premises must be provided for repairs, a member of staff must be made available to demonstrate a fault and verify its subsequent correction, practices must agree to follow operating instructions and prevent negligence
- *Limitation of area of responsibility* – unless so specified, the supplier's responsibility will not extend into third-party hardware or software, communications or consumables
- *Supplier's damage liability limitation* (if not covered by legal statute) in relation to material and personal damages, data loss, consequential loss following system use, third-party action
- *Copyright* – software licence rights to be observed, system not be assigned to others, no copies except for backup
- *Exclusive use* – no consumer modification of hardware or software, no additional hardware or software to be used without approval, no relocation of equipment without approval
- *Supplier's disclaimer of warranty of function* – perfection in software performance is rarely attained, and most suppliers refuse to guarantee it. Nevertheless, system functionality should conform with its specification in the manual, in line with Trades Descriptions legislation.

In the past, some practices have been tempted to cut prices by obtaining hardware maintenance cover elsewhere than from their supplier, or of limiting hardware cover to fileserver, network distribution board, backup and UPS (which is an absolute minimum requirement). While it is true that several suppliers do in fact subcontract hardware maintenance to national electronic engineering repair agencies, it is important from the user's point of view that overall hardware, software and communications maintenance responsibility should be assumed by a single organization, otherwise demarcation disputes are bound to arise. This means, in effect, contracting with the system supplier or the supplier's specified representative for all services.

Maintenance contracts guarantee minimum levels of support, which are often surpassed in practice. Since governmental reimbursement confers some degree of stability on the GP computer market, the NHS can justifiably expect more efficient supplier performance 'as of right' than is specified in most contracts.

Hardware reliability has been greatly improved in recent years and this, coupled with software fault correction through modems, should bring higher support standards well within reach.

27.2 THE HEALTH AND SAFETY EXECUTIVE

The Health and Safety Display Screen Equipment Regulations 1992

When compared with pneumoconiosis in coal miners or cancer in the nuclear industry, the occupational hazards of working with computer terminals look like very small beer. We have had typewriter keyboards and cathode ray television monitors for a considerable number of years during which no-one seems to have thought of suing for occupation-related compensation, but the act of bringing the two pieces of hardware together fired the imagination of potential litigants. Cancer, leukaemia, miscarriage, congenital abnormality and facial dermatitis have all been believed to be sequelae of using visual display units, beliefs now all discounted. Next, upper limb and spinal strain, eye strain and mental stress were attributed to VDU work and, because of the essentially subjective nature of these complaints, it has been difficult to measure them and impossible to discount them. Moreover, successful compensation litigation and the overprotective dictates of the European Commission have ensured them a place in statute and in medical textbooks.

The Treaty of Rome commits the UK to incorporate European directives into the framework of British law, and the deadline by which the directive on VDU and workstation use had to be so implemented was 1 January 1993. The effect of this directive, and the British health and safety legislation that it prompted, was to impose some new, clearly defined responsibilities on employers of VDU operators, designed to reduce the risk of occupational illness. Failure to implement the new measures renders employers liable to prosecution and would be likely to aggravate employees' compensation claims. The regulations discriminate in favour of VDU operators and against conventional typists, who are expressly excluded from the provisions of the law.

The responsibilities of employers

Basically, the ergonomic measures imposed amount to little more than common sense but, as so often happens when an attempt is made to codify the application of common sense, the need to cater for every eventuality, however unlikely, makes for cumbersome documentation. The regulations protect all 'employees who habitually use display screen equipment as a significant part of their normal work', who are designated as 'users'. All new workstations put into service after 31 December 1992 must comply, and workstations that were in operation on or before that date had to be brought up to standard by 31 December 1996. Portable computers were not included.

The risks addressed and the countermeasures stipulated by the Health and Safety Commission (HSC) are summarized in Table 27.1.

Eye and eyesight tests

The HSC's view is that the use of display screens does not cause permanent eye damage but that, like other visually demanding tasks, it can make people with existing visual defects more aware of these, and poor lighting can lead to headaches and tired eyes.

- Users have the entitlement to eye and eyesight tests and, if such tests show them to be necessary, further ophthalmological investigation plus any corrective appliances such as spectacles needed specifically for display work, if normal appliances cannot be used. The term 'normal corrective appliances' is here taken to mean those required for reading or long distance, which must be provided by the user. Spectacles required specifically for display work will have a focal length of approximately 50–60 cm, need provide only basic functionality, and must be paid for by the employer. Eye and eyesight tests must also be paid for by the employer, but specialist ophthalmo-

Table 27.1 The risks and countermeasures associated with display screens and workstations (summarized from the Health and Safety Commission's Regulation Proposals CD 42)

Risk	Preventive measures		
VDU-related risk			
Visual fatigue	Ergonomic planning of workstation and screen quality	Periodic work breaks	Eye tests Regular screen cleaning
Upper limb and spinal strain	Ergonomic planning of workstation	Periodic work breaks	
Mental stress	Ergonomic planning of workstation	Periodic work breaks	Control of noise, temperature, humidity, etc Task training
Other workplace risks			
Electrical and mechanical hazards	Ergonomic planning of office	Correct maintenance of equipment	Health and safety training
Rare risks			
Photosensitive epilepsy	Avoid VDU use		
Discounted or unsubstantiated risks			
Cancer, leukaemia, miscarriage, congenital malformation, facial dermatitis			

logical investigations will normally be obtainable under the NHS.

- The tests must be provided as of right before employment, at any time on request, at 10-yearly intervals or at intervals recommended by the professional adviser, and if visual difficulties are experienced during display screen work.
- Tests are to be undertaken by a registered optometrist or medical practitioner in accordance with the Optician's Act and the Optician's Statement of Good Practice.

The display screen

Screens must achieve minimum standards:

- Characters must be well-defined, clearly formed and given adequate size and spacing. The image on the screen must be stable, with no flickering.
- Brightness and contrast must be adjustable.
- Provision must be made to allow changes in screen height and attitude (swivel and tilt).
- Siting must avoid reflective glare from light sources and shiny surfaces.
- Radiation except for visible light must be negligible. In fact, cathode ray tubes have been shown to produce less unwanted radiation than natural sources.

The keyboard

- The keyboard must be separate from the screen and capable of tilt. In order that the wrists may be supported, a flat surface or purpose-built rest must be provided in front of the keyboard.
- The keys must have a convenient arrangement and a matt surface. The symbols they bear must have adequate contrast and legibility.

The work desk and its equipment

- This must be sufficiently large to allow an adequate flexible arrangement of the workstation and, if present, the document holder, free-standing disk drive, telephone, modem, printer or other peripheral. There must be adequate user workspace around the work desk.
- The document holder must be stable, adjustable, of convenient height, of low reflectance, and must be sited at the same distance and in the same visual plane as the screen.

The work chair

- The work chair must be stable, allow freedom of movement, and provide comfort.

- The seat height must be adjustable.
- The back must be adjustable for height and tilt.
- A foot rest must be provided on request.

Lighting

- There must be a satisfactory general level of lighting, retaining appropriate contrast between screen and background. Window blinds may be needed.
- Direct glare and reflectance on the screen must be avoided by the correct positioning of light sources. (This makes direct light sources either behind the screen or behind the user unsuitable.)

Environment

- Sufficient space must be provided in the office area to allow the user to change position, and vary movements between and around equipment and furniture.
- Noise must not be sufficient to distract attention or disturb speech.
- Temperature must be controlled, including the heat produced by computer equipment.
- Adequate humidity must be maintained.

Work breaks

During otherwise continuous display screen operation, breaks of 5–10 minutes per hour must be provided during which activities other than typing may be undertaken.

Software

Because it is impossible to condense global minimum standards (which would apply to all systems in all circumstances) into a format suitable for the Health and Safety Regulations, the HSC contents itself with generalizations that are so vague as to be of little help to employers or legal authorities. The HSC states: 'Detailed ergonomic standards for software are likely to be developed in future; for the moment, the schedule lists a few general principles which employers should take into account in designing, selecting, commissioning and modifying software.'

The schedule suggests that:

- Software must be suitable for the task.
- Software must be easy to use and, where appropriate, adaptable to the user's level of knowledge and experience; no quantitative or qualitative checking facility may be used without the knowledge of the users.

- Systems must provide feedback to users on the performance of those systems.
- Systems must display information in a format and at a pace which are adapted to users.
- The principles of software ergonomics must be applied, in particular to human data processing.

Assessment

The employer is responsible for ensuring that a formal recorded assessment of health and safety risks is carried out, both on installation of the workstation and when any major modifications are made to it. As the assessment will relate to the matching of the user to the workstation, change in staff should also, in theory, prompt assessment.

Assessment must include enquiries into defects of the user's vision, musculoskeletal system and psyche, the suitability of furniture, screen functionality, electrical and mechanical safety, and environmental factors. Protocols for assessment are published with the HSC Regulations Proposals (CD 42).

Training, information and participation

- Before employment, the user must be provided with suitable task and health and safety training. Training must be renewed if the system is substantially modified.

- Each user must be given comprehensible information on steps taken by employers to comply with their duties under the Health and Safety Regulations, and on the user's entitlement to regular work breaks and eye tests.
- Users should be involved in, and be consulted on, the design of tasks carried out on display screens, and the health and safety measures associated with them.

27.3 THE DEPARTMENT OF HEALTH

The Department of Health has been involved with GP computing since it began, both as sponsor and in a supporting role, notwithstanding that the main thrust of GP system development came from GPs themselves and from the companies that were set up to exploit GP initiatives. The principal areas of Department of Health involvement are shown in Box 27.1.

27.4 NHSE INFORMATION STRATEGY

As part of its campaign to catalyse and direct the development of health service computing, the UK government periodically publishes its strategic plans for health information technology. These projections do not always come to fruition, and they are often

---

Box 27.1 Main areas of Department of Health involvement in GP computing

- Pilot GP systems in the 1960s and 1970s: Oxford, Livingstone, Exeter, Thamesmead
- Micros for GPs Scheme 1982, with Department of Industry
- Communications pilots in the 1980s: Winchester, Wycombe, Links (Devon and Dorset), East Anglia, Kent, Northampton
- NHS Information Technology Branch London (planning) 1984
- Smart cards Wales 1986 Exmouth 1989
- FHS (FHC) Computer Unit Exeter 1988 (FHSA software)
- Racal Healthlink 1989
- NHS Central Registry computerized 1989
- Fundholding 1990
- Reimbursement 1990
- FHSA Computer Facilitators 1990
- Publications: *Security Standards* 1989; *GP Computing* 1990
- Minimum standards specification for GP systems 1991
- All-Wales network 1991
- Communications pilots in 1990s: Surrey, Oxford, Wales, National Links Project
- Surveys of GP computing 1986, 1987, 1988, 1989, 1990, 1991, 1993, 1998

Scottish Home and Health Department
- Scottish Database Initiatives 1982
- GPASS adopted nationally 1984
- Scottish National Network 1984

subject to slippage, but they do inspire a sense of overall direction in a field that would otherwise be one of uncoordinated and piecemeal development.

The NHS Information Management and Technology Strategy was first formulated in 1992, at which time it was inevitably involved in the cost containment exercise of the internal market. Its initial phase can be credited with the following achievements:

- The development and implementation of the new NHS number
- The development of Clinical Terms (Read codes) version 3
- The introduction of the NHS-wide Clearing Service, which rationalizes NHS communications
- Reaching agreement with the clinical community on security and confidentiality of patient data

- Reaching agreement with users on message standards in a number of administrative and clinical areas.

The second phase of the NHS Information Strategy, published in September 1998, covered the years 1998–2005. In 1998, although nearly all GPs were using computers to process clinical data, only 25% of hospitals were doing so, and uptake varied considerably between hospital departments. The strategy could afford, therefore, to be elaborative and futuristic over the developments it recommended for primary care, while still having to confine itself to formulating basic policies for the secondary care sector.

The main aspirations of the document as they affect general practice are listed in Box 27.2.

As will be seen, the changes required extensive reorganization of GP computer record structures.

Box 27.2 Principal objectives of the 1998–2005 NHS information strategy

- Lifelong e-health records for everybody in the UK
- Amalgamation of GP and Community Health Service records (vested in Primary Care Trusts)
- A common minimum data set for GP record summaries, allowing e-transfer between practices
- Merging of primary care and social services databases
- 24-hour secure access to GP e-records by authorized agencies
- The provision of e-information for all clinicians on best clinical practice, to be implemented through the use of computerized protocols and to incorporate local guidelines
- E-facilitated research
- E-requests and e-results for pathology and radiology, e-transfer of referral letters and discharge summaries
- E-data for GPs on hospital waiting lists and times. On-line appointment booking by GPs for patients to attend outpatients, and by patients to attend GPs' surgeries. Hospital admission booking at the time of an outpatient consultation
- Telemedicine for use from nurse practitioners and GPs to consultants, and from consultants to other consultants
- Telecare of vulnerable patients in their homes, with monitoring by community health and social workers
- GP-pharmacy linkages for e-prescriptions, with autoprocessing and autopayment by the PPA
- Data collection for clinical governance at local level, under the supervision of NICE (National Institute for Clinical Excellence), using benchmarks founded on evidence-based practice, audit of clinical and information technology effectiveness, comparison with national data, and data accreditation.
- Local data collection for use by health planners and managers at both local and national levels, to enable them to assess local health needs and inequalities, and to formulate health improvement programmes (with the subsequent assessment of improvements made)
- Provision of health information for patients – NHS Direct, kiosk multimedia terminals, the national gateway site on the Internet, and the NELH (National Electronic Library of Health) on NHSnet. (Topics covered include: lifestyle and condition specific information, self-treatment advice, details of local health services provision and achievement statistics, hospital waiting lists and waiting times, and automated reminders of appointments)
- E-based interactive professional educational programmes targeted at clinical expertise and information technology
- The disjointed and expensive failures that had plagued the development of information technology in secondary care were noted, and more effective progress was to be promoted in three ways:
  - Hospitals must now follow Standards Enforcement Procurement (STEP) procedures
  - NHSE Research and Development Funds would be used to finance and research programmes directed towards refining hospital computer strategy
  - Data accreditation in hospitals will be mandatory by 2001

Apart from this, recommendations were almost all directed towards enhancing the use of communications throughout the NHS. The word used to lubricate acceptance of the changes was 'modernization'.

Some additional points of interest were as follows:

- In 1999 the Clinical Information Management Programme (CIMP), managed by the Clinical Data Standards Board, took over responsibility for:
  - NHS Terms and Coding (the Read codes)
  - the work formerly undertaken by the National Casemix Office
  - the classification of headings and definitions used by the NHS
  - clinical messaging standards
  - condition-specific clinical data sets
  - standard clinical record structures.
- The concept of a National Electronic Library of Health (NELH) was proposed, which would act as a central approved electronic reference source for both health professionals and the general public. The Centre for Health Information Quality would be involved in validating Library data.
- The findings of the Caldicott Report of 1997 on patient-identifiable information were endorsed:
  - All NHS organizations should appoint a senior clinical 'guardian' to ensure that the use of patient identifiable information was effectively governed by appropriate national and locally agreed protocols on patient confidentiality
  - When electronic communications are used, patient privacy should be protected by using the new NHS number as the main patient identifier, and names and addresses should be suppressed
  - In order to support increased reliance on the new NHS number, it would be necessary to establish a National NHS Number Strategic Tracing Service, protected from unauthorized access, which could, when required, match number with identity.
- Central funding was in future scheduled to be applied to locality NHSnet messaging costs to achieve economy of scale and, for the same reason, voice and data transmission were to be tendered together. Central funding was also to be applied to the NHS-wide Clearing Service, the NHS Strategic Tracing Service, Clinical Terms Licences, the Strategic Messaging Service, FHS Exeter core systems, and the development of computer-aided decision support systems for clinicians.
- The government was to sponsor the Public Safety Communications Project, which would build a new digital radio network for the use of all emergency services. This was to be available for voice, data and traditional radio transmission, and would produce a reliable low cost local area network.
- E-mail should be provided for all clinicians, and could employ either the NHSnet, or the Internet through the NHS national intranet – NHSweb.
- Overall responsibility for managing the strategy is vested in the NHS Information Authority (NHSIA). Service quality and effectiveness are monitored through the use of the National Framework for Assessing Performance (NFAP).
- The information management and technology requirements of dentists, opticians and pharmacists will be addressed.
- A target date of the end of 2002 was set for the point at which GPs should routinely be transmitting and receiving e-message referral letters and discharge summaries. The same target date was set for the inauguration of 'beacon sites' to use the newly designed interchangeable GP computer record (designated the electronic health record – EHR).

27.5 REIMBURSEMENT

Phase 1

The Computer Costs Reimbursement Scheme began in 1990 and included repayments for systems purchased in 1989. At that date it covered, unconditionally, the partial costs of outright purchase, leasing, maintenance, and the staff wages needed for setting-up data. Levels of up to 50% were applied, attenuated for those practices with small lists. Payments tended to be on a first-come, first-served basis.

Phase 2

Reimbursement for the period 22 July 1991–31 March 1994 was more closely defined. It applied to general practitioners, restricted principals, partnerships and group practices. Payments were made in respect of purchase, lease, upgrading, maintenance, and setting-up charges. Items covered were software, on-line or off-line hardware for processing, printers, modems, multiplexors, diskettes, tape and communications facilities.

Levels of reimbursement were up to 50% of the cost of the complete system, save that fundholding practices could obtain 75% of fundholding hardware costs and 100% of specific fundholding software and training costs. Proceeds from the sale of anonymized data to collection agencies were matched by deductions from reimbursement. These levels applied to outright purchase, new lease and new maintenance contracts. Purchasers of a hitherto leased system could not claim more than 50% of the original equipment cost (fundholders not more than 75% of original hardware, nor 100% of original software). Initial setting-up costs for staff employed could be reclaimed at the standard 70% rate. Upgrading costs for hardware and software were unchanged from those already in place with the FHSA. All reimbursement was subject to the availability of FHSA funds and that authority's approval.

FHSAs were given the discretion to encourage value for money and efficient service to patients in their reimbursement policies. First priority was always given to fundholding practices, and the casualty practices from the failed AAH Meditel and VAMP data-providing schemes often took second place. For the remainder, available funds were sometimes meagre and might amount to considerably less than 50%. An end-of-year FHSA underspend on computing, or from other types of fund, might produce a sudden loosening of the purse strings. Some FHSAs used their discretionary powers to exert a preference for one or other type of GP system by discriminatory reimbursement. Others negotiated bulk discount with the chosen supplier on behalf of their GPs.

All told, the 1991–94 reimbursement policy proved to be more successful and acceptable than its predecessor and, despite its recognized shortcomings, set the pattern for later payments. However, in 1993 the FHSA reimbursement budgets came under pressure from the demand to upgrade most practice systems in preparation for the GP–FHSA Links scheme. Costs of Links installation, staff training and first-year support costs were met, often in full.

Phase 3

The principles of reimbursement were radically altered at the end of March 1994 with the introduction of accreditation, with which all new systems sold had to comply if they were to attract FHSA payments. Support and some upgrades for older systems were still funded.

Since then, the introduction of the new NHS number, the measures needed to provide Millennium compliance, and the introduction of commissioning, have once again subjected the reimbursement scheme's budgets to severe pressure. To date, practice management system reimbursement has also had to compete with repayments for staff and premises, since all three have been lumped together in a single GMS funds (now PCI) budget. Computing costs for fundholders alone were ring-fenced. The unified PCG+T budgets devolved to practices, and set to include all NHS costs at practice level, will further increase the competitive

pressure on computer refunding, and make it more difficult for doctors to invest in computers. Yet the demands for system upgrades imposed by locality commissioning and the NHS IT strategy will be extraordinary by any standards. There can be little doubt that practice system reimbursement will need to be both ring-fenced and more liberal if the government is to meet its own targets.

The government has unequivocally committed itself to the principle of central funding for a high proportion of NHS IT communication costs to achieve economy of scale. The same principle could be applied to the purchase of PCG+T office systems and intranets.

It is important that GP accounts should show computer expenses as gross, and reimbursement as income, otherwise true costs are misrepresented in review body calculations for GP remuneration.

27.6 ACCREDITATION

The Information Management and Technology Strategy launched by the NHS Management Executive in 1992 included a commitment to develop and agree the minimum requirements for GP computer systems. The Minimum System Specification Project set up to formulate these requirements produced a discussion document running to 1000 pages of highly technical detail, which was circulated to health authorities and to the 109 suppliers then marketing systems to UK general practices. Agreed standards were first published in April 1993 under the title *General Medical Practice Computer Systems – Requirements for Accreditation*. Plans were made for annual revision in accordance with the needs of users, future developments in healthcare, and initiatives from central government and the Department of Health. As from April 1994, coercion was imposed by making computer costs reimbursement for GPs conditional upon the use of an accredited system.

Subsequently, the Family Health Services Computer Unit at Exeter (later the NHS Computer Agency and now the NHS Information Authority) was charged with assessing systems on behalf of the Department of Health. Practice management software testing took place on the supplier's premises, attracted a four-figure fee and, if successful, resulted in the issue of a certificate. Links and fundholding softwares were approved in a two-stage process that involved initial conformity with standard and subsequent beta-testing.

There is a lapse of a year between the publication of the requirements for accreditation (RFA) and the date on which they can be expected to come to fruition. The first RFA, published in 1993, should therefore have been effective as at April 1994, but by the summer of 1994 only eight systems marketed by the 109 suppliers then in business had been accredited, with applications having been lodged for a further 13. It became clear that only the foremost systems were supported by sufficient resources and expertise to produce upgrades in line with the RFA, and that, in any case, only a small proportion of the users of even these systems could afford to purchase the upgrades. A compromise was inevitable, and the Department of Health continued to reimburse a measure of support for what now became known as legacy systems, while the use of local discretion by health authorities produced an increasingly disparate interpretation of the rule book throughout the country.

RFA 1, which became effective in April 1994, dealt with registration, IoS claims, practice annual reports, basic consultation data, Read codes, prevention, prescribing and dispensing, referral, fundholding, back-up, audit trails, Data Protection Agency compliance, and ESCROW.

In April 1995, when RFA 2 became effective, only one supplier had by then upgraded its system to the required standard. RFA 2 introduced wide-ranging enhancement of prescribing and communication functions, data standards, security and confidentiality, the new NHS number, and health promotion with target payments. The importation of a drug product dictionary became inevitable.

RFA 3, which was effective in April 1996, set new standards for confidentiality, prescribing and audit. By this stage it had become clear that some suppliers did not intend to submit their systems for RFA 2 and 3 testing, but would leapfrog to RFA 4. As upgrades required by successive RFA specifications were cumulative, this was simply buying time, and was a reflection of the fact that much developmental effort had been diverted to produce fundholding systems, of which 13 had proved conformable by September 1995.

By May 1998, shortly after RFA 4 should have become effective, only one system (Reuter's Vision) had achieved the necessary level of upgrade. Although 35 systems fielded by a total of 19 suppliers had attained one or other level of either accreditation or conformance, the field of contestants had strung out a long way, and the required improvements had only filtered into a minority of practices. Belatedly, by March 1999, 14 suppliers were able to report that at least one of their marketed systems had passed RFA 4 testing on the bench. Further standards laid down in 1999 resulted in only two systems achieving accreditation by the target date of March 2000.

The principle of accreditation is laudable; it not only raises standards but encourages conformity and thereby interconnectivity. Moreover, the government has every right to specify the quality of the product for which it is paying very large sums of money. It is a pity that the benefits take so long to reach GPs.

27.7 SURVEYS

When marketing a commodity, it is essential to obtain market research and feedback, so that the product can be tailored to meet user requirements. Since computers were first introduced into general practice, a number of surveys have been undertaken by the Department of Health and other agencies that have monitored the uptake, application, and effect of the new technology. The survey results are interesting in that they have served both to guide and chart the development of GP computing in the UK.

The Department of Health commissioned surveys every 1–3 years between 1986 and 1998, which showed that, in the space of 10 years the percentage of computerized practices rose from less than 10% to 96% (Fig. 27.1).

In 1991 the MORI survey of all English and Welsh practices conducted for the Department of Health showed that 112 different systems were then in use, with VAMP, AAH Meditel, AMC, Update, EMIS and Genisyst dominating the market (listed in decreasing order of magnitude). Most responding practices used their computers for registration, repeat medication, partial clinical record keeping and practice annual reports, but less than half had implemented

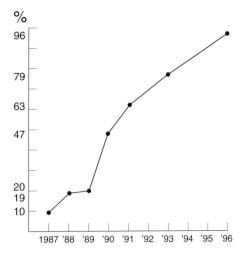

Fig. 27.1 Uptake of computers by UK general practices (data taken from DoH-commissioned and other surveys)

computerized acute prescribing. The main obstacles to computerization in 1991 were reported as being the amount of work involved in setting up a clinical system, the lack of sufficient financial incentive, and the attendant disruption to the working of the practice.

An interesting comparison with the 1991 findings was provided in 1996 by the survey of its readership conducted by *Medeconomics* magazine, to which 1300 practices responded, of which 97% had installed computers. 24% of these used EMIS, 21% VAMP and 15% AAH Meditel. 12% had already changed their system, and a further 11% were planning to do so. 9% recorded consultations exclusively on computer, 62% used their computer together with paper records for consultations, and 28% used paper alone for clinical recording. 82% of respondents had a modem, 70% were linked to HAs under the GP–HA Links scheme, 14% had Pathology Links, 3% Hospital Links, 50% had business and accounts packages, 33% used DTP, and 11% used laptop computers for home visits. 8% of practices had had computers stolen, and 6% had contracted a computer virus. Surveys from other sources showed that, by 1996, most practices were using computers for all acute and repeat prescribing.

The 1996 *Medeconomics* survey showed a dramatic increase in the versatility with which computers had come to be used during the previous 5 years. The growth in market share achieved by the EMIS system during this period is noteworthy.

In 1998, a survey instigated by the Department of Health addressed the effect that computers had had on the 5000 practices that responded. Only half the practices believed that computers had improved consultations but the great majority of both doctors and practice staff thought that there had been an improvement in the delivery of clinical care in terms of administration, management of clinical records, research and audit. Nine out of 10 practices found their systems easy to use, secure and functionally efficient in support of clinical work. Most were also happy with the way systems enabled information to be amended and updated, the way clinical histories were displayed and the way prescriptions were generated. Respondents showed somewhat less satisfaction with levels of support and training provided by suppliers, and the value for money that these represented.

27.8 THE PRIMARY HEALTH CARE SPECIALIST GROUP

The Primary Health Care Specialist Group (PHCSG) of the British Computer Society was formed in 1981 when a number of small localized groups of comput-

er enthusiasts amalgamated. It holds several meetings each year and circulates a quarterly newsletter and magazine in order to exchange ideas, and update members on the latest computer developments. Small working groups undertake projects of special interest.

The group's meetings are rotated geographically to ensure convenient attendance for all members at at least one meeting each year. Meetings commonly incorporate lectures, practical workshops and demonstrations of marketed systems, and are approved for PGEA accreditation. The group also holds training courses from time to time, which doctors and practice staff may attend. The group has cooperated with the Department of Health in the preparation of several publications on GP computer topics, and its officers are regarded by the press and public as spokesmen for the profession on GP computing affairs. (Contact: The Group Administrator, Hop Kiln Offices, Kiln Lane, Leigh Sinton, Worcs WR13 5EQ, tel: 01886 833848.)

27.9 THE ROYAL COLLEGE OF GENERAL PRACTITIONERS

The college has taken an active interest in GP computing since development began, and publishes articles on computing in its journal, the *British Journal of*

Box 27.3 Royal College of General Practitioners computing activities

1972	Birmingham Research Unit
1978	Computer Working Party (medical records)
1980	Joint Computer Policy Group (working party with GMSC)
1981	Central Information Service computerized (phone or postal GP enquiries, access to remote research data bases such as Medline or NHS Data)
1981	MESH; Prestel-based live study groups (with Wellcome Foundation)
1983	Information Technology Group
1983	Computer Fellowship (ICI Sponsorship), N. Stoddart
1985	Computer Appreciation Courses (PGEA approved). Permanent display of prominent marketed GP systems. Directory of current user practices. Central information service on GP computing (post or phone)
1997	RCGP website launched

General Practice. Its principal activities in the computer field are listed in Box 27.3.

27.10 THE BMA GENERAL MEDICAL SERVICES COMMITTEE

In 1979 the GMSC set up an advisory service on GP computing, and in 1980 it formed a computer sub-committee to monitor and make recommendations on the medicopolitical aspects of computing. Broadsheets are issued on an occasional basis.

In 1981 a Joint Computer Policy Group was set up with the RCGP, which represents the profession politically in computer affairs.

A series of publications explaining the medical implications of the DPA has been published by the GMSC (see Chapter 26).

27.11 USER GROUPS

Most marketed systems have their own individual user groups, within which local members meet to exchange experiences and give mutual support. Recommendations on system functionality should be funnelled from local user groups through national user representation to the supplier, who needs feedback to produce useful system modifications. A regular newsletter should be produced to chart the progress of the cycle of feedback and system enhancement.

As with most amateur enterprises, user group enthusiasm tends to wane, and attendances fall after a time. Add to this the difficulty of raising money for running costs from sources other than the supplier in order to maintain political independence, and the reasons for failure to thrive become clear. Because the momentum of the user group depends upon a handful of enthusiasts, it is not truly representative. If it were, a consortium formed from the chairmen of the user groups of all the main systems would constitute a strong political lobby for GP computer interests, possibly under the banner of the PHCSG.

27.12 OTHER AGENCIES

The Data Protection Commissioner

See Chapter 26.

Degree courses in medical informatics

Degree courses related to medical information technology are run by Manchester University, the University of Wales and jointly by London's City University and the United Medical and Dental Schools of Guy's and St Thomas' Hospitals (see also Chapter 22).

The Committee on Standards of Data Extraction in General Practice (COSODE)

This committee approves and monitors the activities of the data collection agencies.

The General Practice Computer System Suppliers Group

This group meets to promote marketing interests, to disseminate information about products, to consult with the Department of Health on policy and encourage funding improvements, to establish operating ethics and standards, to consult and cooperate with user groups, and to liaise with professional bodies. The group is formed by representatives of the foremost system suppliers.

REFERENCES AND FURTHER READING

Department of Health 1990 A survey of GP computing March/April 1990. Bulletin 4(7) 90

Department of Health 1990 GP computing: information for GPs on practice computer systems. HMSO, London

Health and Safety Commission 1992 A guide to the Health and Safety (display screen equipment) Regulations 1992. HMSO, London

Herd A 1990 User groups put GPs in the driving seat. Practice Computing, May: 14

Johnson K 1992 How a computer facilitator could help you. Practice Computing, September: 13

Medeconomics Magazine 1996 You and your computer. Medeconomics, June: 76–77

Practice Computing Magazine 1992 Maintenance: the low-down on the small print. Practice Computing, May: 22

NHSE 1997 Evaluation of GP computer systems 1997: Summary report for GPs (E5407), National Report (E5409) and System reports (E5410) (published January 1998). NHSE, London

NHSE 1998 Information for health: An information strategy for the modern NHS 1998–2005. NHSE, London

28 Selecting, funding, upgrading or changing a system

28.1 OVERVIEW

This chapter summarizes those points that must be borne in mind when purchasing or upgrading a system. It is placed at the end of the book because a background knowledge derived from the chapters that proceed it must be acquired before an informed choice can be made.

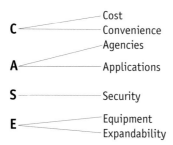

Fig. 28.1 The criteria by which to judge a general practice computer system may be considered under seven broad headings

The criteria by which the prospective user may judge a system fall into three categories – system functionality, supplier support and minimum data requirements. While embellishments will continue to appear, the principal application areas and accompanying functionality of GP systems can be defined, and are displayed in the following pages as summarizing diagrams, which can be photocopied so as to act as check lists for assessment. Important aspects of supplier support are also listed in the diagrams.

Minimum requirements in all categories of data used by general practice proliferate as computer systems acquire greater sophistication. Many of these categories were not used prior to computerization, and so their data are not obtainable from manual records, but must be acquired either opportunistical-

ly or as a separate exercise. Definitive minimum data sets for patient registration and administration (Chapter 7), locality commissioning (Chapter 17), prescription statements (Chapter 11) and procedures associated with HA claims (Chapter 8) have already been established, but in other areas are still evolving. For this reason, detailed check lists which focus on minimum data sets are rapidly outdated, and must be reviewed at least every year.

The Standards Committees will in future regularly review minimum data requirements for GP computers, and all responsible suppliers will incorporate data category upgrades as and when the committees' recommendations are published.

28.2 SUPPLIER AND BRAND

There are currently more than 30 brands of GP system in the UK that have achieved various levels of accreditation. They are marketed by 13 different system suppliers, whose details are listed at the end of this chapter. While many of the less well known system houses have been efficient and innovative, it is inevitable that a small supplier with minimum financial backing will lack the investment capital required to develop a large package such as that needed for locality commissioning, and may find it difficult to provide nationwide call-out support. On the other hand, large suppliers experience scale-related difficulties if they decide to make fundamental changes to their system functionality, file structure, or term coding system, which must then be transferred across to practice level. System suppliers are under considerable pressure from their competitive situation, from the dictates of government policy and changes to that policy, and from discriminatory reimbursement by HAs who, for reasons of economy or uniformity, may wish to promote the use of a particular system. Many casualties among suppliers have already occurred, and it is

SYSTEMS COSTS

Initial hardware and upgrades ☐

Initial software and new modules ☐

Sockets, wiring, conduits, furniture, lighting, windowscreens, security measures, nightsafe ☐

Telecommunications charges
HealthLink fees
NHSnet fees ☐

Maintenance of hardware and software ☐

Staff training and new posts ☐

Staff wages for take-on of practice data, and reconciliation with HA register ☐

Insurance ☐

DPA registration ☐

Paper, labels, printer ribbon or cartridge, electricity ☐

HA download (or upload check) ☐

Local database licence fees
Drug database
Read codes, protocol library ☐

Remote database enquiry charges ☐

Fig. 28.2 Costs to the practice – at purchase and with ongoing use

SYSTEM CONVENIENCE

Consistent design principles throughout system for navigation, macro, function key, menu and protocol use ☐

Easy control for data input point and mouse cursor ☐

Toggle between appointments and clinical screens ☐

Data entry validated from dictionary whenever possible ☐

Comprehensive drug, morbidity, protocol dictionaries, and practice formulary easy to use ☐

Data presented clearly, concisely, with visual appeal and without crowding ☐

Data entry quick and easy: default option used wherever possible, otherwise minimum number of key depressions to be used ☐

Sensible arrangement of function keys/icons ☐

Entry selection from short menus or protocols whenever feasible ☐

Refer to look-up data in a small enclave on screen (window) while retaining main record display in background ☐

Facility to rescind latest command ☐

Facility to 'escape' to main menu from any part of system ☐

Clear and unambiguous user instructions given at each decision point in progression through software as prompts, error messages, then fresh options. Every eventuality must be covered ☐

Easy transfer from one part of system to another
Easy change from one part of record to another for same patient, or change of patient while viewing same area of record ☐

Data entered once can be assigned to multiple subrecords if required ☐

Links between diagnosis and prescription ☐

Easy export of data from one file to another, e.g. payroll to accounts ☐

Help screens raised in relation to all parts of the system ☐

Impossible to be trapped in a 'vicious circle' of key sequences ☐

Impossible to 'crash' system by miskeying ☐

User designed screen format option ☐

Record links between individual patients living in same household ☐

Search routines easy to specify: allow to search on up to 3 variables at a time ☐

Simple archiving facility ☐

Screen dumps from any screen ☐

Fast system response time under heavy load in demonstrator practice ☐

Fully automatic fast back-up ☐

Printers fast, quiet, easy to use; ease of ribbon or cartridge change ☐

Interruption and resumption of print run without loss of data or other penalty ☐

Printer buffer ☐

Automatic dial-up and data transfer through e-mail on NHSnet ☐

Fig. 28.3 Convenience – factors affecting a system's ease of use

AGENCIES – SUPPLIER AND MAINTENANCE CONTRACTOR

How long in market?

Track record in developing efficient new software modules

How many systems in field?

What commercial backing does supplier receive from financial institutions?

Sufficient hardware and software support teams to give national coverage

On-line software support through modem

Hotline with fast response and adequate hours of manning

Supplier maintains hardware, software and communications

Adequate training on-site

Training as software package

Member of GP computer suppliers group

Organized user groups who have power to enable design improvements

Watertight maintenance agreement to include software enhancement, guaranteeing no loss of data in process

Fast call-out in emergency

All equipment used is from well established manufacturer

Supplier keeps equipment spares for 7 years after sale

Lends alternative equipment up to full replacement during repairs

Good user manual

Source code in ESCROW

Fig. 28.4 Agencies – support is a vital consideration

SYSTEM APPLICATIONS

Total record reform: entry of all consultation data on computer

Summary history records (dictionary validated entry)

Surveillance shared care clinics and records

Preventive records, target calculations, call or recall and opportunistic screening

Pathology records, test requests and reports with automatic filing

Repeat medication

Acute prescribing using prescribing monitor Prescribing audit for PPA E-PACT

Appointments

Encounter forms to show summary records, repeat medication, allergies and opportunistic reminders

Commissioning

Word processing, mailmerge and standard letters

Locally held databases – drugs and morbidity

Protocol library for histories, diagnoses and patient management

Desk-top publishing, printed patient instructions, practice brochures

Automated referral letters and log, with hospital appointment-making

Reference displays – national, local and individual

HA upload reconciliation with practice patient registers

Electronic mail with HA, pathology laboratory and hospital. Interrogation of remote databases

'Search and list' on up to 3 defined parameters from any part of the patient record with statistical and graphical output

Business packages – spreadsheets for ledgers, payroll, accounts, claims. Electronic banking

Automated PMA insurance questionnaire completion

Provision for remote access to server

Dispensing

E-drug response recording and reporting

Educational packages

Research, Audit, Practice Annual Reports

Electronic summarisation of incoming hospital reports, subsequent scanning of full report. If e-reports, then autofile

Provision for incorporation of cooperative initiated data

Patient-held monitoring devices can be downloaded

Fig. 28.5 Applications – the specification should be based on current and future needs of the practice

---

SYSTEM SECURITY

Entry and depth of access to system controlled by password. Repeated false password attempts temporarily disable the system ☐

On-line uninterruptible power supply ☐

Unique computer symbol for each user is attached to all data entries so that authorship can always be traced (symbol derived from password) ☐

Automatic back-up by reduplication of recorded data as security copies on secondary hard disk or magnetic tape. Physical removal to fireproof lock-up safe of back-up data, copies of system program, dictionary diskettes and unused EC 10 comp . at night ☐

Content, time, date and authorship of all data amendments logged (audit trail) ☐

Antivirus software ☐

Premises in which the computer is kept are locked. Increased security if user must physically unlock terminal by key as with cash tills ☐

In networked systems, record being amended by one user must not be alterable by another ☐

Software safeguards to ensure data are incorruptible and preserved intact in the event of system failure ☐

Network management and security software ☐

Prompt hardware repair or else replacement contract. Software patch via modem ☐

Data amendment must always be subject to two key depressions, one to propose change and other to confirm (prevents accidental action) Miskeying should never be able to crash system or destroy data ☐

Internet access and e-mail restricted to NHSnet, challenge handshake authentication protocol for electronic mail ☐

Fig. 28.6 Desirable security features built into systems – users have additional responsibility for DPA registration, insurance, exterior lightning conductor installation, protection of equipment during relocation, antivirus discipline, backup, UPS provision, and for requiring guarantees of confidentiality from practice staff, visitors, system maintenance engineers and Data Collation Schemes

---

EQUIPMENT

Fileserver: IBM-PC compatible, Pentium circuitry, RAM requirement determined by sum of application, communication, workstation and printer loading ☐

Floppy disk drive for double-density double-sided diskettes, CD-ROM drive or multidrive ☐

Modem or CODEC ☐

Distributed workstation or Network stations using visual display units with not less than 20 lines of 80 characters, colour, graphics; adjustable for tilt, contrast and brightness. No flicker ☐

On-line uninterruptible power supply ☐

Data back-up facility: magnetic tape (tape streamer) or supplementary hard disk ☐

Local area network with appropriate distribution of storage and processing power between terminals ☐

Printers – one quiet running for each prescriber. One or more batch mode machines in secretaries' office ☐

Alphanumeric keyboards with adequate function keys, 'Mouse' input ☐

Scanner, shredder ☐

Storage (hard disk) not less than 5 Gb, more for large practices ☐

Fireproof safe ☐

Fig. 28.7 Equipment – the basic hardware specification for an adequate system

---

inevitable that more will either be bought out by a larger competitor or just cease trading. When buy-outs occur, practices with legacy systems are put under pressure to convert to the new supplier's product. When a supplier goes to the wall, the practice must obtain ESCROW facilities and face the severe disruption of changing systems at short notice. While all major suppliers field teams of staff skilled in conversion from other systems to their own, the degree of success they achieve will largely depend upon any

similarities that exist between the data categories and file structures of the two systems. Inevitably, extra work, sometimes of considerable magnitude, will be required by practice staff to make good the record deficits that conversion creates.

It is not at all easy to reach a rational decision as to which system to buy. All too often, the uncomputerized practice bases its choice on the immediate applications it wishes to implement, only to find that its requirements change once the computer has become

SYSTEM EXPANDABILITY

Add applications without reorganization of files, re-entry of practice data, or need to change processor ☐	Add more storage ☐
Add more workstations and printers without degradation of performance ☐	Add more processor memory ☐
Accept software enhancements; add new software modules ☐	Access remote databases ☐
Accept full suite of locally held databases – drug, morbidity, protocol, travel medicine, etc. ☐	Change single CD-ROM drive to multidrive ☐
Incorporate cooperative initiated data ☐	Upgrade back-up equipment to on-line configuration ☐
Add new off-the-shelf packages ☐	Accommodate split-site landlines and radio transmission for remote portable access ☐
Access NHSnet ☐	Audio and video ☐

Fig. 28.8 Expandability – again, the long-term needs of the practice should be anticipated

operational and the machine's full potential, together with its limitations, become clear. The situation is made more difficult by the fact that all GP computer systems are still going through a phase of active development, and that purchase remains to some extent an act of faith. A critical look at the supplier's track record for developing new and efficient software modules, his stake in the market and the strength of those investing in him, will provide the best available indication of his ability to honour future developmental obligations. Coupled with this, an assessment of maintenance support must be made. In the past, some companies that provided vigorous development lacked adequate field support, and those with efficient maintenance operations were not always innovative, or else made poor strategic decisions.

28.3 FUNCTIONALITY

- The definitive general practice computer system must now be regarded as being based on a local area network configuration, with the instalment of workstations or network stations on all staff desks, with quiet printers beside all prescribers, and with a batch printer in the reception area. It must be possible for the system to run all record-keeping and prescribing functions and, for these, a Read-code morbidity dictionary and comprehensive drug database such as Multilex will be necessary. The drug database must not only support the printing of a prescription statement, but provide electronic matrices for automated checks on the suitability of drugs, and a textual lookup facility for drug product attributes. A protocol library for patient management must be integral.

- The appointments system must be integral and interleave with access to patient records.
- Communications must be provided that connect with the PCG+T, with the HA, laboratory, radiology department and providers. While a locality intranet may support these connections, ISDN and NHSnet access will ultimately be needed for e-mail and the interrogation of the Internet and other remote databases. Linkages with the community health, local mental health and social services must also be available.
- Options must be available for remote access to the practice server from portables, and it should be possible to import 'dawn report' data directly from cooperatives to the practice system, with subsequent autofiling.
- Tapestream backup and an uninterruptible power supply must be provided.

This is an exacting specification, but any general practitioner who cannot see his way clear to attaining all these goals, when negotiating with a prospective supplier, should reconsider his choice.

28.4 STEPS TAKEN IN REACHING A DECISION

Because some factors in the selection process take precedence over others, the following order of priorities in decision making is suggested:

1. Is system choice limited by the need to accommodate a distinctive practice activity?
   - Locality commissioning and the creation of PCG+T intranets will impose constraints of compatibility, but will also provide the

opportunity for bulk purchase of systems for the PCG+T office and its member practices.

- Dispensing practices must choose a system with specialized dispensing software, backed by a comprehensive drug database that includes stock control data, in order to provide for all the refinements that automation can offer the integrated prescribing and dispensing processes.
- Private practices require a billing system linked to consultation, pathology and treatment records in the patient files.
- Split-site practices should choose a supplier with experience in landline management or, if the branch surgery is used relatively infrequently, in providing file reconciliation between portable computers and the main system.
- Very large practices with multiple partners have special logistical problems in running computer systems, and should opt for a supplier with extensive experience in dealing with these. Single handed, or other small urban practices, while retaining discrete patient record files, may wish to share the facilities and costs of a single central fileserver, accessed through landlines – a speciality configuration offered by some suppliers.
- Practices in remote locations may have special communication requirements to accommodate the use of portables or telemedicine.

2. All practices must now opt for a system that employs a graphical user interface with mouse or touchscreen. Text-based systems and multiuser configurations based on dumb terminals must now be regarded as obsolete, since they cannot access NHSnet.

3. Draw up the initial list of applications that the practice will use, trying to allow for those revisions that the next few years might bring. You will find that the most prominent suppliers will be able to cater for the majority of these applications. If not, ask what other modules are under advanced development. List the applications in the order in which you propose to implement them, and ask the prospective supplier to comment on the order and grouping that you plan.

4. Familiarization with market products is needed.
- Study suppliers' paper-based and website brochures carefully.
- Familiarization with rival systems can be obtained by attending displays arranged by some HAs, by the PHCSG, or by the GP Computer magazines.
- Courses with hands-on experience are run by the PHCSG and some colleges of technology.

5. Seek impartial advice. Involve your HA's Computer Liaison Officer. Visit other practices that have installed system brands in which you are interested – the HA may be prepared to provide a list of local practices willing to offer their colleagues demonstrations.

6. Finally, ask for on-site demonstrations from shortlisted suppliers and use the sequence of summary diagrams as check lists to draw comparisons between them.

7. Cost each item carefully, determining what is included in the purchase price and maintenance contract, and what will be charged as an extra.

28.5 FUNDING PRACTICE SYSTEMS

As HAs are now intimately involved in the purchase, maintenance and security of GP systems, their advice and approval must always be obtained before decisions on choice and timing are made. Many suppliers are prepared to set up tripartite meetings between themselves, the practice and the HA. It is also important to seek the advice of the practice accountant.

There are four ways of funding computer purchase:

- *Outright cash payment* – tax relief on 100% of the written down value applies (formerly 25% annually)
- *Bank or finance company loan* – tax relief is granted on interest and repayments
- *Hire purchase* over a fixed period, during which tax relief will be allowed on both interest and capital repayments, but repossession follows default in premiums – this method tends to be of the order of 10% more expensive overall than either bank loans or leasing
- *Leasing.* Most suppliers have arrangements with leasing companies so that divided payments may be spread over 3–5 years. An initial deposit of around 25% is paid to the supplier by the practice. The first actual lease payment must be made when the computer is installed, and customarily covers the first 3 months. After this, monthly payments are instituted, the supplier is paid in full by the leasing company, and the deposit is returned to the practice. The equipment remains the property of the leasing company during the tenure of the lease but, when most of the debt has been paid off, it is usual for the equipment to be formally sold to the user for a small nominal sum. Leasing payments are allowable for tax purposes.

BMA Services offer a range of methods of financing computer purchase and can be contacted on Freephone 0800 716167.

- Heavily discounted prices on new PCs, bundled with mobile telephone packages and internet services, are offered by such firms as Time, Tiny and PC World.

Other ways of contributing to the cost of computer systems should also be considered. These are:

- Combining with other practices to arrange joint purchase and bulk discount from a supplier – this is best done in conjunction with the HA
- Using savings made from prescribing incentive schemes
- Enrolling for participation in a Data Collection Scheme
- Using advertising to fund kiosk terminals in the waiting room
- Portable computers, like co-op systems, may attract funding from the out-of-hours development fund
- A scheme has been proposed by BT whereby practice systems may be part-funded by commercial organizations. It is not yet clear to what extent advertising will be involved, and whether this would be acceptable on an NHS facility, but the proposal is worth watching.
- As locality commissioning unrolls, some form of incentive payment to upgrade practice systems in line with PCG+T compliance, and overt funding for PCG+T office systems, seem inevitable.

28.6 SYSTEM UPGRADES

The practice system needs to be upgraded if:

- the software will not provide all the applications that the practice or the RFA require
- software is inconvenient to use, contains significant 'bugs', or crashes
- the secretarial staff have to queue to use terminals
- the speed of data processing by the system slows significantly.

Upgrades may be made to hardware or software, or both. Software streamlining and debugging are undertaken continuously by suppliers, and new versions of software designed to pass on these improvements are usually referred to as enhancements. There should be no extra charge for these, as provision for them should be included in the maintenance contract. When software is extensively rewritten, or new functionality is introduced, a new software module will have been created for which most suppliers reserve the right to charge afresh. Software upgrades often follow the uprating of requirements for system accreditation. When a system's software has previously been customized at practice level, upgrades will frequently prove more difficult to implement.

Hardware upgrades may be obviously necessary to the practice – more terminals may be required for desktop record keeping by doctors, or more printers may be needed to cope with acute prescribing. If, however, the speed of reactivity of the system becomes significantly reduced, then either the hard disk or processor functionality may be proving inadequate. The possibility of hard disk saturation can be checked by 'housekeeping' programs available to the user that report the percentage of unused storage, and rationalize its use (see also Chapter 1). Although some economies may be made by expunging obsolete files (such as old search operations), a larger hard disk will need to be installed if the old one is approaching saturation.

If the hard disk is not saturated, then system slowing is nearly always a sign of inadequate processing power. This is most likely to show itself after software upgrades, the addition of new users, the implementation of new applications, or the loading of new dictionaries. Although extra RAM can be added to a processor, this will not upgrade the basic processor circuitry and a new processor is usually required.

Some system suppliers (such as EMIS) have a policy of selling customers more processing power than they need at system inauguration, in order to avoid frequent processor upgrades. Other suppliers warn customers that new processors are likely to be needed every few years. The current pace of technological development brings with it the promise that, before too long, processors will cease to be overstretched by the expanding demands of general practice.

Backup copies of all files should be taken before all upgrades.

28.7 CHANGING SYSTEMS

A small proportion of practices become dissatisfied with their original system and change it. There are even a few practices that have changed twice. Change carries the penalties of expense (both of purchase of the new system, and data conversion), inconvenience and the possibility of data loss. A practice that made an incorrect first choice should refine its selection procedure very carefully before purchasing a second time. Reasons for changing will include a supplier's demise or sell-out, a supplier's repeated inability to meet practice requirements or to produce upgrades in line with other suppliers or the RFA, and overpricing of upgrades or maintenance.

Choice of a replacement will be limited by any incompatibilities that exist between the old practice system and its proposed alternatives. The following problems may exist:

- The employment of different operating systems by the old and the new computer used to be an absolute bar to the transfer of data between systems. This obstacle has, in most cases, been overcome by compilation (the use of software translation programs).
- File format and data category standards have still not been introduced into GP system development, so that it is easy for data to be 'posted to the wrong address' on transfer. Portability of software, files and data between systems will be markedly improved by the recommendations of the standards committees as these become available.
- Standard codes for essential clinical, pharmaceutical and administrative terms are essential if data are not to be corrupted or lost through mismatch on transfer. Only now, through general adoption of Read codes, is this problem being solved, but difficulties may still exist if four- and five-byte Read sets have both been employed, either in the past or between the new and old systems. Converting practices have also reported data losses resulting from the use of personalized abbreviations, ampersands, recall markers, mileage units, and incompatible appointment systems. The expertise of the new supplier's conversion team is vital to success, and the use of a postconversion audit module, if available, will demonstrate exactly where data have failed to convert.
- Hardware may have to be scrapped. Some suppliers are only prepared to service their own recommended brands of equipment. If transfer is made from a multiuser to a local area network configuration, extensive terminal repurchase will be necessary. There is no trade-in on old equipment.

Suppliers' claims to be able to convert practice systems to their own brand are rife, but should be viewed with due scepticism. The steps to be taken are:

1. Ask the new supplier for the name of a practice that has already converted to the new system, if possible from the same old system. Visit the practice, go through a formal preselection check, and investigate all conversion problems that arose.
2. Ask the new supplier for a test conversion on your backup data, a specimen data conversion contract, a quote for system conversion, and a specification and quote for all new equipment that will be required. Ask your practice solicitor to check the new contracts.
3. Check that the HA will reimburse for data conversion, all new equipment, and changes in staff duties required by the conversion process.
4. Ask the HA to check the new supplier's claims to be able to convert. Ask the HA's Computer Liaison Officer to oversee the process.
5. Plan the logistics of conversion. Some suppliers will convert at weekends. Arrange staff retraining, any necessary overtime, and any new appointments required.
6. Take and retain at least two security copies of all data on the old system, plus specimen printouts from each category of file. After conversion, check the new with the old data in detail. Do not complete payment until satisfied.
7. Use printed-out encounter forms taken from the old system while data are being converted.

Costs for conversion

Costs incurred in the conversion process are for:
- new hardware
- new software
- data conversion
- training
- extra staff time.

These can in part be set against system and staff wages reimbursement, and may to some extent be rationalized if an upgrade would have been due anyway.

28.8 MINIMUM DATA SUBSETS

Every category of general practice activity uses its own subset of the overall medical vocabulary to formulate the subset of data that is particular to it. As medical record data are descriptive and scientific, the statements within them consist of a succession of data categories (parameters such as 'systolic blood pressure' or 'cough') linked to the values (such as '150' or 'productive, present for 3 weeks') assigned to them. The list of data categories that pertains to a given practice activity is called its *data subset*. In order to produce conformity between records, it is necessary to define a minimum agreed array of those data categories which are required to describe each particular activity, and this is known as the activity's *minimum data subset* (MDSS).

The evaluation of a system should include an assessment of how adequately it has incorporated both those MDSSs that are by now well established, and those that are still only partially defined.

The following minimum data subsets are now well defined:

- Registration
- IoS claims – proforma completion (Chapter 8)
- Prescription statements (Chapter 11)
- Dispensing line reorder (Prescription Pricing Authority Database) and reimbursement data
- Immunization
- Cervical cytology
- Notification of infectious disease
- Adverse Drug Reaction Report (Committee on Safety of Medicines)
- Child Health Surveillance checks (Department of Health)
- Locality commissioning accounts (Chapter 17).

The following minimum data subsets have been defined in principle, but not in a sufficient degree of detail to meet with unanimous acceptance:

- Referral letter

- PMA Insurance Report
- New patient check
- Geriatric screening
- Asthma and diabetes review
- Reviews of other forms of surveillance
- Synopsis of manual record
- Synoptic pathology recording
- Practice brochure.

The standards committees periodically review the degree of definition that minimum data sets and sub-sets have reached. An up-to-date check list of the Primary Health Care Specialist Group Standards Working Party may be obtained from the Administrator, Mrs J Hayes, 3 Beech Avenue North, Worcester WR3 3PX.

All responsible system suppliers will incorporate new MDS subset categories in their systems as and when they are defined by the standards committees.

28.9 SUPPLIERS OF ACCREDITED GP SYSTEMS

These are listed in Table 28.1. At least one product from each supplier had achieved RFA 4 status by 29 March 1999. This list is subject to change without warning.

Table 28.1 Suppliers of accredited GP systems

Supplier	Former names associated with products	Tel. number
Aremis Soft	AmSys, Genisyst, LK Global	01462 755100
Chime UCL MS	Paradoc	(020) 7288 5209
ECL Medical		(020) 8654 9000
EMIS		01132 591122
Exeter Systems		0121 248 1234
In-Practice Systems Ltd	VAMP, Reuter's, GP Plus, MicroSolutions	(020) 7501 7000
ITS Wales Ltd		01792 818270
Microtest Ltd	G and G Software	01208 73171
Pennine Medical Systems	Phenix	01422 886171
PMY Solutions Ltd		0117 9886501
Seetec Ltd		01702 201070
The Computer Room		01773 718578
Torex Health Ltd	Micro-Doc, Meduser, Update, MCS AMC, ARH Meditel	01865 373797

Source: NHS Information Authority Exeter (formerly FHSCU)
Updates obtainable on http://www.fhs.org-uk/gpservs/accred/list.asp

29 Preparing for the computer

This chapter is primarily intended for those few practices that have not yet embarked on computerization. It also deals with organizational methods, which may be helpful to those who are not yet fully paperless.

Installing a computer in the practice is not merely a question of selecting and taking delivery of a suitable system. It also requires:

- fundamental organizational changes to data handling at all levels and to staff duties
- significant capital outlay and increased practice running expenses
- a planned progression from preliminary preparations through to total computer implementation.

29.1 ORGANIZATIONAL CHANGES REQUIRED WHEN PREPARING TO INSTALL A COMPUTER SYSTEM

The need to confer

Every member of the practice team must be prepared to accept the change to electronic data processing and to adopt a strictly disciplined approach in using the system. All those involved in formulating computer policy should assemble periodically to decide objectives and methodology, and to monitor progress. It is best to keep informal minutes of these meetings for future reference.

New appointments

New posts will be required:

- Computer Manager

The *Computer Manager*, who assumes overall responsibility for computer operations, must designate and allocate tasks, supervise all aspects of security and confidentiality, and implement the provisions of the Data Protection Act (including subject access to data). S/he must ensure that backup procedures are adhered to punctiliously, will be responsible for training all members of staff in computer use and discipline, and will liaise with the PCG+T/HA's IT officer and with the supplier when system problems occur. A time/date log and description of all computer faults and actions taken should be kept. Backup tapes, diskette security copies of drug, morbidity and protocol dictionaries and unused prescription stationery should be stored overnight in a fireproof secure cabinet or safe under the computer manager's control. Specific computer insurance must be put in place.

- Records Officer

A *Records Officer* must be appointed (see also Chapter 5). Field studies show that an intelligent and carefully trained Records Officer proves capable of reliable summarization of records. All output should be scrutinized by a doctor before it is transferred to a computer, and the summarizer must always seek medical expertise in case of doubt.

The induction of the Records Officer should be progressive, with training beginning on the daily hospital and pathology reports received by the practice before these are read and checked by the doctors, highlighting first pathology, then X-ray reports, later surgical, and finally medical reports. From the start the Records Officer must learn to recognize when to ask for help, for there will always be times when s/he needs to do so. Having achieved proficiency, s/he then transcribes summary from old records on to take-on cards, and here initially every card completed must be counterchecked by the doctor against its manual record. When word perfect, the Records Officer is entrusted first with small records, then large ones, with the doctor reading the take-on cards for obvious errors. When fully proficient, the skilled Records Officer attains a higher level of accuracy in record abstraction for summary than is achieved by most doctors.

The Records Officer will be responsible for ensuring that the new methods of manual data support required by the computer system are properly maintained (see below).

With the implementation of computer records, the Records Officer must ensure that all practice-generated data and all continuing hospital-based summary data are recorded on the system. This vigil cannot be relaxed until all GPs enter all data directly on to the system, and all summary data from hospital reports are automatically transferred to the practice records from incoming electronic mail.

Intelligence, training, and self discipline are necessary qualities in a Records Officer, but a nursing qualification is not essential.

- Update Clerk

The *Update Clerk* requires typing skills and must be trained to use the system's special data entry protocols (such as 'shoehorn' techniques for keying-in details of all family members resident together without the need to repeat the address). The Clerk's work is supervised by the Records Officer. The computer's facility for earmarking all entries with the author's identity proves to be an incentive for accuracy of input.

The posts of Computer Manager, Records Officer and Update Clerk may be combined in small practices.

Training

The most important training will be that provided by the system supplier before, during and after installation, and it is vital that all staff members should be present when this is taking place. Although a good user manual should also be provided by the supplier, and should be read by all members of staff, it is common for some systems' features to remain undiscovered by a practice unless the system has been demonstrated in depth during the supplier's training sessions.

Most GP supplier software, and some off-the-shelf commercial packages, now incorporate tuitional modules for staff training using dummy documents.

HAs appoint members of staff with specialized computer knowledge who are prepared to offer practices technical support, especially as regards Links, security and funding. Nearby practices with longer experience of computers may also be prepared to help.

PGEA approved courses of computer training are occasionally run by the Primary Health Care Specialist Group of the British Computer Society, some of the regional colleges of technology and the postgraduate educational centres.

Business-orientated training courses (not usually PGEA-approved) are of limited value but will provide experience in word processing, financial applications, desktop publishing and computer maintenance. Such courses tend to be expensive.

Distance learning courses on network use and the Windows operating system are available from Microsoft and these may attract PGEA accreditation.

Defining responsibility

All staff responsibilities for operations connected with the computer should be strictly defined and written down. There is a case to be made out for displaying a notice in the reception area that reminds staff of their security obligations. Important responsibilities such as those relating to data confidentiality, backup, the Data Protection Act, and unauthorized computer use should be built in to staff contracts. On pain of instant dismissal, some practices forbid staff to take extraneous diskettes into the medical centre.

Siting the terminals

The positioning of terminals, printers, wiring, telephone and lighting should be planned in advance, bearing in mind that display units should not be placed either facing or in front of direct light sources (including windows). Electricity sockets should be located with care so that computer equipment cannot be switched off accidentally, and the hazards of loose cabling are avoided. Detailing faults to a supplier will require a telephone next to the terminal. Acute prescribing requires that each prescriber has a printer. Noisy printers disturb consultations.

Registration under the Data Protection Act

All practices must notify to be entered on the DPA register. Applications should be made to the Data Protection Commissioner, Wycliffe House, Water Lane, Cheshire SK9 5AF (see also Chapter 26).

Accountant advice

The decision as to whether a system is leased or purchased, and the implications of the timing of purchase for tax and cash flow, should be reviewed with the practice accountant.

Liaison with the health authority and supplier

It is important to secure the HA's prior approval for computer purchase so as to ensure that reimbursement will be available, and that the timing and choice of system purchased will be such as to obtain maximum reimbursement. Suppliers will usually provide a practice with a quotation for the cost of the system it is proposing to purchase, and this quotation should be sent to the HA so that funds can be earmarked in advance. The date of registration file download to, or upload from, the practice should be pre-arranged with the HA. If the practice wishes to begin cross-checks of practice and HA registers before the computer's arrival, the HA will usually provide a printout of practice patients registered with them.

29.2 SUMMARIZING AND TRANSFERRING MANUAL DATA TO THE COMPUTER

The four main obstacles to the introduction of full computerization into general practice have been:

- Error-prone hardware and software design
- Expense
- The need to convert doctors to keyboard use
- The need to summarize manual records (and, on a continuing basis, further incoming reports from hospital) and load summary data on to the computer.

Advances in computer design and improved supplier support are overcoming the first obstacle, and reduction in real term cost of systems, coupled with partial reimbursement, have made practice computing relatively less expensive. Newer and more convenient methods of data entry are being developed and introduced which should resolve outstanding objections to the use of keyboards. There remains the problem of data conversion.

Manual records are grossly inefficient. The unstructured contents of the general practice manual record wallet develop into a cumulative chaos in which the important synoptic data, essential to future patient management, are scattered throughout a larger quantity of obsolete material, rather like flowers in a garden overgrown by weeds. Any reform on or off computer requires a process of abstraction or summarization. The general practice record is tripartite, containing GP notes, hospital letters and pathology test results. It is the first and second of these elements that need summarizing by text sifting – pathology results are not obscured by outdated verbiage, although many historical test results may prove subsequently irrelevant. Retained pathology results must be classified and ordered, and some may be requoted synoptically.

The abstraction process must be applied, both during the initial preparation of manual records for transfer to computer, and also after practice computer records have become operational, but hospital reports continue to be received on paper. A typical procedure is for GP notes and hospital reports to be summarized on to 'take-on' or 'transfer' cards in preparation for loading, and for pathology test results to be transcribed in synoptic form to their own dedicated take-on card. After computer records have become operational, GP notes will be entered directly on to the visual display unit at consultation, while hospital reports that are still paper-based will need summarizing and summary transcription to computer. Pathology test results on paper will need transcription in synoptic form.

In both initial preparation for take-on and in continued updating after take-on there are two separate operations:

- Record summarization
- Data entry to computer.

The first operation requires the appointment of a Records Officer. The second, being a transcription process, is given to the Update Clerk, who need only possess typing skills. Both processes may, of course, be undertaken by the same individual. There is no reason why existing practice staff should not be employed for these tasks, but training in their new duties will be required.

29.3 THE EFFORT INVOLVED

Continuous updating of the established computer record will take up to half an hour per day for hospital report summarization, and pathology and hospital report data input, and this may be absorbed into existing hours of work. Historical record take-on, however, requires a concerted and extra effort on the part of the practice staff. Here, record abstraction takes 6–12 minutes for an average record, and loading takes a further 6 minutes.

The cost of record preparation for computerization depends upon the amount of staff wages reimbursement that is made available. Some HAs have gone so far as to provide total refunding for summarization.

29.4 TAKE-ON CARDS

Surveys have shown that the general practitioner wishes to retrieve data for the purpose of later patient management in a totally different form from that in which it was entered. The computer, with its ability to manipulate text, effects this transformation between input and output formats.

The design of the take-on cards (see also Chapter 5) secures a preliminary sorting of data. The cards cannot, of course, achieve the computer's ability to present the same data in a variety ways, nor can they sort entries in chronological order as the computer does. Summary data from both general practice and hospital, labelled according to source, are taken jointly on to one card because they refer to the same illnesses. This card gives precedence not only to summary history but also to allergies, and to repeat medication in synoptic format. The same card makes provision for the recording of all necessary patient identification details (including such items as hospital and NHS numbers) and also for immunizations. Long-term follow-up of chronic disease such as hypertension or diabetes is accommodated on its own take-on card, and pathology synoptic recording is also housed on a separate card. Obsolete material from general practice and hospital documents is not transcribed to take-on cards. When take-on cards have been completed, they are stored in the manual record wallet until take-on to computer.

29.5 PLAN AHEAD FOR TAKE-ON

Record take-on to computer will proceed more smoothly if preparations are begun several months in advance of the take-on date. This will allow adequate time for the training of staff, for the preparation of the take-on cards, and for the detection of gross deficiencies in the manual records by the use of the take-on cards at consultation. Take-on cards are updated with new consultation data until the card's contents are transferred to computer.

29.6 PROCEDURE AT TAKE-ON

At the time of take-on to computer, the take-on cards are removed from the record wallets a few at a time, and the details they contain are keyed into the computer. Thereafter all patient record details will be accessed through the computer, other than for the very exceptional recourse that is needed to old full-length hospital reports. The update clerk must always take care to enter new hospital summary material to the correct file, whether this be take-on card or computer, during the interim period of take-on.

29.7 THE RECORD OFFICER'S PROTOCOL

By following a simple agreed protocol the harvesting of summary material becomes an organized exercise. The end result is a nutshell synopsis of past and ongoing morbidity – a precision instrument used in the provision of future patient management.

When abstracting a summary from past records, the Records Officer (for the sake of simplicity, let's suppose that she is female) must use guidelines set by the practice. These are likely to include the following points:

- When summarizing, the need is for painstaking accuracy in following the practice protocol, with recourse to medical advice when the protocol is not explicit in dealing with a problem.
- The Records Officer keeps on her desk the three categories of take-on card (summary card, condition orientated card and pathology synopsis – if used), the summarization protocol, a dictionary of medical terms for secretaries, and a list of abbreviations and synonyms frequently used in medical note keeping.
- She has centrally in front of her the take-on cards ready for completion, and on one side of these the contents of the record wallet she is about to summarize. After she has summarized a document, she transfers it to the other side of her desk.
- The three components of the wallet, GP notes, hospital reports and pathology tests, are best summarized separately, so these three types of document must first be segregated. When this has been done, it is common practice to order all hospital reports and all pathology test results by date. Some practices further subclassify hospital reports by department, and pathology tests by type of investigation, but this confers little advantage. The three separate bundles of documents are now each secured by a treasury tag or splay rivet for ease of handling. The proportion of practice records that have been processed in this way is a factor taken into account when performance-related practice bonuses are allocated. Strictly speaking, it is not necessary to order documents chronologically when transferring summary data to take-on cards, as the computer can be programmed to order all entries chronologically after key-in.
- Each manual document within the wallet must be checked for the correct patient identity – names, address and date of birth – in case a document was previously misfiled. When the date of birth is not given, special care must be exercised to avoid confusion between two patients with the same name.

- Care must be taken to avoid entry reduplication of an episode, which might result from its occurrence both in GP and hospital notes, or in multiple hospital reports. As many as seven hospital documents can be received in relation to a single surgical episode.

- Summarized statements must always be complete and explicit in their content. Terms such as EUA or colectomy are insufficient in themselves and must be accompanied by summarized indications and findings. With surgical procedures, precision in recording what was removed and retained are important – e.g. ovaries at laparotomy for endometriosis, appendix at laparotomy, or cervix at hysterectomy. Incidental findings at operations – e.g. old duodenal ulcer or gallstones at nephrectomy – must also be included. If histology is available, it too must be summarized.

- The Records Officer must be conscious of the problems of double meanings for terms like cervical, rectal, tubercle or CDH. She must be alert to certain terms that signal potentially important episodes – e.g. haemoptysis, haematemesis, melaena, diplopia, jaundice, hemiplegia and haematuria. She must distinguish with certainty the difference between immunized disease and diseases suffered, between toxoids and antitoxins, between drugs prescribed and allergies to drugs.

- The criterion for the selection of a record statement for summary must be whether it is relevant to further patient care months or years after the event. For most practices this will result in a telegram style of statement, which, although unambiguous and complete in itself, owes its clarity to economy of words. A simple recording convention uses an oblique stroke to punctuate between statement components of equal weight, and a hyphen to punctuate before an elaboration of a statement. (Commas and stops may not show up well on the VDU.)

- Clarity and economy in recording data on take-on cards are assisted by the introduction of a few well-chosen symbols that classify certain categories of data. Although there is general agreement as to the need for these symbols, there is no consensus as to what their identity should be, and rival conventions conflict. The records officer must be familiar with her own symbol convention, and be aware that others may be at variance when she receives printout from other practices on patient transfer. Hospital or X-ray statements should be distinguished from GP-originated data by the use of single character symbols. Immunizations, drugs, and other idiosyncrasies, and repeat medication may also require distinctive symbols on take-on cards.

At take-on, the identity of these data categories must be rigorously observed. Computer systems allocate most data classification through specific data fields, function keys or menus. The Read morbidity dictionary allows a term to be entered by progression through a succession of sub-classifying menus to narrow the choice until the target term is reached. Alternatively, Read terms may be selected by keying in the whole term, or the first few letters of the term, whereupon a short list of alternatives will be presented, from which final choice must be made. Read term selection may also be facilitated by techniques such as data entry through graphical images, or the presentation of limited picking lists based on frequency of occurrence (see Chapter 6). Each term has its own unique place in the classification, which obviates the need for the user to allocate a physiological system but does not remove the need to distinguish between hospital, X-ray or GP output.

- The take-on card usually makes special provision for recording the latest normal, and all abnormal, blood pressure readings and urine albumen and sugar tests. At take-on, these will appear in the consultation log and will be reduplicated into the prevention (screening) record. Hypertensives, who have too many abnormal readings to be accommodated in this way, have their own condition-orientated take-on cards and records, as do patients suffering from other chronic diseases under regular surveillance by the practice.

- Pathology test results, whether quoted in pathology reports, hospital reports or GP notes, are recorded on the pathology take-on cards. Synoptic recording allows compaction and clarification of entries. It is usual to omit pregnancy tests, normal swab results, and historical tests taken as a result of monitoring anticoagulants, lithium or immunosuppressive therapy.

- Special hospital procedures such as lumbar puncture, ECG, EEG, endoscopy, diagnostic manipulations, X-rays or scans will be shown, whether normal or abnormal. Medical specialty reports are more difficult to summarize than surgical ones from the point of view of future general practice use. Much output from hospital departments of medicine needs heroic surgery, but must never be doctored. Some hospitals already accompany their reports with separate general-practice-type summary statements, and the general adoption of this policy is highly desirable for both the immediate provision of GP summary records, and the long-term needs of electronic mail.

The degree of economy and standardization used in selecting statements for summary, and the convention used for recording summary, must vary from practice to practice. The more experienced a practice becomes in summary methods, the more economy is exhibited.

29.8 STRATEGY FOR RECORD CONVERSION AND COMPUTER IMPLEMENTATION

Conversion of a practice from manual records to computer records, and from paper-based to terminal-based working procedures involves a transitional period lasting many months. The rate and strategy of conversion will be matters of practice policy. During the transitional phase it is inevitable that both manual and computer systems will be operating concurrently, and confusion will arise unless this is pre-empted by careful planning and strict staff discipline. It is essential that those manual record wallets whose data have been transferred to computer should be clearly identifiable. For this purpose, indelible ink should be used in preference to adhesive labels, since the latter may become dislodged. The following transitional procedures all have their exponents:

- Conversion in alphabetical order of surname of all manual patient record data which are ultimately to be required for computer use. Computer records will be accessed at consultation if data have been converted to them, manual records if data have not yet been converted.
- New data before old. With registration data already housed on the system, new clinical data are keyed in as they are generated, but old data must be accessed from the manual record. The watershed is the date at which the system began to operate but, even so, both records will always need to be accessed in tandem.
- 'Top-up' encounter forms. While the conversion of all practice records to computer storage is in the process of taking place, the partial data stored for each patient are printed out in time for each doctor–patient consultation. The doctor endorses the printout with handwritten details of the current consultation and any historic data needed to complete the computer record. These data are later keyed-in by the secretary.
- 'Task-by-task' record conversion. Simple tasks are undertaken initially by the computer and, as staff gain confidence, so further applications and categories of data are transferred. At consultation, the task to be performed determines which record will be used. The method's disadvantage is that the practice manual records must be reprocessed for each new application.

Top-up encounter forms may be combined with task-by-task conversion. Records of the tasks already converted will then be printed out on the encounter form at patient attendance.

All transitional systems fragment data in one way or another between manual and computer records. Double systems are error-prone and labour-intensive, It is imperative that the point that record conversion has reached between patients or within individual records should be readily identifiable, otherwise the doctor does not know which field to access, nor the secretary which field to update. The alphabetical and encounter form methods of conversion solve this problem reasonably easily, but the other methods do not, and symbols marked on manual wallets must clearly show which categories of data have already been converted.

Encounter form systems result in transcription delay and transcription errors and, with summary and preventive medicine encounter forms, the shredding of computer stationery that follows each session seems wasteful. With surveillance encounter forms linked to repeat prescriptions, only the blank area that accompanies the FP10 (comp) prescription is subsequently destroyed.

29.9 STEPWISE IMPLEMENTATION

Conversion policies vary from practice to practice, and the larger the practice, the more difficult will be the logistics of converting more than one application at a time to the computer. In consequence, a stepwise conversion is usually adopted. Perhaps the most important decision to be made is to select the application that should be used as a starting point for conversion. The following four applications have all been used in this context:

- *Repeat medication.* Undoubtedly the most successful of the preliminary applications, the repeat medication file can be built as and when re-authorization of the prescription is due. Having installed repeat medication on computer, doctors might proceed to enter all prescriptions through a VDU on their desk at consultation. Ultimately, full record take-on would follow.

- *Pathology test results.* The setting up of terminals to receive pathology test results in general practice has been the first step in data automation in many US and Australian practices. Over time, the results build into a practice pathology test result database.
- *Surveillance and preventive medicine records* may initially be transferred to computer, and accessed either on the visual display unit or as printed encounter forms to support clinics. Conversion for other tasks will follow later.
- *Summary details* may be transferred to computer (see Chapter 5). These prove to be sufficient in themselves to support clinical decision making at 50% of all consultations.

Historically, most practices have chosen repeat medication as their preferred initial application. Stepwise implementation will then often occur in the following order:

- Registration download from, or upload check with, the HA
- Registration through GP-PPSA/HA Links
- Computerized repeat medication
- Submission and checking of Item of Service claims on-line
- Conversion of cervical cytology and immunization records, with subsequent e-entry of new data relating to both, and link-up with e-IoS claims and target calculations: call and recall clinics
- Surveillance of chronic disease, using e-records linked to repeat medication
- Conversion of historical pathology records: GP–Pathology Links implementation, with autofiling of results
- Conversion of summary records, including patient-drug idiosyncrasies: ongoing summarization of incoming paper hospital reports, with summary data keyed in by practice
- Acute prescribing with prescribing monitor software functions
- Scan and archive of historical hospital reports
- On-line hospital reports, with on-screen summary extraction and autofiling.

Appointments and non-clinical applications such as book-keeping or locality commissioning can be introduced at any stage of clinical implementation.

29.10 VARIANTS OF THE SUMMARIZATION PROCESS

- In the early days of computerization, some system suppliers insisted that all summarization was undertaken by doctors. As s/he checked the contents of the manual wallet, the doctor entered summary history, immunization, idiosyncrasy and repeat medication data directly into the system via the keyboard and VDU. As a rule, the secretary had already entered details of the patient's identity on to the computer. This method avoided the use both of take-on cards and records officers, but was onerous for the doctor. Instead of checking the validity of take-on cards at consultation, the doctor was asked to check details on the computer record when s/he next saw the patient.
- Some practices do not load data from the paper-based pathology reports that preceded take-on, and therefore do not use pathology take-on cards. As the majority of historic pathology reports are no longer relevant to patient management, other practices frequently discard those that are obsolete, but take on all previous abnormal results and the latest normal result of each test. All incoming paper pathology reports that follow computerization will have their results keyed in to the practice system unless or until electronic reporting through Links is available.
- Summarization with or without take-on can be undertaken on all patients who have booked consultation appointments for the following day. This method has the advantage that all patients attending for consultation will have summarized, and perhaps computerized, records, but the attendant disadvantage is that staff dealing with incoming hospital and pathology mail will need constantly to check the symbols marked on manual wallets to determine whether a patient's records have been processed for computer or not.
Piecemeal conversion of records from appointment lists can be augmented by the processing of records when PMA insurance reports are prepared, or when repeat medication for a patient is transferred to computer.

29.11 MODIFICATIONS TO PRACTICE MANUAL DOCUMENTATION

Conversion of patient data from paper records and reports to computer takes place over a prolonged period, and during this transitional phase it is essential that foolproof methods should be adopted to ensure that no item that should be entered on computer is omitted. Other than by the use of take-on cards, data control is materially assisted by the following manual procedures.

Date status change reported to practice	Source of amended registration details	Code letter of change	Present surname or new surname if changed	Former surname if changed	Forenames	Date of birth	Present address or new address if changed	Former address if changed	Transferred to patient record – date and initials of clerk

Code letters of status change

A. Change of address

B. Birth

*C. Transfer to another doctor within HA area with previous doctor's consent

*D. Death

*E. Embarkation

M. Marriage

*N. Transfer to another doctor within HA area after giving notice

O. Change of name other than by marriage

*R. Removal to another HA area

*S. Enlistment

*X. On removal. Transfer to another doctor within HA area

Z. Card signed and left at practice

T. Notes recalled by HA but removal believed temporary

* These codes are already in use between the HA/PPSA and practices for recall of patient records

Fig. 29.1 Deskbook for change of patient status

The deskbook for change of patient status (Fig. 29.1)

This is a record of all new patient registrations, all removals from the list, or changes of name or address, as notified to the practice. At regular intervals these amendments will be transferred to the computer record (see also Chapter 7).

The new patient questionnaire

All patients who register with the practice must be asked to fill in a medical history questionnaire, which includes identification details; past diseases; preventive procedures; family, occupational, social and lifestyle factors; medication, allergies and current health problems. Completion of this form and the consequent transfer of its data to computer will be coupled with a health check and claim, which the computer should coordinate (see also Chapter 8).

The referral log

A log of patient referrals to hospital, which will initially be kept manually by each doctor, but which will later be transferred to the doctor's desktop computer terminal (where it will integrate with locality commissioning procedures), must show the patient's and GP's identities, consultant and hospital department, and type of referral. As the categories of referral data that will be required by practice and management will increase with time, some computer systems have already made provision for the inclusion of diagnosis, presenting symptoms, and pathology test requests by investigation and department. The referral log must be available to the PCG+T during the report phase of commissioning.

Disposal of incoming reports from hospital

All hospital reports are initially read in full by the recipient practice. During the following 3 months, a proportion of these reports will be reread in full as patients attend the practice and the consultant's recommendations are implemented. At the end of 3 months, the full report is only read again at one in 250 consultations, provided that a summarized alternative is available. The report should be summarized in the form of a term or chain of terms, and this reduced form of the report will be used for inclusion in the patient's computerized summary history.

A patient's summary history is accessed as a self sufficient data source at 50% of all consultations, displaying a greater frequency of use than any other record subset. If summary records are available on computer, together with a log of GP consultation entries, then old hospital reports become redundant after 3 months, except at a small minority of consultations.

Procedures for managing hospital reports within 3 months of their receipt

While hospital reports continue to be received on paper, provision must be made for access to them during the first 3 months after their receipt, and this can be done either by scanning them in to the practice system as image files, or by adopting a manual 3-month holding bank with subsequent archive to the manual record wallets.

A manual bank stores all incoming hospital reports in ring files by month. Within each month's input, reports are ordered by sex and date of receipt. When the receptionist asks the reason for a patient's request for a GP appointment and learns that it is to discuss the consultant's recommendations following a recent hospital attendance, she is able to retrieve the report from the holding bank and place it on the GP's desk prior to the appropriate consultation session. The report is subsequently returned to the bank. At the end of the 3-month holding period, all paper reports are filed in the manual record wallets.

As an alternative to the manual holding bank, incoming hospital reports can be scanned in to the practice system as images, and accessed in this format when the patient visits the medical centre following a hospital attendance. Images are extravagant of storage space, but do not have to be edited by practice staff during the scanning process as digital storage using OCR does. The image scanning method allows the paper hospital report to be filed in the manual wallet on receipt. The practice using this method must determine whether it has sufficient storage space to retain image scans permanently as archives, or whether to use manual wallet retrieval for the occasional access to the full length hospital report when the 3 months of initial retention has elapsed.

Some practices will opt to scan all hospital reports using OCR, which, because of its errors, has to be edited before storage, but this hardly seems worth while. When all hospital reports are received electronically, they are already digitalized and do not need further editing, other than that summary history statements must still be extracted if provision for this has not already been made by hospital staff.

Practices are still legally required to retain patients' manual record wallets, but the day will dawn when electrification renders them redundant. Antique full hospital reports received prior to practice record conversion, which very few practices scan into their systems, will then be left in limbo.

30 A brief history of GP computing

30.1 GENERAL COMPUTER DEVELOPMENT

Charles Babbage (1792–1871) is generally held to have been the originator of computer science. A native of Devon, he became Lucasian Professor of Mathematics at Cambridge. Babbage set out to invent an advanced calculating machine based on mechanics, using a sequence of rotating drums, cogs and gears activated by a crank handle. In effect this was the mechanical equivalent of the spreadsheet with its rows and columns. Government funding for the project, which was called the 'Difference Engine', ran out in 1842 before it could be built, and it was left to Babbage's successors to construct a working model from the original drawings.

Babbage's second brainchild was even more advanced, using data from punch cards, and having a mechanical memory capable of linear programming. This was called the 'Analytical Engine'.

The principle of using cogs and gears to represent interactive data surfaced again in the Enigma machine used by Nazi Germany to send coded messages to its armed forces. The need to crack these codes led the Cambridge mathematician Alan Turing (1912–1954) to pioneer a sophisticated calculating machine, which used the variable strengths of electric currents to represent numbers, and used valve technology. This machine was the original analogue computer, and was used at GCHQ Bletchley Park, where it played a dominant role in Allied war intelligence.

In 1944 Von Neumann and his team at Philadelphia University built the first machine to use electronic memory. Called ENIAC, it had no less than 18 000 valves. The Americans have retained the lead in hardware and generic software development ever since, throughout the 1950s and 1960s pioneering electronic binary text processing (digital computing), ASCII, magnetic storage, and the mainframe configuration.

By 1970, IBM controlled 70% of the world market in computers. In the 1980s the microchip and microcomputer were introduced. During the 1990s, Microsoft and Intel became the dominant influences in, respectively, software and processor design.

30.2 MEDICAL COMPUTING

Medical computing began in the late 1950s with attempts to set up all-embracing hospital systems in the USA (Kaiser Permanente) and Sweden (Karolinska). These attempts failed, because technology at that time was too primitive. Even when hardware became more powerful, software development was hampered by the inability of computer staff to appreciate the needs of the medical profession, and by the inability of medical staff to appreciate what computers might achieve in the healthcare field. Stalemate led to extravagant failure in the hospital sector where for many years, even in America, the most successful applications were purely administrative and commercial. In the UK, prior to 1999, a significant level of computerization had only been achieved by 25% of hospital trusts, a deficit that is set to be redressed by the NHSE's IT strategic plans.

30.3 GENERAL PRACTICE COMPUTING

- During the 1960s, on both sides of the Atlantic, primitive attempts were made to use punch cards and mark sense cards in order to batch process individual categories of data derived from general practice. As the turnaround time from data recording to printed output was usually 6 weeks, the resultant document was always 6 weeks out of date, and therefore useless for day-to-day patient

325

management at consultation, although it was able to support research.

- In the late 1960s, the Department of Health and Social Security began to take an interest in the uses computers might have in the medical field, and they set up research bases at Exeter and Oxford. Both project teams were tasked with producing a unified computer record for each patient, which could be stored on a central mainframe at the health authority, and accessed remotely by all health professionals with whom the patient came into contact. This simplistic proposition was soon found to be totally impracticable, because healthcare is essentially compartmentalized. Each healthcare department paddles its own canoe and creates its own speciality-orientated record subset, which it has neither reason nor desire to share with other departments. The only data invariably shared across boundaries are the summary past history, idiosyncrasies, immunizations and repeat medication (the components of the GP system's principal screen).

- In 1969 IBM was attracted by the potential of the global medical market and saw the defined structure of the NHS general practice as a suitable starting point for medical system design. It chose a single handed practice in Whipton, Exeter, to launch a prototype known as the IBM Desktop Pilot, which was to be the world's first point-of-care GP computer system. Medical records were abstracted, transferred to computer and used in this format for patient management at all medical consultations. VDUs with keyboards in the doctor's and secretary's offices communicated through landlines with a remote mainframe computer. Patient records were viewed and updated on the local terminals with 4-second response times. Printout was used for backup and home visits, and tetanus immunization recall was enabled by search and list. The exercise demonstrated and quantified the outstanding advantages of electronic GP records and served to define the main subsets of the GP e-record which are now in general use and which will eventually become the basis for the Electronic Patient Record of the NHSE's information strategy (Preece et al 1970, Lippmann & Preece 1971).

- The design of the GP e-record was further refined, and adapted for multidoctor use at the Ottery St Mary Health Centre, Devon, whose system became operational in 1976. Again using VDUs with keyboards, landlines and a remote mainframe, but with ICL technology and DHSS funding, this practice was the first in the UK to achieve paperless status. Its early work became the basis for the currently marketed Exeter System (Bradshaw Smith 1976).

- In 1981 many GP enthusiasts became interested in using the newly developed microcomputer at the point of care, and two forums were provided for them with ICI sponsorship: The Primary Health Care Specialist Group of the British Computer Society was formed to hold periodic meetings, and *Practice Computing* magazine was launched as a free service to all UK practices.

- In 1982 the Department of Industry funded the 'Micros for GPs' Scheme to foster the uptake of electronic health systems. 150 UK general practices were provided with subsidized 'back of office' systems implementing registration, age–sex registers and repeat medication.

- In 1982 the ABPI–Whipton Project was launched to construct an electronic drug database and computerized prescribing support for GPs (Preece 1984). With further development this became Philex, then Multilex.

- In 1983 James Read's codes were initially developed in association with the ABIES GP system, later to become independent and adopted as a comprehensive classification of medical terms for use throughout the NHS.

- In 1983 the Scottish Home and Health department opted to use Glasgow GP David Ferguson's successful system designs as the basis for the GPASS software that is offered freely to all Scottish practices. In the same year, Dr Alan Dean's designs, incorporating large internal dictionaries and fast search routines, became the basis of the VAMP system, and Drs David Stables and Peter Sowerby launched the EMIS system.

- In 1987 'no-cost options' campaigns were launched by VAMP and Meditel. These schemes effectively gave free computer systems to practices in return for anonymized consultation and prescribing data. The data were then used to fuel a database that provided sponsors with epidemiological and market research facilities.

- In 1991 the UK government became more closely involved with the development and propagation of GP computing, recognizing the potential use which could be made of the GP system as a fulcrum both for the improvement of patient care and for the implementation of administrative and political control. Department of Health intervention took the form of system accreditation, the computer reimbursement scheme, fundholding, HealthLink and plans for the NHSnet.

- In 1997 the GP cooperative strategy was instigated by Dr Krishna Korlipara of Bolton and rapidly gained acceptance throughout the UK, bringing with it the need for the rapid development of cooperative support software.

- In 1998 fundholding was disbanded, to be replaced by locality commissioning as a means of apportioning NHS funding for patient care. Tasks formerly undertaken by practice fundholding software were extended by commissioning, and were split into two levels of activity and responsibility. Practices remained responsible for providing data, but PCG+Ts became responsible for collating them and reporting to the HA.

REFERENCES AND FURTHER READING

Abrams M E 1972 Health services and the computer – real-time computing in general practice. Health Trends 4: 18–20

Bradshaw Smith J H 1976 A computer record-keeping system for general practice. British Medical Journal 1: 1395

Ferguson D 1983 Repeat performer. Practice Computing, April: 18–19

Gillings D B, Preece J F 1971 An analysis of the size and content of medical records used during an on-line record maintenance and retrieval system in general practice. International Journal of Biomedical Computing 2: 151–165

Linacre J 1985 Evaluation of the micros for GPs scheme (interim report). Nottingham Family Practitioner Committee, Nottingham

Lippman E O, Preece J F 1971 A pilot on-line data system for general practitioners. Computers and Biomedical Research 4: 390–406

Preece J F 1972 The computer file in general practice. Update, July: 155–166

Preece J F 1984 A new interaction. Practice Computing, April: 14–15

Preece J F, Lippmann E O 1971 Record design for the computer file in general practice. Practitioner (Supplement), August 3–12

Preece J F, Gillings D B, Lippmann E O, Pearson N G 1970 An on-line record maintenance and retrieval system in general practice. International Journal of Biomedical Computing 1: 4; 329–337

Schmidt E C, Schall D W, Morrison C C 1974 Computerised problem – orientated medical record for ambulatory practice medical care. Medical Care 13(4): 316–327

Tanner S 1982 Computers in care. Practice Computing, October: 18

Appendix A
Internet sources

Interesting medical URLs and databases

Alzheimer's Disease Society	http://www.alzheimers.org.uk
American Medical Association	http://www.ama-assn.org/
Audible Heartsound Library (multimedia)	http://www.medlib.com/spi/coolstuff2.htm
BMA Library Services (access to Medline)	http://ovid.bma.org.uk
BT Health	http://www.bthealth.com
Centre for Evidence-Based Medicine	http://cebm.jr2.ox.ac.uk/
Centers for Disease Control and Prevention (free US chronic disease, injury and disability data)	http://www.cdc.gov/
CliniWeb (categorized US medical site)	http://www.ohsu.edu/cliniweb/
Cochrane Collaboration Database (comprehensive compilation of clinical abstracts)	http://www.cochrane.co.uk/abstracts http://www.Doctors.net.uk
Coronary Prevention Group	http://www.healthpro.org.uk
Department of Health	http://www.coi.gov.uk/coi/depts/GDH/GDH.html http://www.doh.gov.uk/
Dermatology Atlas	www.dermis.net/bilddb/index-e.html
Doctor's Guide to the Internet Medical News (free)	http://www.pslgroup.com/MEDNEWS.HTM
DoH guidelines on clinical management of drug misuse and dependence ('the Orange Book')	http://www.tsonline.co.uk
DoH National Service Framework for coronary prevention	http://www.doh.gov.uk/nsf/coronary.htm
ECG Tracings Library	http://homepages.enterprise.net/djenkins/ecghome.html
Health on the Net (categorized, partly selective medical site)	http://www.hon.ch/
Hospital Waiting List Data (UK)	http://www.open.gov.uk/hmis/waitime.htm
Imperial Cancer Research Fund	http://www.icnet.uk/public.html
Internet Mental Health (free: Java required)	http://www.mentalhealth.com/
Macmillan Cancer Relief Data for Patients	http://www.macmillan.org.uk/

Mayo Clinic	http://mayohealth.org/
Medical Information on the Internet (Kiley)	http://www.hbuk.co.uk/kiley/
Medical Matrix (free US clinical site with good links)	http://www.medmatrix.org/index.asp
Medical Research Council	http://www.mrc.ac.uk
Medscape (URL for 18 medical specialties)	http://www.medscape.com
National Electronic Library of Health	http://194.129.181.161/buildng.htm
National Institute of Health (free site of biomedical research)	http://www.nih.gov
National Society for Epilepsy	http://www.epilepsynse.org.uk
NHS Information Zone (also interactive discussions)	http://www.inform.nhsweb.nhs.uk
NHS PCG Alliance	http://www.nhsalliance.org/
OMNI (categorized biomedical site)	http://omni.ac.uk
OncoLink (free US oncology site)	http://cancer.med.upenn.edu/
PCG Resource Unit	http://strauss.ihs.ox.ac.uk/pcgru/index.html
PCG-UK Mailing List	http://www.healthcentre.org.uk/hc/staff/peg-uk_list.htm
PHLS (regional information on infections)	http://www.phls.co.uk
PubMed-Medline on the Web (free Web interface to Medline – the world's most important biomedical database)	http://www.ncbi.nlm.nih.gov/PubMed
RCGP Research Pages	http://www.rcgp.org.uk/college/activity/research/index.asp
Reuters Health (toll: daily medical news)	http://www.reutershealth.com/
Shoreland Travel Health Information	http://www.tripprep.com/index.html
Toxbase Poisons Information	http://www.spib.axl.co.uk
Travax Travel Health Information (free in Scotland)	http://www.axl.co.uk/scieh
University of Dundee Palliative Care Data	http://www.dundee.ac.uk/meded/help/indexb.htm
The Virtual Hospital (peer-reviewed books and booklets)	http://www.vh.org
Web Doctor (comprehensive medical URL)	http://fs.dai.net/ac/232481/N01.html?http://www.gretmar.com.webdoctor
Web Med Lit (research data culled from 23 English language medical journals: free)	http://www.webmedlit.com/
Wisdom 2000 (Department of General Practice, Sheffield University	http://www.wisdom.org.uk
World Health Organization (WHO publications: free)	http://www.who.ch/

Interactive medical programmes

Global Textbook of Anaesthesia	http://gasnet.dundee.ac.uk/gta/
The Interactive Patient (US consultation simulation)	http://medicus.marshall.edu/mainmenu.htm
MedWeb Automated Assessment Service (University of Birmingham Medical School)	http://medweb.bham.ac.uk/caa/mcq/
Merck Manual of Diagnosis and Therapy (the most widely used US medical textbook)	http://www.merck.com./
On-line Course in Biocomputing	http://www.TechFak.Uni-Bielefeld.DE/techfakengl.html
Supercourse: Epidemiology, the Internet and Global Health (available in eight languages)	http://www.pitt.edu/~super1/main/
Trauma Moulage	http://www.trauma.org/resus/moulage/moulage.html
Virtual Autopsy	http://www.le.ac.uk/pathology/teach/va2/titlpagl.html/

Healthcare journals, magazines, and journal clubs

Bandolier (free abstracts and good links)	http://www.jr2.ox.ac.uk/bandolier/
British Medical Journal	http://www.bmj.com/index.shtml
CMO's Letters	http://www.open.gov.uk/doh/cmo/cmoh.htm
Doctor Magazine	http://www.healthnews.co.uk/doctor
Family Net Doc	http://www.famnetdoc.com/index.html
Journal of Family Practice	http://jfp.msu.edu/
The Lancet	http://www.thelancet.com/index1.html
MEDNEWS (Medical News Update)	http://www.pslgroup.com/MEDNEWS.HTM
New England Journal of Medicine	http://www.nejm.org/content/index.asp
Web Med Lit	http://www.webmedlit.com/

Chat forums

Free doctors' discussion groups and personal e-mail boxes	http://www.doctors.net.uk
NHS Information Zone	http://www.inform.nhsweb.hns.uk
Virtual Nurse	http://chat.virtualnurse.com

Validated patient sites

NHS Direct on-line	http://www.nhsdirect.nhs.uk
Validated sites for health information	http://www.patient.co.uk
	http://www.surgerydoor.co.uk
	http://www.docres.co.uk
	http://www.netdoctor.co.uk

Medical societies and organizations

British Medical Association	http://web.bma.org.uk/homepage.nsf
Commission for Health Improvement	http://www.doh.gov.uk/chi/index/htm
Dr Lowe's PCG website	http://e-nhs.org/hollandhouse/ITlinks/ITlink.htm
General Medical Council	http://gmc-uk.org/
Junior Doctors' Website	http://web.bma.org.uk/homepage.nsf/htmlpagevw/juniors
Locum Directory (GMC and defence organisation membership required)	http://www.locum.org
Medical Defence Union	http://www.the-mdu.com/
Medical Protection Society	http://www.mps.org.uk
Medical Research Council	http://www.mrc.ac.uk
National Association of GP Co-operatives	http://www.nagpc.org.uk/
National Association of NonPrincipals	http://www.nanp.org.uk
National Institute for Clinical Excellance	http://www.nice.org.uk
Royal College of General Practitioners	http://www.rcgp.org.uk
Royal Society of Medicine	http://www.roysocmed.ac.uk

Sites of general interest

BBC weather reports	http://www.bbc.co.uk/weather
RAC road conditions and route planner	http://www.rac.co.uk/
How Stuff Works (science education)	http://www.howstuffworks.com/

Medical services

Cancer BACUP	http://www.cancerbacup.org.uk
Marie Curie Charity Nursing Care	http://www.mariecurie.org.uk/
National Council for Hospice and Palliative Care Services Directory	http://www.hospice-spc-council.org.uk/indexf.htm
Patient UK (patient self-help groups and links to patient health information)	http://www.patient.co.uk/
Data on setting up PCGs	http://www.ManchesterHealth.co.uk
Lists of residential homes and care services	http://www.intercarenet.co.uk

Computer system data

Program to convert Adobe Acrobat files into html before they are downloaded	http://access.adobe.com/
AltaVista (search engine)	http://www.altavista.digital.com
Antivirus software reviews	http://www.microsoft.com/office/antivirus/
BT Internet (ISP)	http://www.bt.com/internet/index.htm

Demon Internet (ISP)	http://www.demon.net
Dell (computer supplier)	http://www.dell.co.uk
Doctors' Guide to the Internet	http://www.pslgroup.com/DOCGUIDE.HTM
Encryption information website	http://www.ftech.net/~monark/crypto/
Gateway 2000 (computer supplier)	http://www.gw2k.co.uk/
Lycos (search engine)	http://www.lycos.com
Microsoft UK	http://www.microsoft.com/uk
Northern Light (search engine)	http://www.northernlight.com/
Tesconet (ISP)	http://www.tesco.net
Yahoo! (search engine)	http://www.yahoo.co.uk/

Conferencing

Medscape Video Conferences	http://www.medscape.com/home/news/Medscape-News.html#conference
Permanent e-mail address (despite change of ISP)	http://www.doctors.net.uk
Wisdom 2000 (Department of General Practice, University of Sheffield)	http://www.wisdom.org.uk

Financial and purchase advice

Bargain airfares	http://www.airnet.co.uk
Financial Services Industry Directory (compares insurance quotations and investments)	http://www.find.co.uk
Interactive Investor International (support for investment decisions)	http://www.iii.co.uk
Investment advice	http://www.invest-faq.com
Share prices	http://www.share-aware.co.uk
Ticketmaster (ticket details and bookings for theatres and events)	http://www.ticketmaster.co.uk
What Car? On-line	http://www.whatcar.co.uk

Book purchase

Amazon (discounted books)	http://www.amazon.co.uk
Books On Line	http://www.booksonline.co.uk
Books Out Of Print	http://www.waterstones.co.uk
Harcourt Health Sciences	http://www.harcourt-international.com
Medscape Bookshop (world's largest medical bookstore)	http://www.lb.com/medscape
MicroInfo (also CD-ROM)	http://www.microinfo.co.uk

Appendix B
Some CD-ROMs of importance to central practice

This list contains CD-ROMs chosen for their utility and value for money. Extensive lists of titles available on general release can be obtained from retailers such as Computers Manuals (tel: 0121 706 6000), Focus 77 (tel: freephone 0500 947177), MicroInfo (tel: 01420 86848) and RCSG Medical CD-ROM Shop (http://rcgp.org.uk/cdrom/cdshop.html).

Anxiety self-help CD-ROM. Glasgow Community and Mental Health Services NHS Trust. Assessment and two treatment sessions of 40 minutes each.

Akusoft Acupuncture patient records, needle sites, invoicing system. Source: SEIRIN Medical Systems GmbH, Germany, fax: +49 (0)6 01 23 13 40

Basic Ophthalmology CD-ROM — Price code A

Beating the Blues: Cognitive Behavioural Therapy. Institute of Psychiatry. Source: Ultramind (tel: (020) 7660 6777)

Body Works. Human anatomy graphics. Source: PC Connections Direct (tel: 0706 222888) — Price code A

Cancer BACUP: 52 booklets and 73 fact sheets, contact http://www.cancerbacup.org.uk — Price code A

CD Atlas of Allergy. Mosby — Price code B

Forbes C D, Jackson W F. *CD Atlas of Clinical Medicine* (Windows or Macintosh versions). Mosby, 1200 hypertext and cross-references, 2000 colour photographs — Price code A, general release

Dorland's Electronic Medical Dictionary, 28th edn — Price code A, general release

EBNF and Drug and Therapeutics Bulletin, on one CD (flags preparations considered to be less suitable for prescribing). Published each March and September. Source: Drug and Therapeutics Bulletin (tel: 0645 830082) — Price code A

The Electronic Red Book (Windows). Radcliffe Medical Press — Price code A, general release

E-MIMS (60 Mb available hard disk if run directly from CD-ROM, otherwise 600 Mb) — Free to approved GP users

Gray's Interactive Anatomy 38th edition — Price code B

McMinn's Interactive Clinical Anatomy. 200 dissections and 124 radiographs, interactive 3D reconstruction — Price code A, general release

The Medical Directory. Source: Cartermill, tel: (020) 7896 2401 — Price code B

Kneebone and Schofield, *Minor Surgery and Skin Lesions*. RCGP, 450 subject areas, 150 training areas. Minimum requirement: PC, Windows 95. Source: RCGP, tel: (020) 7247 3680	Price code A
Mosby's Comprehensive Review of Nursing (core nursing information and principles)	Price code A
New Phased Evaluation Program (PEP) Interactive. Source: RCGP, tel: (020) 7247 3680	Price code A
Oxford Clinical Mentor (searches text taken from three Oxford Clinical Handbooks and analyses combinations of symptoms, signs and test results). Updates (Windows) on Internet. Source: tel: 01865 267979	Price code B
Oxford PILs (patient instruction leaflets). Comprehensive collection for printing out, including self-help group addresses. Updates (Windows) on Internet	Price code A
Oxford Textbook of Medicine (electronic equivalent of over 5000 pages of text)	Price code B, general release
PhysioTools (physiotherapy exercises and advice handouts). Source: PIP Professionals, 8 Culverwell Cottages, Pilton BA4 4DG, tel: 01749 890870	Price varies with package – A & B
QuickBooks 6.0 (accounting software). Source: Intuit, orders tel: 01932 578522	Price code A
Quicken 2000 DeLuxe (personal finance package). Source: Intuit, orders tel: 01932 578522	Price code A
Quicken 2000 (Accounts). Source: Intuit, orders tel: 01932 578522	Price code A
Requirements for Accreditation 99 (October 1999). A consolidation of RFA4 with additional requirements of training mandatory pathology reporting, MIQUEST and PRODIGY integration. Source: NHS Information Authority, Exeter, helpline: 0121 625 2711	
Stedman's Electronic Medical Dictionary (over 100 000 medical terms; synchronous extraction from any Windows file with hotkey toggle)	Price code A, general release

Price code A = below £100; price code B = £100–200 at time of writing

Index